Trauma, Autism, and Neurodevelopmental Disorders

Jason M. Fogler • Randall A. Phelps
Editors

Trauma, Autism, and Neurodevelopmental Disorders

Integrating Research, Practice, and Policy

Springer

Editors
Jason M. Fogler
Developmental Medical Center
Boston Children's Hospital
Boston, MA, USA

Randall A. Phelps
Oregon Health & Science University
Eugene, OR, USA

ISBN 978-3-030-00502-3 ISBN 978-3-030-00503-0 (eBook)
https://doi.org/10.1007/978-3-030-00503-0

Library of Congress Control Number: 2018962963

This Springer imprint is published by the registered company Springer Nature Switzerland AG
The registered company address is: Gewerbestrasse 11, 6330 Cham, Switzerland

Dr. Phelps dedicates this book to friend and colleague, the late Dr. Debra Eisert, who planted the seed for this project. Dr. Phelps would also like to thank his mother, Jean Phelps, who, as executive director of the Relief Nursery, first taught him about TSRD; mentors Dr. Heidi Feldman and the late Dr. Bill Cohen, who taught him about neurodevelopmental disabilities; wife, Liz Phelps, and mother-in-law, Dr. Judy Tanner, who helped with editing suggestions; and his many wonderful colleagues, patients, and families at the Child Development and Rehabilitation Center of Oregon Health and Science University, who have generously shared their stories, time, and wisdom.

Dr. Fogler dedicates this book to his family, friends, colleagues, mentors, and students who shine a light in the darkness so that we can keep a light burning for the families who seek our help. These good souls – too many and too special to do justice in a list – live, work, and attend school throughout most of the 50 states (with particular recognition to those in New England and the tri-state area, Pennsylvania, Missouri, Mississippi, Georgia, Oregon, Ohio, Wisconsin, and California); Ottawa, Canada; Yokosuka, Japan; and Vienna and Linz, Austria.

Contents

1 **Introduction** 1
Jason M. Fogler and Randall A. Phelps

2 **Tangled Roots and Ramifications: The Early Histories of Autism Spectrum Disorder and Reactive Attachment Disorder** 5
Randall A. Phelps and Jason M. Fogler

3 **Posttraumatic Stress Disorder: From Neurobiology to Cycles of Violence** 19
K. M. McCullough and K. J. Ressler

4 **Trauma and Neurodevelopmental Disorder: Assessment, Treatment, and Triage** 55
Lisa Prock and Jason M. Fogler

5 **The Challenge and Importance of Differentiating Trauma and Stress-Related Disorders from Autism Spectrum Disorders** 73
Amanda Van Scoyoc, Melissa B. Marquardt, and Randall A. Phelps

6 **Fetal Alcohol Spectrum Disorders: Diagnostic Considerations for Children with a History of Trauma** 93
Prachi E. Shah, Danielle Shapiro, Tedi Milgrom, and H. Eugene Hoyme

7 **Interventions for Trauma- and Stressor-Related Disorders in Preschool-Aged Children** 123
Kelley Munger, Elizabeth C. Loi, and Amelia Roth

8 **Reactive Attachment Disorder and Autism Spectrum Disorder: Diagnosis and Care in a Cultural Context** 149
Jorge Benavides-Rawson and Roy Richard Grinker

9 **Special Population Consideration in ASD Identification and Treatment** 161
Alison Chavez, Lark Huang-Storms, and Katharine Zuckerman

10 Challenges with Transition to Adulthood 195
Ami Bear, Raegan Smith, and Charlotte Alverson

11 Trauma and Neurodevelopmental Disorders from a Public Health Perspective 205
Sarah R. Lowe, Kate L. Walsh, Emma Opthof, and Petty Tineo

12 From the Outside In: Using a Whole-School Paradigm to Improve the Educational Success of Students with Trauma Histories and/or Neurodevelopmental Disabilities 241
Michael Gregory and Emily Nichols

13 Assessment and Recommendations 269
Randall A. Phelps and Jason M. Fogler

Afterword: Precision Mental Health and the Twilight of Categories 277

Index 281

Contributors

Charlotte Alverson College of Education, University of Oregon, Eugene, OR, USA

Ami Bear Child Development and Rehabilitation Center, Oregon Health and Science University, Eugene, OR, USA

Jorge Benavides-Rawson Department of Anthropology, The George Washington University, Washington, D.C., USA

Alison Chavez Department of Psychology, University of Massachusetts, Boston, MA, USA

Jason M. Fogler Developmental Medical Center, Boston Children's Hospital, Boston, MA, USA

Michael Gregory Harvard Graduate School of Education, Cambridge, MA, USA

Roy Richard Grinker Department of Anthropology, The George Washington University, Washington D.C., USA

H. Eugene Hoyme University of Arizona, Tuscon, AZ, USA

Lark Huang-Storms Department of Pediatrics, Oregon Health and Science University, Portland, OR, USA

Elizabeth C. Loi Department of Psychology, University of Oregon, Eugene, OR, USA

Sarah R. Lowe Department of Psychology, Montclair State University, Montclair, NJ, USA

Melissa B. Marquardt University of Oregon, Eugene, OR, USA

Oregon Health and Sciences University, Portland, OR, USA

Department of Psychiatry, University of New Mexico, Health Sciences Center, Albuquerque, NM, USA

K. M. McCullough Department of Psychiatry, McLean Hospital, Harvard Medical School, Belmont, MA, USA

Tedi Milgrom University of Michigan, Ann Arbor, MI, USA

Kelley Munger Early Intervention Program, University of Oregon, Eugene, OR, USA

Emily Nichols Medstar Georgetown Center for Wellbeing in School Environments (WISE Center), Child and Adolescent Program, Department of Psychiatry, Medstar Georgetown University Hospital, Washington, DC, USA

Emma Opthof Department of Psychology, Montclair State University, Montclair, NJ, USA

Randall A. Phelps Oregon Health and Sciences University, Eugene, OR, USA

Lisa Prock Division of Developmental Medicine, Boston Children's Hospital, Boston, MA, USA

Harvard Medical School, Boston, MA, USA

K. J. Ressler Department of Psychiatry, McLean Hospital, Harvard Medical School, Belmont, MA, USA

Amelia Roth OHSU Child Development and Rehabilitation Center, Eugene, OR, USA

Prachi E. Shah University of Michigan, Ann Arbor, MI, USA

Danielle Shapiro University of Michigan, Ann Arbor, MI, USA

Raegan Smith Child Development and Rehabilitation Center, Oregon Health and Science University, Eugene, OR, USA

Petty Tineo Department of Psychology, Montclair State University, Montclair, NJ, USA

Amanda Van Scoyoc University of Oregon, Eugene, OR, USA

Oregon Health and Sciences University, Portland, OR, USA

Yale School of Medicine, Yale Child Study Center, New Haven, CT, USA

Kate L. Walsh Ferkauf Graduate School of Psychology, Bronx, NY, USA

Katharine Zuckerman Division of General Pediatrics, Oregon Health and Science University, Portland, OR, USA

About the Editors

Jason M. Fogler, MA, PhD is a Staff Psychologist and the Co-Director of ADHD Services at Boston Children's Hospital's Division of Developmental Medicine. At Boston Children's, he is the Attending Psychologist on a multidisciplinary team devoted to the complex developmental and mental health issues of children in foster care and various phases of adoption, both domestically and internationally. After graduating from Boston University's Doctoral Program in Clinical Psychology, he completed clinical training and a postdoctoral clinical research fellowship in a joint appointment at the VA Boston Healthcare System's National Center for Posttraumatic Stress Disorder and Boston Medical Center's Center for Medical and Refugee Trauma. During this period, he served as training faculty for the National Child Traumatic Stress Network's Learning Collaborative. Dr. Fogler is an Assistant Professor of Pediatrics and Psychiatry at Harvard Medical School, has taught nationally and internationally on the topics of trauma-focused treatment and assessment, and published articles on comprehensive treatment for traumatized children and clergy-perpetrated sexual abuse. He is one of the editors of *Trauma Therapy in Context: The Science & Craft of Evidence Based Practice* (APA Publications: 2012).

Randall A. Phelps, MD, PhD is a developmental and behavioral pediatrician and associate professor of pediatrics at the Child Development and Rehabilitation Center, Institute on Development and Disability, Oregon Health and Science University. He completed MD and PhD degrees at the University of Washington, residency in pediatrics at the University of Michigan, and fellowship in developmental-behavioral pediatrics at the University of Pittsburgh. He attends on interdisciplinary teams to provide diagnostic assessments and care to children with developmental disabilities and/or behavioral conditions throughout the state of Oregon and surrounding states. He created an outreach clinic to provide developmental-behavioral pediatric consultation to the relief nursery, a therapeutic preschool program for children at high risk of trauma. Dr. Phelps has been a co-investigator, with the relief nursery, on several demonstration grants to improve care coordination for children utilizing multiple community resources. He has given lectures and workshops regionally, nationally, and internationally on differential diagnosis of autism, including the diagnostic confusion between autism and reactive attachment and related disorders.

Chapter 1
Introduction

Jason M. Fogler and Randall A. Phelps

> When we feel weak, we drop our heads on the shoulders of others. Don't get mad when someone does that. Be honored. For that person trusted you enough to, even if subtly, ask you for help.
>
> –Lori Goodwin: science fiction author, Operation Iraqi Freedom veteran, trauma survivor

For centuries, we have known that war, abuse, natural disasters, and unexpected loss and death profoundly changes people and that women, children, the elderly, and, of particular relevance to this book, children with developmental disabilities are the ones who are most likely to be victimized. Yet it is only within the last 25 years that we have begun to explore the overlapping features of what are currently known as trauma- and stressor-related disorders (TSRD) and neurodevelopmental disorders (NDD)—a category that subsumes the highly prevalent and widely known attention deficit hyperactivity disorder (ADHD), autism spectrum disorder (ASD), intellectual disability (ID), learning disabilities (LD), and disorders of speech, communication, and motor functioning. At first glance, these diagnostic families seem to have a mirror-image relationship: Both have pervasive effects on the brain and development; but NDD are assumed to be present from birth (and thus mostly hereditary), whereas TSRD require an external traumatic event (or events) to activate a characteristic storm of reexperiencing, emotional avoidance and numbing, hyperarousal/hypervigilance, negative cognitions about oneself and one's future, disordered attachment, and even dissociation—the psychic defense of disconnecting from reality.

In many ways, the publication of the 5th Edition of the Diagnostic and Statistical Manual of Mental Disorders (DSM-5) marked an important shift in our field's approach to diagnosis and conceptualization [1]. Informed by advances in

J. M. Fogler (✉)
Developmental Medical Center, Boston Children's Hospital, Boston, MA, USA
e-mail: Jason.Fogler@childrens.harvard.edu

R. A. Phelps
Oregon Health & Science University, Eugene, OR, USA
e-mail: phelpsr@ohsu.edu

J. M. Fogler, R. A. Phelps (eds.), *Trauma, Autism, and Neurodevelopmental Disorders*, https://doi.org/10.1007/978-3-030-00503-0_1

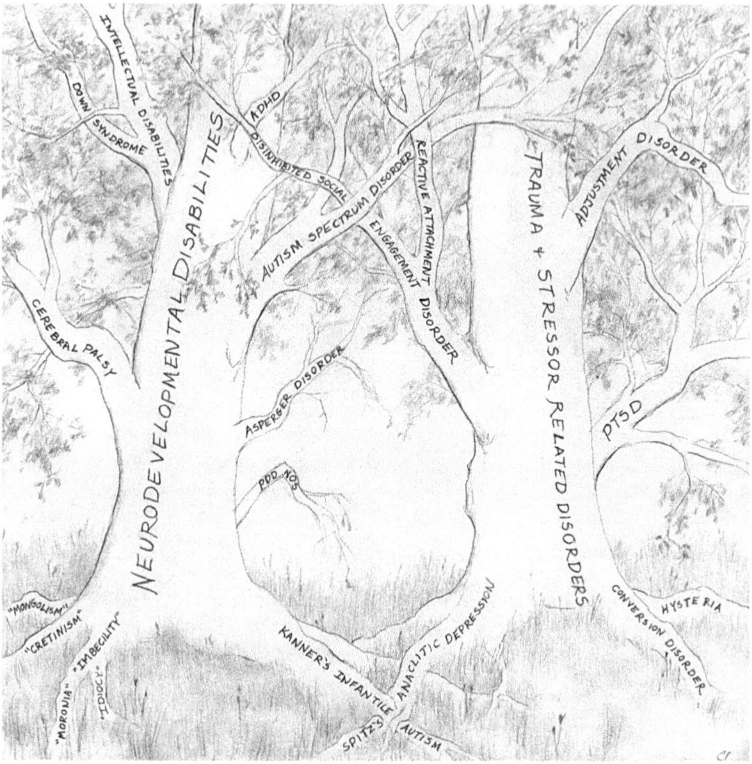

Fig. 1.1 Illustration by Elizabeth Phelps

neuroscience, psychiatric genetics, and biostatistics, clinician-scientists were increasingly modeling psychiatric phenomena as continuous variables rather than hand-sorted into a priori categories [2]; and surprising shifts began to occur in how disorders were clustered into superordinate groups. Perhaps the most dramatic of these shifts occurred among the disorders that are the focus of this book: the newly coined neurodevelopmental disorders and the trauma- and stressor-related disorders. Both of these new families of disorders represented a substantial reshuffling and reorganization of conditions from DSM-IV to 5 (Fig. 1.1).

At first glance, the emergence of trauma- and stressor-related disorder as a new category appears to be the more dramatic case of divergent evolution from previous diagnostic families, most notably anxiety disorders; but the neurodevelopmental disorders category includes some equally striking changes that could perhaps be likened to the massive mergers of corporations or states. The most widely publicized and anxiety-provoking change was the merging of several categories of autism—autistic disorder, Asperger's disorder, pervasive developmental disorder, and childhood disintegrative disorder—into a single autism spectrum. The other change was no less profound in its implications but received far less publicity: the recasting of schizophrenia spectrum and other psychotic disorder as having common genetic and neurobiological features with neurodevelopmental disorders.

Taken together, these two families of mental disorders affect millions of children and their families (see Chap. 11 of this volume) and are far from mutually exclusive. Indeed, children with neurodevelopmental disorders are 2–3× more likely to be bullied, victimized, and maltreated than typically developing children [3, 4]. The costs of these conditions, in direct care of primary and secondary illness, special education, and lost productivity and wages, are exorbitantly high—hundreds of billions if not trillions of dollars [5–9]. Anyone who works with these children feels an incredible sense of mission to do right by them and fight for their care. We co-edited this volume with these unsung heroes in mind: clinicians, educators, advocates, and policy-makers at all levels of training and career. Whether you are a veteran of this rewarding and challenging field, or a student considering it as your calling, this book is for you.

We met at the 2015 annual meeting of our professional society, The Society for Developmental Behavioral Pediatrics (SDBP), presenting on very similar work (and very similar approaches) with children who were both severely traumatized and struggling with co-occurring neurodevelopmental disorders. In short order, we were approached by Garth Haller, a wunderkind associate editor from Springer, to write this book; and, perhaps not realizing what we were really getting into, we dived headfirst into this daunting and exhilarating project. Unsurprising to us from his steady at the helm/there when you needed him approach to managing his newly contracted bicoastal team, Garth was promoted to editor in Springer's Clinical Medicine Division and handed over the reins of our project to senior editor, Judy Jones, and assistant editor, Michelle Tam—both equally a pleasure to work with. In addition to Garth and Judy, a wide network of friends, family, and colleagues helped to make this book possible. Colleagues stepped up to write chapters or recommend others who could if they didn't have time. Family members loved and supported us while putting up with cloistered writing sessions and strangely timed phone calls. Friends provided fresh ears for our ideas and/or needed distraction when they had their fill.

Two years later, nearly to the day when we first met, we are bunking together and putting the finishing touches on this book in a hotel room at the SDBP Annual Meeting in Cleveland, Ohio. Co-editing this book has been incredibly fulfilling and validating to the work we do—with the added bonus of being able to assemble an extraordinary team of professionals working in this relatively new area of integrated mental health care and clinical research. We of course hope that veteran clinicians will find the book useful to their clinical practice and supervision, but perhaps more so, we hope to expand the horizons of clinicians entering the field and to motivate those in a position to shape policy and the healthcare system to increase their efforts and investment in the service of our most vulnerable children.

References

1. American Psychiatric Association. Diagnostic and statistical manual of mental disorders. (DSM-5). 5th ed. Washington: American Psychiatric Association; 2013.
2. Brown TA, Barlow DH. Dimensional versus categorical classification of mental disorders in the fifth edition of the diagnostic and statistical manual of mental disorders and beyond: comment on the special section. J Abnorm Psychol. 2005;114(4):551–6.

3. Mandell DS, Walrath CM, Manteuffel B, Sgro G, Pinto-Martin JA. The prevalence and correlates of abuse among children with autism served in comprehensive community-based mental health settings. Child Abuse Negl. 2005;29:1359–72.
4. Sullivan PM, Knutson JF. Maltreatment and disabilities: a population-based epidemiologic study. Child Abuse Negl. 2000;24:1257–73.
5. Doshi JA, Hodgkins P, Kahle J, Sikirica V, Cangelosi MJ, Setyawan J, Erder MH, Neumann PJ. Economic impact of childhood and adult attention-deficit/hyperactivity disorder in the United States. J Am Acad Child Adolesc Psychiatry. 2012;51(10):990–1002.e2. https://doi.org/10.1016/j.jaac.2012.07.008.
6. Fang X, Brown DS, Florence CS, Mercy JA. The economic burden of child maltreatment in the United States and implications for prevention. Child Abuse Negl. 2012;36(2):156–65.
7. Lavelle TA, Weinstein MC, Newhouse JP, Munir K, Kuhlthau KA, Prosser LA. Economic burden of childhood autism spectrum disorders. Pediatrics. 2014;133(3):e520–9.
8. National Center for Learning Disabilities. The state of learning disabilities: facts, trends, and emerging issues. 3rd ed. New York: National Center for Learning Disabilities; 2014.
9. Salvador-Carulla L, Symonds S. Health services use and costs in people with intellectual disability: building a context knowledge base for evidence-informed policy. Curr Opin Psychiatry. 2016;29(2):89–94. https://doi.org/10.1097/YCO.0000000000000237.

Chapter 2
Tangled Roots and Ramifications: The Early Histories of Autism Spectrum Disorder and Reactive Attachment Disorder

Randall A. Phelps and Jason M. Fogler

Vignette

Emma, a 3-year-old girl, was brought by her mother to our regional diagnostic center for a developmental assessment. Mom's chief concerns were speech delays and frequent screaming. Emma was never a cuddly baby, but she was always stiff and squirmy whenever her mother would try to hold her. On the rare occasions when she did allow her mom to hold her, Emma would avoid eye contact, and she would tend to poke her mother in the ears and neck and fiddle with her earrings. Mom reports that Emma often screamed, with no apparent triggers. She only used a few words consistently to obtain basic needs and wants. Most of Emma's verbalization was completely unintelligible and repetitive or consisted of echoing things she had heard in a singsong voice. She spent most of her time lining up objects by size or throwing objects to watch how they fell.

On observation in the clinic, Emma avoided eye contact. She didn't turn to look when the examiner entered the room, nor did she respond to verbal overtures by the examiner. She flapped her hands frequently, and she had a flat affect. Most of her vocalizations consisted of repetitive sounds, such as "diga-diga-diga-diga." One recognizable word was "puh-lease," said over and over, out of context. When the examiner demonstrated pretend play with dolls and cars,

R. A. Phelps (✉)
Oregon Health & Science University, Eugene, OR, USA
e-mail: phelpsr@ohsu.edu

J. M. Fogler
Developmental Medical Center, Boston Children's Hospital, Boston, MA, USA
e-mail: Jason.Fogler@childrens.harvard.edu

J. M. Fogler, R. A. Phelps (eds.), *Trauma, Autism, and Neurodevelopmental Disorders*, https://doi.org/10.1007/978-3-030-00503-0_2

Emma showed no interest. Instead, she threw, banged, and lined the toys up. Of note, mom also had a flat affect. When holding Emma and being poked in the face, mom looked very tired and sad, and she didn't seem to make an effort to divert or engage Emma.

Based on detailed history, structured observations, and direct assessments, Emma was diagnosed with autism. Appropriate referrals were made for treatment and family support. Emma was already enrolled in public early intervention services. Recommendations included referrals for enrollment in applied behavior analysis, county developmental disabilities services, and supplemental speech/language therapy and occupational therapy. In addition to recommendations made for Emma herself, it was also clear to the team that mom also needed referrals for her own emotional health support. Mom was given information about resources, and a public health nurse was brought on board to help facilitate these referrals.

To our contemporary eyes, this vignette illustrates a rather classic presentation of autism. In this scenario, it would be a fair assumption that mom's apparent depression may well have resulted from 3 years of exhausting and dispiriting efforts to try to connect and communicate with her daughter. On the other hand, one could perhaps argue that Emma's mother was prone to depression anyway. Certainly, there are parents of children with autism who do not become depressed. Perhaps mom has a history of depression that predates Emma's birth? To modern diagnosticians in the United States, it is unfathomable that mom should be blamed for Emma's autism, yet, strangely, tragically, inconceivably, 50 years ago in this country, the arrows of causality would have been reversed, and Emma's autism would almost certainly have been blamed on her mother's apparent emotional inaccessibility. This error in the understanding of the etiology of autism was once greatly influential in the United States, is still the prevalent viewpoint in some countries, and continues to impact parent-professional communication around the world to this day.

Confusion between reactive attachment disorder and autism spectrum disorders can be traced back to the 1940s, when these disorders were first described. Bruno Bettelheim first ascribed the cause of autism to cold, distant parenting—the archetypal "refrigerator mom" [1]. Specifically, Bettelheim hypothesized that a child confronted with such a parenting style would internalize a sense of not being loved by the parent and would thus *negate* himself or herself by turning inward, not communicating, not interacting, and engaging in repetitive self-stimulatory behavior. This concept was eventually adopted (after some initial resistance) by Leo Kanner, the person credited with coining the term "autism," thus establishing the "refrigerator mom" concept as the orthodox explanation for the etiology of autism for more than a generation [2].

Subsequently, as described in more detail below, the use of the diagnostic label of "autism" was disengaged from the notion that autism was caused by inadequate parenting of any sort, and we have come to understand that autism is a neurobiological disorder with a complex set of genetic etiologies. Over the last several decades, the use of the diagnosis "autism" has been expanded and applied to a broader range of presentations, ranging from severe, classic "Kanner's" autism, to individuals with much milder impacts on social and communication skills and milder symptoms of repetitive behaviors and movements or intrusive interests [3].

Interestingly, as Bettelheim, Kanner, and others endeavored to understand autism and its causes, other investigators were simultaneously describing the impact of severe, institutional neglect on children's development. For example, Rene Spitz described the delays in development of children who lived in institutional orphanages where basic physical needs such as food, clothing, and shelter were provided but affection and physical contact were absent. Even though physical needs were met, these children had stunted physical as well as social-emotional growth, and many of these children died. This condition was initially termed "anaclitic depression" and later reactive attachment disorder (RAD) [4]. In the subsequent decades since these initial descriptions of the impact of institutional care on children's development, it has been recognized that RAD exists in a spectrum of severity, from the most extreme RAD, associated with institutional care as described above, to milder forms, resulting from chronic disruptions to the caregiver-infant relationship (such as may be seen in cases of severe depression or substance addiction in the caregiver). In milder manifestations, physical signs such as growth stunting or severe delays in achieving developmental milestones may not be seen, but children may be conditioned to making escalating and negative bids for attention due to chronic inaccessibility of the caregiver [5].

Overview and Disclaimer

The diagnostic confusion between ASD and TSRD has undermined the credibility of professionals in the field and contributes to challenges in professional-caregiver collaboration to meet the needs of children and youth with these conditions. In this chapter, we describe how the diagnostic and etiological confusion between autism spectrum disorder (ASD) and trauma- and stressor-related disorder (TSRD) stems from the early efforts to understand each of these conditions. The chapter is not a comprehensive history of ASD and TSRD, but an attempt to understand their confused and entwined histories. We hope that this understanding will put us in a better position to suggest some potential ways of dealing with this problem.

Historical Context, Part 1: The Ideological/Intellectual Conflict Between Nazi Naturism vs. Freudian Nurturism—Influence on Kanner, Bettelheim, and Asperger

Historical context is important in understanding the evolving professional consensus about these conditions. This story begins with Leo Kanner and Bruno Bettelheim. Both men were personally and deeply affected by the Holocaust and by the cruelty of Nazism. Kanner and Bettelheim were both Austrian Jews. They worked out their understanding of autism during World War II and in the years immediately following the war. Bettelheim was interned at Buchenwald, and he attributed his insights about the impact of traumatic experience on the psyche to his own experiences there. Bettelheim "describes observing the impact of cruelty on the psyches of his fellow inmates—e.g. cruel guards, withholding permission to visit latrines, induced infantile regression in the inmates" [1]. Kanner left Austria in the 1920s to advance his career in America, so he did not experience the war or the Holocaust firsthand. However, as Steve Silberman illustrated in his book *NeuroTribes*, Kanner did lose many relatives in the Holocaust, and he personally intervened to save the lives of hundreds of Jewish colleagues by sponsoring them for positions in the United States [6]. The point is that both men were personally and deeply affected by the Holocaust and by the cruelty of Nazism. The fact that both Bettelheim and Kanner were personally impacted by Nazism is important to understanding this whole story, because Nazism was the culmination of the Eugenic movement.

The Eugenics movement was characterized by policies promoting segregation, disenfranchisement, and sterilization of people with disabilities along with ethnic minorities and immigrants. Its influence increased steadily throughout Europe and America, reaching its zenith when the Nazis came to power in Europe. The Nazi perspective regarding people with disabilities was that they were "polluting" the gene pool, and therefore they must be "purged" from the gene pool. Whereas the American and European Eugenicists who preceded the Nazis pursued policies of segregation, institutionalization, and sterilization, and discussed but (generally) discarded the option of "euthanasia," the Nazis embraced "euthanasia" as a central component of their Eugenics program. The Nazis' rationalization underpinning this brutal policy was the belief that disabilities result from impurities of genes, thus that disabilities are inherent and irreparable and that individuals with disabilities must be eliminated for the greater good of preserving a healthy gene pool. Nazi thinking thus tended to err on the side of attributing pathology to heredity. This philosophy held true on the individual level (attributing various personal traits to family or origin) as well as on the larger, societal level (attributing traits of a whole people to racial origin). This bias caused Nazis to neglect the contribution of environmental factors to their understanding of psychopathology. In other words, mental illness was understood as the result of flawed genes. Nazis were not interested in the impact of parent-infant bonding or of the result of traumatic experiences on child mental health. This approach, overemphasizing the role of genetics and underemphasizing the role of environment, is often termed biological determinism or "Naturism" [7].

In contrast to the Nazis and Eugenicists, Jewish thinkers of the time, including Kanner and Bettelheim, were heavily influenced by Freud. They were intrigued by the impact of the parent-child relationship on mental health and illness, as well as on development. This approach of emphasizing the role of environment over that of genetics is often termed biological potentiality or "Nurturism" [8].

The Nazi bias against Nurturism and toward Naturism was strengthened by the fact that Nurturism was championed at that time by Freud and Freudians, the vast majority of whom were Jewish. Naturism was also championed by other enemies of the Nazis, the socialists and communists. In summary, the Nazis' and other Eugenicists' inclination was to attribute parents' influence on their children's mental health to the genes they bequeathed and not to their parenting practices. This inclination was only strengthened by the association of Nurturism with Jewish thinkers, like Freud. Even if Freud's ideas had not been diametrically opposed to Naturism, they would have been rejected by the Nazis as inferior, flawed Jewish science.

A parallel process of polarization occurred with the Freudians. The inclination of Freudians like Kanner and Bettelheim was to favor Nurturism. This bias was only strengthened by the Nazis' embrace of Naturism and rejection of Nurturism. The impact of Nurturism on postwar American thinking was bolstered by the flood of Jewish, Freudian refugees, rescued by the heroic action of Kanner, among others, and by the fact that the non-Jewish anti-Freudian types were more likely to remain behind in Europe [6]. In addition to these more dogmatic influences, there were implications for the young field of psychiatry. As asserted by Silberman in *NeuroTribes*, "To a generation of erudite intellectuals who had barely escaped extermination, [the] suggestion that the fate of these children was sealed at birth seemed nearly traitorous to the profession. If autism was rooted in disturbed family dynamics, however, there was still reason for hope" [9]. In other words, Silberman seems to imply here that psychoanalysts may have been biased toward Nurturism out of self-interest, to preserve their own job security, because with the philosophy of biological potentiality, there is a hope for cure through psychoanalysis. Maybe it is our own bias, as pediatric clinicians, but this seems like an excessively cynical viewpoint to us. At the very least, job security was probably not the only consideration. Just as plausibly, we would argue that the large number of Jewish refugees in the profession may also have wanted to get as far from Nazism and Eugenic ideas as possible.

In this context then, we can understand why Bettelheim promoted and Kanner later embraced the tempting but flawed notion that autism was caused by cold, distant mothering. To our modern eyes, which can see clearly that physical and mental pathology is a product of an interaction of genes and environment,and that Naturism and Nurturism are both extreme viewpoints (clouded by ideology and thus missing the mark), Bettelheim and Kanner seem at best hopelessly naïve. At worst, when we reflect on the terrible impact their theory of autism had on the parents of their patients—casting blame on these parents already beleaguered by challenging behavior and frustrated attempts to communicate with their own children—Bettelheim and Kanner seem cruel. Indeed, parents today tend to demonize these pioneers, if they think of Bettelheim and Kanner at all. This reaction from parents today is completely understandable. In the past, many parents brought their children to Bettelheim and Kanner, and to the generation of professionals trained by these men, for help. Instead, the parents were blamed and berated, and the children were placed in institutions, as was the standard of care in this country from the 1940s into the 1970s. However, if we examine the historical context and understand that Bettelheim and Kanner were reacting to an extreme and cruel ideology of Naturism/Nazism, we can at least understand why they let themselves be blinded by their own extreme ideology of Nurturism.

Historical Context, Part 2: Implications for Current Care of ASD and TSRD, "Fictitious Epidemics," and Families' Expectations of the Mental Health System

The histories of our understanding of ASD and TSRD are important for a two reasons. First, by examining this history, we can better understand the dynamics of mistrust that parents might have of professional diagnosticians in the area of childhood mental health and development. We, as autism and mental health diagnosticians, inherit a mantle associated with deeply flawed diagnostic processes, disparagement of parents, and careless inflicting of pain on the parents who came to our forebears for help. Secondly, as has been said many times before, if we do not study our history, we are doomed to repeat it. We need to study errors of the past to better understand how to avoid errors in the present and future.

When we meet with families of children or youth with developmental and/or behavioral problems, our goal is clearly to help these families. The purpose of performing diagnostic assessments is to help to better understand developmental and behavioral problems so we can better direct effective therapy for children. We try to do our diagnostic assessments with great care, empathy, and professionalism, in attempt to provide the most accurate and meaningful assessments possible. Thus, while the goal is to provide compassionate care, we aim for precision and scrupulousness, as well as kindness, in our clinical approach. Our point is that because we care, we take care to be accurate. The quality of our recommendations for interventions depends on the quality of the diagnostic assessment. The quality of this assessment, in turn, is highly dependent on the quality of the information gleaned in the diagnostic interview. We also do some direct assessment, observation, and examination of the child. The challenge is that for the diagnosis of ASD or TSRD, there are no reliable "biomarkers," no brain imaging or laboratory testing, which can confirm or rule out the diagnosis. We rely on clinical interview and examination. A very large component of the assessment is the interview of the caregiver because, for one thing, children often behave differently than they usually do while in the artificial setting of the clinic. For that reason, we also gather data from teachers and other reporters, to supplement interview data. We may even do observations in the community. Nevertheless, we still rely heavily on caregiver reports describing a child's behavior and developmental progress in order for us to form our diagnostic impressions.

In addition to relying on interview of caregiver for data to help us form a diagnosis, we interview the family extensively to make sure that we understand caregiver goals for treatment. While there may be certain evidence-based interventions for any given diagnosis, different families may and will select different treatment options. In the family-centered model in which we practice, clients and professionals are equal partners in treatment planning. They have different roles, but, in the ideal scenario at least, decision-making power is shared.[1] Without a partnership,

[1] Even as we write this, we appreciate that we are speaking about an ideal scenario. Many families with whom we work with are profoundly disempowered by socioeconomic circumstances, the legacy of oppression of "non-majority groups" (broadly defined), and the increasingly dehumanizing and confusing healthcare system. We believe strongly that these families need assistance to feel that they can engage in the diagnostic process on equal footing.

goals of accurate diagnosis and assessment of appropriate treatment cannot be achieved. Although there is power sharing in an ideal diagnostic assessment, there are rules and roles. The caregivers' obligations are to disclose accurate information to the best of their abilities. This is challenging, as caregivers may be influenced by stigma, embarrassment, or shame, which might inhibit the disclosure of information that could be crucial to the diagnostic process. The diagnostician's obligation is to put the available data together into an accurate diagnosis. This too is challenging, as the diagnostician may be influenced by cultural biases, dogma, interpersonal interactions, or work pressures. These might lead the diagnostician to disregard some bits of data or to overemphasize other bits of data, thus skewing the diagnostic picture. Once the diagnosis is established, there are again roles for all participants. The professional provides a menu of evidence-based treatment options and explains the potential pros and cons of various choices. The caregiver selects treatment options that fit with the family's values and preferences from this slate of choices.

This delicate balance of roles and responsibilities, already beset by the challenges posed by emotional vulnerability and by bias, is further undermined by the power imbalance inherent in the doctor-patient relationship. Furthermore, the belief that the actions of parents are the cause of autism, which was engrained in a generation of diagnosticians, has exacerbated this imbalance by heaping blame on the parents of children with autism. We now know autism to be a neurodevelopmental disorder, with neurodevelopmental etiology, not the result of indifferent parenting. Unfortunately, Bettelheim's original mistake contributes to mistrust, undermining honest, open communication between patient and provider even today.

More problematic still is that the current realities of resource allocation further increase the tension between needing to correctly identify and communicate diagnoses and feeling compelled to advocate for children and families. To understand how resource allocation has evolved over time, we again have to review some history. Back in Bettelheim's and Kanner's day, the diagnosis of autism was rarely made. Only the most extreme presentations, in which children had profoundly impaired social interaction and communication skills, *and* had intrusive fixations and repetitive self-stimulatory behaviors, met diagnostic criteria. Even when a child had a rather classic presentation, if no evidence could be found to support that parenting quality could be called into question, a formal diagnosis was deferred, and the child was merely said to have "features of autism." This was the case because the implication of a diagnosis of autism was that the parents were at fault; thus, the treatment was removal of the child from the parents, placement of the child in an institution, and subjecting the parents to protracted courses of psychoanalysis. The end result of this hesitancy to use the diagnostic label of autism meant that children were rarely diagnosed with autism, and there was little need to allocate resources to autism. Autism was a clinical curiosity, not a public health issue.

With the advent of effective, evidence-based intervention for autism (e.g., applied behavior analysis) and with the rise of an autism parent advocacy movement in the 1970s led by Bernard Rimland, a psychologist and parent of a child with autism, the resistance to the use of the diagnosis of autism began to weaken. With an effective treatment available, and with a gradual lessening of parent blaming, providers slowly became more comfortable with identifying autism. In the 1990s, the work of Hans

Asperger was disseminated by Dr. Lorna Wing, a British physician and parent of a child with autism. Her background as a parent gave her clarity that parents are not to blame for autism. Living and working in Britain, she was free from the history of parent-blaming bias of Bettelheim and Kanner. Parallels between the histories of ASD and TSRD are equally notable in this case: Bettelheim's error in understanding the etiology of autism may have stemmed from his lack of understanding about reactive attachment disorder. Bettelheim and his wife adopted a girl named Patsy, who had an emotional disturbance. Patsy reportedly experienced significant improvement in their home, and much of this improvement was no doubt attributable to the care given to the girl by Bettelheim's wife, the primary caregiver. The story told at the time is that Patsy had autism and that Bettelheim had discovered parenting interventions which were effective in ameliorating the symptoms of the condition. At the time, Patsy's behavioral difficulties were attributed to autism. However, with the benefit of hindsight, and with the knowledge that Patsy was a girl with emotional disturbance who was adopted, one wonders whether Patsy's behavioral difficulties might have been more accurately attributed to disrupted attachment [6].

Thanks to Asperger, Wing, and others, the realization that autism is a spectrum,[2] including even mild, very high-functioning presentations, became widespread and was codified among professionals in the DSM-IV, in 1994. Also in the 1990s, autism was included as a qualifying eligibility for special education services under Individuals with Disabilities Education Act (IDEA). Over the last quarter century, autism awareness has increased substantially, and the crucial importance of early detection of autism and referral for treatment has enjoyed widespread acceptance. With this burgeoning of autism awareness, we now experience an interesting paradox: we have a public health success—heightened autism awareness, producing increased screening, referral, and diagnosis, allocation of resources to treatment—with a simultaneously occurring public hysteria about a fictitious "epidemic."

Kanner lived into the 1990s, long enough to see the application of his diagnosis broadened. This prompted his complaint, in a review for Rimland's book, that "his concept of early infantile autism….had been applied so broadly that 'the term was used as a pseudodiagnostic wastebasket for a variety of unrelated conditions'" [11]. Frankly, we have little sympathy for Kanner in this regard. As pointed out in *NeuroTribes*, "by overturning [Kanner's] conception of autism as a rare, inevitably devastating, and homogeneous disorder, [Wing] made it possible for tens of thousands of children, teenagers, and adults to gain access to the educational placements and social services they deserved, for the first time in history" [12]. However, though "Wing's goal was to help 'make it possible for children who would have been excluded from support services to get them'…by the end of the decade…the startling rise in diagnoses…and the alarms in the media that autism had become an epidemic—took even Lorna by surprise… I have felt like Pandora after she opened the box" [13].

[2] Before and during World War II, Hans Asperger sought to protect his patients from the gas chambers by emphasizing his charges' exceptional giftedness in the topics of their intrusive interest; thus Asperger disorder would eventually be coined to describe individuals with autism spectrum disorder with typical to advanced language and intellectual development [10].

Interestingly, such false epidemics have occurred previously in the history of our understanding of developmental disabilities. For example, in 1859, after Dr. Langdon Down first described the syndrome that would later bear his name, an epidemic of the syndrome was described, with alarm, in London. The medical profession of that time and place attributed Down syndrome (what they called "Mongolism"—literally, not figuratively) to tuberculosis infections, which were thought, ludicrously, to be inducing racial degeneration, causing English children to actually turn into Mongols! Of course, there was no epidemic of Down syndrome in Victorian London. Rather, as we now understand with the benefit of hindsight, once "Mongolism" was described and medical professionals knew what to look for, Mongolism awareness was heightened, and the prevalence was skyrocketed [14].

Forty-five years later, the French government commissioned Alfred Binet and Theodore Simon to create a developmental assessment which would allow early detection of developmental delay in children, to improve timeliness of referral of these children to France's new invention, early intervention. Binet and Simon created the world's first "IQ test." Again, the goal was to improve identification of children in need of early intervention, in order to improve outcomes in these children. Unfortunately, this test was imported to the United States by the Eugenicist, Henry Goddard, who employed it in his effort to detect children with subtle developmental delays (children he termed "Morons"—a new diagnostic category!), in order to expedite the segregation and sterilization of these unfortunate children. The test itself, of course, was deeply flawed, resulting in overdiagnosis of "Moronia," frantic and alarmist heightening of Moronia awareness, and the creation of another "epidemic" [8]. This, tragically, led to the involuntary institutionalization and sterilization of many people with developmental disabilities and also of immigrants (who failed the test due to lack of familiarity with English and with American culture) and impoverished people (who lacked legal advocacy and/or educational opportunity) [7].

Finally, a third example of fictitious epidemics, cited by Silberman in *NeuroTribes*: "In an eerie preview of the autism epidemic to come four decades later, the prevalence of childhood schizophrenia started spiking in the mid twentieth century...In fact, if Kanner's syndrome was defined too narrowly, childhood schizophrenia had the opposite problem: its boundaries were so diffuse that it included too many different types of patients" [15].

The Unexpected Consequences (and Ramifications) of Heightening ASD Awareness

As autism awareness has grown, so has allocation of services and resources. Services through mental health clinics, developmental disabilities agencies, and schools have expanded markedly. Allocation of resources into research and into improving diagnosis, treatment, and accommodation has also increased greatly. However, we still have much room for improvement. Children and their families wait far too long for diagnostic assessments. Once diagnosed, children and their families wait far too long to access treatments and services, or they meet various barriers or interruptions to receiving services. Services are often still inadequate. We still lack much of the knowledge and resources that children with autism and their families need. As children grow up, entitlements vanish and are not replaced, and there can be yet more waiting in line to access adult services, if they exist. Nonetheless, while there is tremendous room for improvement, progress has been made.

Meanwhile, progress toward the treatment of trauma and stressor-related disorders is slow. Unlike autism, which has been unshackled from the stigma of parent blaming, TSRDs still implicate parental roles in abuse or in inadequate protection of children from trauma, disrupted attachment, and/or chaotic homes and neighborhoods. Given this dynamic, parents are inhibited from self-advocacy. Without the advocacy, pressure to advance research and to increase availability of treatment and other resources for these children lags behind. Certainly, there are high-quality interventions and high-quality programs which serve the needs of children with TSRDs [16]. There is some funding for these services; however, because of the stigma, biological parents of children suffering from TSRDs tend not to clamor for recognition or for services for these conditions. Also, by the nature of these conditions, affected families tend to be saddled with chronic stress and everyday chaos; they are not in a position for effective self-advocacy.

So, we find ourselves in the position in which we are today. Autism awareness is heightened. Resources are allocated to children with autism. Stigma has been lessened; in fact, autism self-advocates have reduced stigma to the point that autism is often embraced or celebrated. Meanwhile, children with TSRDs and their families, seeing their neighbors receiving intensive in-home services (such as applied behavior analysis and respite supports through developmental disabilities services), often seek assessments at our diagnostic referral centers. Often, these parents aren't just requesting comprehensive diagnostic assessments. They are pointedly requesting diagnoses of autism, in order to access the services they see their neighbors, relatives, and friends accessing with this diagnosis. Also, the autism diagnosis may be seen as an absolution, as autism, by definition, does not implicate parenting in the etiology, in contrast with TSRD. So, the great irony here is that autism used to be blamed, falsely, on parents. Now, we often encounter parents, who may be struggling to provide adequately safe or nurturing homes to their children, actively seeking a diagnosis of autism. Today, a diagnosis of autism provides an explanation for problem behaviors that does not implicate parents or parenting, and it provides access to valuable services.

Identifying that an aspect of parenting might be contributing to a behavior problem or a developmental delay is hard, in part, because parents are often loath to accept that. Conveying such a conclusion to a parent at the end of a diagnostic assessment is also extremely difficult. It is painful to have to look someone in the eye and to share such an opinion. And it is painful for a parent to hear it. Nevertheless, it is a fact that parenting matters and that there are parenting behaviors that can shape child behaviors [5]. There are parenting practices that can and do influence the achievement of developmental milestones. There are social circumstances in which some families find themselves, which are greatly detrimental to the development and mental health of children. To deny this would be folly. That doesn't make it any easier to diagnose TSRDs and to share this conclusion with parents.

Complicating matters further, we often encounter parents who are not just hoping for absolution from blame in their children's behavior problems; they are also seeking services. Injury is added to insult, as parents feel blamed and criticized, and simultaneously they lose anticipated access to particular services or supports. Providers, well steeped in a professional culture of family-centered care, often justify avoiding conversations about environmental contributions to a child's condition; often they hedge and defer a definitive diagnosis, or they just go ahead and give a diagnosis of autism when the available clinical data do not support this conclusion. In medical anthropologist Roy Grinker's book, Judith Rapoport, former chief of child psychiatry at the NIMH, admitted to Grinker, "I am incredibly disciplined in the diagnostic classifications in my research, but in my private practice, I'll call a kid a zebra if it will get him the educational services I think he needs" [17]. This example illustrates how a professional diagnostician, motivated only by the highest, purest reasons, such as compassion and a drive to advocate for families struggling to find help for their children with special educational and/or behavioral health needs, may justify adjusting the burden of proof for confirming a particular diagnosis if that is likely to improve access to care. For better or worse, some diagnoses have more stigma attached to them than others. As of this writing, in 2017, ASD is a less stigmatized diagnosis than conditions like conduct disorder or reactive attachment disorder. We are not calling out Dr. Rapoport or picking on her here. Again, we attribute to her only the highest, most selfless motives: the desire to help people who need help. Yet she, like many of our compassionate family-centered colleagues, is contributing to the problem of inappropriate usage of the autism label. This, in turn, makes it harder to efficiently and effectively serve both children with autism and children with TSRDs. As we explore further in the conclusion, it behooves us, as a society, to find better ways of helping children than falsifying diagnoses.

Full Disclosure: Our Reasons for Writing this Book

When we started writing this book, we were prompted to do so by our independent observations that a large number of children were being referred to our diagnostic centers for autism assessments whose presentations did not remotely resemble autism. That in and of itself is not a problem; we are strongly in favor of robust programs for autism screening. The purpose of any screening program is to pick up all people who may have a condition and to refer these people for further testing to determine whether they have the actual diagnosis. When screening is done well, there should be no false negatives, and there should be many false positives. The false positives are then screened out in secondary screening or diagnostic testing. However, one cause for concern has been that over the last several years, we have been receiving referrals of large numbers of children and youth who are not coming for our diagnostic opinions. Rather, we commonly encounter parents who communicate that they "already know" their child or youth has autism. Less frequently but still regularly, we encounter parents who state unequivocally that they "already know" that their ex-spouse or partner inflicted the trauma that caused their children's presumptive posttraumatic stress. In either case, they view the referral to our clinics as a mere formality, a tedious process that they must go through to get their rubber stamp of autism (or TSRD) so that they can access various supports and services. This leads to a significant amount of pain and frustration for all parties during feedback sessions, no matter what the final diagnosis. When parents are expecting their child to be diagnosed with autism, we meet resistance no matter what our diagnosis is, be it TRSDs or something else, such as of intellectual disability, anxiety, ADHD, or Tourette syndrome. However, for the reasons described above, it is the communication of a diagnosis of TSRD, either positive or negative, that can be most painful for the parent and for the provider, which is why this dynamic is the focus of this book.

As our waitlists get longer and longer—families routinely waiting over a year for a comprehensive diagnostic assessment!—this problem has become more than just a frustrating experience for families and professionals. It has become a major public health problem. Families of children and youth with autism wait intolerably long intervals for the diagnosis they need to be able to access appropriate interventions and supports. Meanwhile, families with children with other conditions wait intolerably long times for autism assessments, only to be told that their child doesn't have autism and that they will need a referral to the mental health system. Attempts to expedite diagnoses and shorten wait times by doing cursory diagnostic assessments run the risk of misdiagnosis. This leads to further overburdening our systems for autism treatment, misallocation of resources, and further delay in identification of the correct diagnosis and treatment for children without autism. As this issue has become more and more of a problem in our respective clinics, we have reached out and communicated with our colleagues around the country, only to find that we are not alone in our experience or perception; this is a problem familiar to many in the field. So, we decided to write this book to focus on this problem, which seems not to be receiving as much attention as it should.

As mentioned above, historical context is important. We started writing this book in 2015, which was not that long ago, but was, frankly, a different era in the United States. In 2015, the government's policy was that autism and other developmental disabilities were areas in which robust research was needed and to which substantial funds were allocated. Now, in 2017, the current administration makes irresponsible, ill-informed tweets and public statements about vaccines causing autism, threatens drastic cuts to research funding, and generally casts aspersions on the scientific method as a valid approach to understanding life on Earth. In 2015, there was a general acknowledgement in the federal government that depriving people with "pre-existing conditions" of healthcare is cruel and dangerous. In 2017, although lip service is paid to the concept that people with pre-existing conditions should be able to maintain access to healthcare, both the US House of Representatives' American

Health Care Act and the US Senate's Better Care Reconciliation Act included giant loopholes to enable insurance companies to charge more for those with pre-existing conditions or simply to not fund services and treatments for those conditions. By 2015, the Department of Education had enjoyed years of expansion, and, nationwide, we had seen years of augmentation of educational services for students with special educational needs. In 2017, the current administration favors a voucher system that allows for the diversion of education funds to schools that admit that they do not have the capacity to serve those with special needs, in violation of both Individuals with Disabilities Education Act and the Americans with Disabilities Act. In 2015, public support providing respite to families with children with developmental disabilities had grown immensely, thanks to the Affordable Care Act, and had helped to keep families together. In 2017, the same politicians who most vociferously promote "family values" threaten to cut these supports in order to give giant tax breaks to billionaires and, much like the Eugenicists of the last century, demonize immigrants, refugees, non-Christians, and people with disabilities.

The situation in clinic which prompted us to write this book has not changed significantly since 2015. We still see a large number of people seeking autism diagnoses for their children who have TSRDs, and sometimes we see the opposite, i.e., children with developmental disabilities referred for a question of TSRD in the context of a legal dispute between the child's parents. We seek to shine light on this phenomenon, to try to understand it, and to try to improve the situation. However, we also want to emphasize that we do not wish in *any* way, consciously or inadvertently, to adversely impact any aspect of autism advocacy. Autism is a common neurodevelopmental condition that has a substantial impact on lifelong functioning. Even those with milder autism often require a high level of support in order to be successful. However, as Asperger pointed out to a previous short-sighted (and short-lived) government, people with high-functioning autism can contribute greatly to the community, nation, and world. Children with more severe autism symptoms may need a high level of intervention to try to improve communication and behavior but can also contribute to society when their needs are met with proper supports. Their families need a high level of respite support in order to maintain parental employment, preserve marriages, and maintain nurturing and safe homes for siblings. We certainly do not advocate for any lessening of support for people with autism and their families. Quite the contrary, we need to continue to increase funding for autism research, educational supports, medical services, and social services. Additionally, it is also our goal to advocate for more visibility for other disabilities, including TSRDs, and to increase supports to prevent and ameliorate the effects of these disorders. In brief, we wish for a world in which all children are given their due: the appropriate services for their specific challenges. Children and families in need of support, whether the children have ASD or TRSD, should not have to fight over resources and should not feel that they must "work the system" to get what they need, and clinicians should not feel like they have to "call a kid a zebra" to get that child appropriate services.

In this volume, we seek to clarify this diagnostic confusion, which arises from the origins or the "tangled roots" of the understanding of ASDs and TSRDs. We then explore its ramifications for today's practice. Toward these ends, we have assembled a set of very fine contributors with diverse voices and perspectives. We begin with our "in-the-trenches" perspectives on what we see in our respective clinics. We describe how we have independently come upon very similar ways to navigate these thorny diagnostic issues. Next, we turn to the neurobiological aspects of the conditions, followed by [We are no longer dividing the contents by sections] treatment in preschool-aged children, cultural context, and transition to adulthood. The book concludes with some modest proposals toward some potential solutions.

References

1. Fleck C, Muller A. Bruno Bettelheim and the concentration camps. J Hist Behav Sci. 1997;33(1):1.
2. Sanua V. Leo Kanner (1894-1981): the man and the scientist. Child Psychiatry Hum Dev. 1990;21(1):3.
3. Wing L. The history of ideas on autism: legends, myths, and reality. Autism. 1997;1(13):13–23.
4. Emde RN. Individual meaning and increasing complexity: contributions of Sigmund Freud and Rene Spitz to developmental psychology. Dev Psychol. 1992;22(3):347–59.
5. Center on the Developing Child at Harvard University. The science of neglect: the persistent absence of responsive care disrupts the developing brain. Working Paper No. 12. 2012. www.developingchild.harvard.edu.
6. Silberman S. NeuroTribes: the legacy of autism and the future of neurodiversity. New York: Avery, Penguin/Random House; 2015.
7. Cohen A. Imbeciles: the Supreme Court, American eugenics, and the sterilization of Carrie Buck. New York: Penguin Press; 2016.
8. Gould SJ. The mismeasure of man. New York: Norton; 1981.
9. Silberman S. NeuroTribes: the legacy of autism and the future of neurodiversity. New York: Avery, Penguin/Random House; 2015. p. 197.
10. Frith U. Autism and Asperger syndrome. Cambridge: Cambridge University Press; 1991.
11. Silberman S. NeuroTribes: the legacy of autism and the future of neurodiversity. New York: Avery, Penguin/Random House; 2015. p. 270.
12. Silberman S. NeuroTribes: the legacy of autism and the future of neurodiversity. New York: Avery, Penguin/Random House; 2015. p. 41.
13. Silberman S. NeuroTribes: the legacy of autism and the future of neurodiversity. New York: Avery, Penguin/Random House; 2015. p. 381.
14. Hickey F, Hickey E, Summar KL. Medical update for children with Down syndrome for the pediatrician and family practitioner. Adv Pediatr. 2012;59(1):137–5715.
15. Silberman S. NeuroTribes: the legacy of autism and the future of neurodiversity. New York: Avery, Penguin/Random House; 2015. p. 196.16.
16. Hodas GR. Responding to childhood trauma: the promise and practice of trauma informed care. 2017. http://www.childrescuebill.org/VictimsOfAbuse/RespondingHodas.pdf. Accessed 24 Nov 2017.
17. Grinker RR. Unstrange minds. New York: Basic Books; 2008. p. 131.

Chapter 3
Posttraumatic Stress Disorder: From Neurobiology to Cycles of Violence

K. M. McCullough and K. J. Ressler

Introduction

Case Study

A 45-year-old male. Multiple lifetime trauma exposures, with the most significant being childhood trauma. He also endured a serious accident, assault by a family member and a stranger, military combat, imprisonment, and even torture experiences. He referred often to his time in prison, where he said he spent many years. While going through the PTSD Diagnostic Scale, he was surprised by how accurately the hyperarousal questions described what he's been going through as a result of his traumas.

"I've been trying to figure out what was wrong with me all this time. All these days of just … acting the same … I can't sleep, my head has all this junk in it.

To get by, I kind of blended in, I did really bad things. But … I see I'm not normal. I'm not like other people, I don't react and respond the same way that most people react and respond. If somebody, say something you don't like, you may respond and kind of let it go. I can't. I go on and on and on and then in my head I tell myself, why am I not stopping? Anyone else could just stop. For me it just goes on and on and on.

"… how the violence was first portrayed on me. I can definitely see how that's gotten me into so much trouble. There's a lot of people who suffer …. A lot of us have been labeled as being, as having an anger disorder. And it's

(continued)

K. M. McCullough · K. J. Ressler (✉)
Department of Psychiatry, McLean Hospital, Harvard Medical School, Belmont, MA, USA
e-mail: kmccullough@mclean.harvard.edu; kressler@mclean.harvard.edu

J. M. Fogler, R. A. Phelps (eds.), *Trauma, Autism, and Neurodevelopmental Disorders*, https://doi.org/10.1007/978-3-030-00503-0_3

not an anger disorder.... The type of person you become after being battered. Many of us become defensive. Many of us learn how to defend ourselves. And a lot of the things we believe is for self-defense is not always for self-defense. But it was only for self-defense in that situation. But you can't just drop these behaviors once you get out of the situation. It becomes a part of who you are."

"I forget initially why I became an aggressive person. I realized that the aggression I used then—it helped me to establish a sort of fear amongst others. And so they say, "I ain't gonna mess with him." And they labeled me crazy. And crazy was the key to get me out of, or protect me. But I wasn't crazy, I was tough, I was scared. And only I knew that. I was the only one who knew I was scared so what I'm gonna do is, because it worked before, I'm going to do something really extreme so that ... you don't want to mess with me.

A lot of guys say, "I'm tired, I'm tired. I'm not coming back." But I see them all coming back (to prison). And I knew they were sincere. I sat there and I look in his eyes and he said to me, crying, "I'm so tired of this. I've been doing this all my life." And would go home, and then come back (again). What happened? Being sick and tired is not enough to keep you out. You have to know what keeps you coming back".

The words of the patient in this case study strongly give a sense of the psychological stress he lives with and the extent to which his life has been affected by his history of trauma. Trauma and stressor related disorders (TSRD) such as posttraumatic stress disorder (PTSD) are among the most prevalent of all psychiatric disorders worldwide. PTSD is characterized by having experienced at least one strongly distressing event and four primary symptom clusters: re-experiencing (intrusion), avoidance, changes in arousal and reactivity, and negative changes in cognition or mood [1]. In the testimony of this patient who had a series of traumatic experiences, we see a variety of PTSD and defensive-aggression symptoms, notably hyperarousal. Notably, as a young child this individual experienced several types of physical and psychological abuse, illustrating the fact that childhood trauma is one of the greatest risk factors for later development of PTSD. Beginning with his testimony we may explore the symptoms and potential causes of PTSD knowing that children who experience trauma are much more likely to grow into the adults whose case studies we discuss.

In the Unites States the average lifetime prevalence of PTSD is around 8%; however, women are diagnosed at a rate twice that of men (10% vs. 5%, respectively) [2, 3]. Among at-risk populations, rates of PTSD are much higher. Soldiers returning from the wars in Iraq and Afghanistan exhibit PTSD at a rate of almost 14% [4]. Among Vietnam war veterans, rates of PTSD are equally high with 15.2% of men and 8.5% of women who served suffering from PTSD at the time of the study, more than 15 years after the end of service with substantially higher rates among war-zone respondents (35.8% of men and 17.5% of women) [5]. Finally, civilians who lived through large-scale disasters like Hurricane Katrina or September 11th or live in certain high crime inner-city areas also exhibit remarkably high rates of PTSD [6–11]. Thus, PTSD is not exclusively the domain of veterans; it occurs at high rates among many US populations exposed to chronic stress and trauma.

While lifetime rates of PTSD among at-risk populations are quite high, only about 10–30% of people who experience a single traumatic event will develop PTSD [11–13]. This demonstrates that people are not equally susceptible to development of TSRD. Some people have "risk" while others have "resilient" traits modulating whether they will develop TSRD after trauma. A myriad of factors play a role in determining risk for development of PTSD including genetic risk factors, developmental or environmental traumatic experiences, and the interaction between these two factors (so-called gene by environment or G × E factors). Childhood maltreatment is an especially important environmental risk factor. Although children develop PTSD at lower rates than adults, childhood trauma is a major risk factor for PTSD later in life following adult trauma. The intricate balance between genes and environment during development plays a critical role in setting up an individual's stress response system, which will determine whether they are resilient to trauma or at risk of development of TSRD (Fig. 3.1).

While the costs to individuals with TSRD symptoms are often discussed, the public health costs of TSRD, specifically PTSD, are less recognized. People with PTSD are at increased risk for a number of negative life outcomes such as

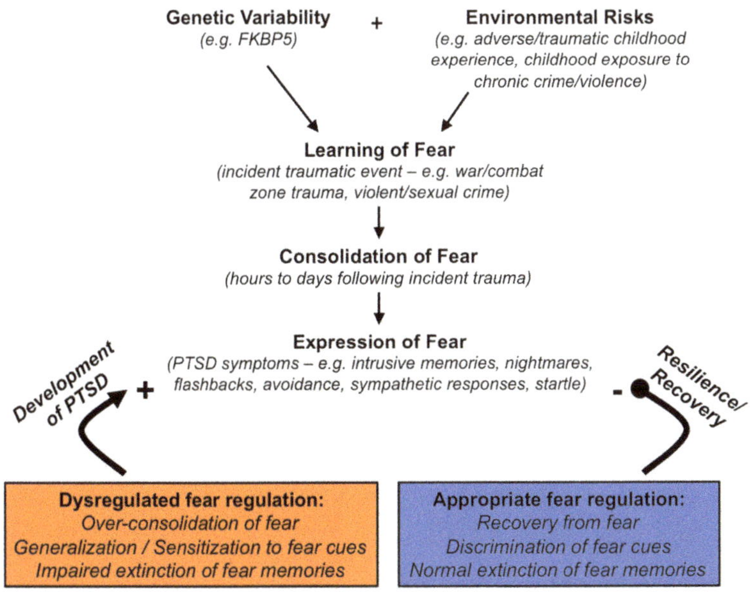

Fig. 3.1 Risk and resilience for development of PTSD depend upon many factors including environmental factors and genetic predisposition

substance abuse, including alcohol and illicit drug abuse, violent altercations and entrance into the criminal justice system. While these variables are generally inter-connected, there is convincing evidence that one significant contributor to the high rates of incarceration seen among inner-city men is the concomitantly high rates of childhood trauma and PTSD. Studies examining the benefits of emergency room and community therapy programs demonstrate that even minimal intervention at the time of trauma can greatly improve mental health outcomes later in life [14, 15]. Greater investment in public mental health resources may be efficacious at reducing the rate of PTSD, violent crime, and incarceration in the United States.

Given the enormous costs in life-quality and to the economy associated with lost productivity and direct costs of treating TSRD, it is unsurprising that much effort has been spent researching the causes, risk factors, and neurobiological underpinnings of these disorders. Accordingly, great gains have been made in our understanding of PTSD and other TSRD. Researchers have identified the major elements of neural networks controlling threat and anxiety behaviors and have made progress towards discovering how pathological alterations in the activity balance or function of these networks results in symptoms observed in PTSD.

Evolutionarily, the neural networks involved in threat and anxiety were likely some of the first to evolve, since maintaining homeostasis is proximally contingent upon avoiding destruction by a predator or other malign force [16]. Likewise, neural networks involved in the production of threat responses are some of the best conserved across species from fish to mice to humans [17]. This conservation intuitively makes sense as the nature of responses to threatening stimuli is maintained across the animal kingdom: increased arousal and avoidance of threatening stimuli. Appropriate threat responses in all animals are adaptive; however, in humans and other animals, dysregulation of neural circuitries governing threat responses may lead to maladaptive behaviors where threat responses are exhibited at inappropriate times or in inappropriate situations. Importantly, in PTSD, which is by definition caused by one or more specific traumatic events, symptoms are associated with the inability to suppress threat responses or to learn when stimuli are no longer threatening, rather than the de novo generation of unassociated threat responses [1, 18]. This suggests that interventions diminishing initial trauma responses or augmenting emotional regulatory systems, such as enhancing fear extinction, may have great efficacy at decreasing rates of PTSD.

In this chapter we will (1) review the basic neurocircuitry of threat responses and anxiety in humans and rodent models, (2) examine genetic and environmental variables that may determine neurodevelopmental trajectories setting up risk and resilience, and (3) discuss the roles childhood trauma and PTSD may play in the current mass incarceration crisis in the United States.

Neural Networks Involved in Threat Responses

Rodent Models

Examination of the neural networks involved in threat responses has benefited greatly from research using rodent models of threat behavior. It is impossible to model the subjective experience of fear in rodents, thus we will refer to responses to threatening stimuli by rodents as threat responses. The primary method for uncovering neuronal circuitry in rodents involves ablating or manipulating activity of specific brain areas or cell populations, and then observing the effects on the rodent's expression of fear or anxiety-like behaviors. Tasks such as Pavlovian threat conditioning and fear-potentiated startle are popular models for aversive learning in rodents because subjects acquire learned threat associations. In the auditory threat conditioning paradigm, an initially innocuous conditioned stimulus (CS, e.g., an auditory tone during auditory threat conditioning or the context of training during contextual threat conditioning) is paired with an aversive unconditioned stimulus (US, e.g., a mild foot shock). Following several CS-US pairings, the subject will exhibit threat response behaviors or conditioned responses (CRs) to presentations of the CS alone. The most common threat responses investigated are freezing (the cessation of all non-homeostatic movement) and fear-potentiated startle (FPS, in which the amplitude of an animal's startle to a noise burst is potentiated upon combined presentation of the CS and noise burst) [19, 20]. The use of these paradigms provides researchers with easily quantifiable and translationally robust techniques for probing the basic threat response circuitry in model animals.

For both rodents and humans, threat responses are adaptive only as long as the CS clearly predicts the US. When the two stimuli are no longer paired it is adaptive to modify behavioral responses to the CS. During extinction training in rodents, which closely mirrors exposure therapy for humans, a previously threatening CS is repeatedly presented in a safe environment. Multiple unpaired exposures to the CS gradually cause a decrement of CRs. Importantly, extinction is generally considered to be a new learning event that modulates rather than "erases" the original learned fear association [21]. In both animal models and humans pathological threat responses are often caused or accompanied by a failure to extinguish threat associations or by an over-generalization of associations between the original trauma CS to CSs divergent from original threat-paired CS [22, 23]. Animal models of threat learning and extinction closely resemble aspects of human fear learning and extinction allowing close examination of the systems which contribute to adaptive and pathological human behaviors.

Rodent Fear Circuitry

Animal models have allowed researchers to identify, in a causal manner, regions of the brain involved in threat responses. Broadly, the amygdala is canonically known as a hub of emotional processing; it is involved in flight, anxiety, and aversive behaviors as well as approach and appetitive behaviors [24–26]. Made up of 15 subnuclei, the diverse connections of the amygdala are known to mediate many aspects of emotional regulation and responding [27]. The main output nucleus of the amygdala, the central amygdala (CeA), has diverse connections to the brainstem and other regions directly responsible for symptoms of fear and panic. For example, connections to the *Reticularis Pontis Caudalis* mediate startle responses, connections to the *Central Grey Nucleus* mediate freezing responses, and connections to the *Paraventricular Nucleus* mediate corticosteroid release (Fig. 3.2) [25, 28–32]. The amygdala is known to mediate a large variety of threat and anxiety-like responses in both humans and rodent models.

Rodent models have allowed tracing of emotionally relevant circuitries to a high level of precision. Generally, learning related stimuli such as CS and US information are processed separately and converge on the amygdala from the auditory cortex/auditory thalamus and the somatosensory cortex/somatosensory thalamus, respectively. This information is also relayed to other regions such as the hippocampal complex (HPC) and the medial prefrontal cortex (mPFC), which in turn make reciprocal connections with the amygdala and each other. In rodents, the dorsal elements of the HPC encode contextual elements of threat learning while the ventral aspect encodes valence specific information [33, 34]. The mPFC, the infralimbic (IL) and prelimbic (PL) cortices, are intimately implicated in fear extinction and fear acquisition and expression, respectively [35]. The bed nucleus of the stria terminalis (BNST), with projections to the CeA, plays an important role in anxiety-like behavior and contextually driven fear [36]. Finally, the nucleus accumbens (NAc) is strongly connected to the amygdala and mediates many elements of motivated learning especially appetitive learning [37–39]. Together, rodent models allow for the in-depth causal dissection of neural circuitries mediating distinct elements of behavioral learning.

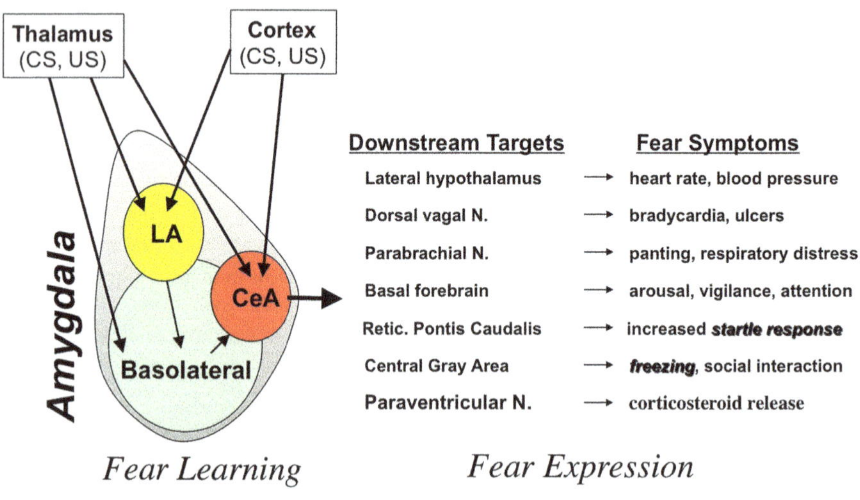

Fig. 3.2 Schematic illustrating basic circuitry of the amygdala involved in fear learning

Human Fear Circuitry

Model organisms provide an important platform from which to explore the neurobiology of fear in humans; however, the human experience of fear is a complex subjective event that cannot be solely encapsulated by a model behavior. Therefore, examination of human biological responses to fear is necessary. Determining the neural substrates of fear in humans is more difficult as researchers must generally rely exclusively upon non-invasive and *post mortem* sample collection techniques. Most common among these is functional magnetic resonance imaging (fMRI), which takes advantage of the fact that activity in a brain region is correlated with blood-flow to that region, to reveal broadly which areas of the brain experience increases or decreases in activity in response to a stimulus [40, 41]. Using brain imaging techniques researchers have determined many of the brain regions involved in fear processing and examined the changes to this circuitry that accompany TSRD (Fig. 3.3) [42].

The central elements of fear circuitry found in humans largely correlate with those found in rodent models, thus further validating the use of these animal models for translational research. Across research platforms the primary regions involved in emotional regulation, especially fear, are found within the limbic system. Convergent with animal models, human imaging studies have found a prominent role for the amygdala in the learning and expression of fear in humans. Training paradigms similar to those used in animal models are likewise useful in humans, for example, specific stimuli or contexts (using virtual reality, VR) (CSs) may be paired with

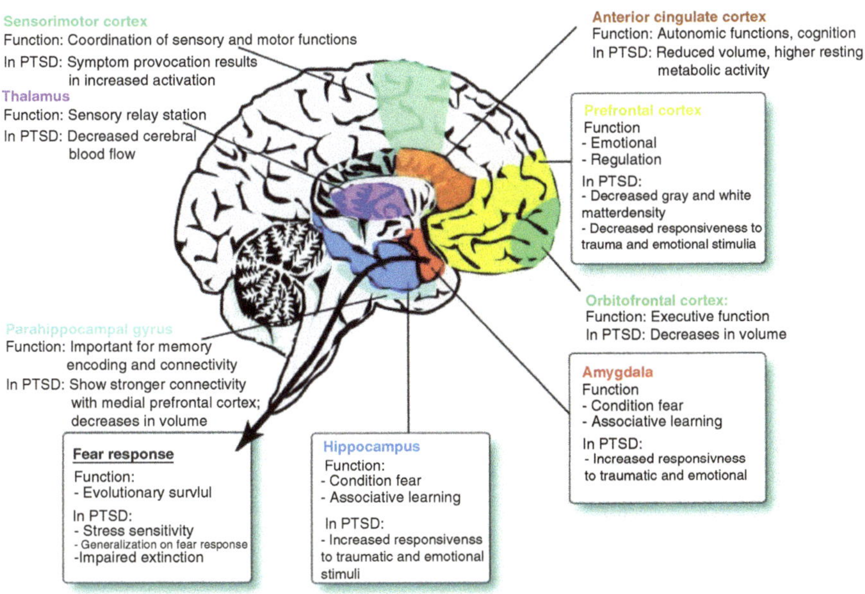

Fig. 3.3 Schematic illustrating limbic regions found to be involved in PTSD

noxious stimuli such as aversive air blasts (USs) to form specific fearful associations. Using these techniques many researchers have demonstrated increased activation of the amygdala during fear conditioning [43–46]. Interestingly these increases in amygdala activity are observed even when the subject is consciously unaware of the presence of the CS [47]. Importantly, amygdala activation is also correlated with other psychophysiological measures of fear responses such as changes in skin conductance, changes in heart rate variability (HRV), and changes in fear-potentiated acoustic startle [48, 49]. In humans, increases in amygdala activation reliably correlate with fear expression and other physiological indictors of fear.

The human experience of fear is complex and not easily equated to a unitary emotional output as is often done in animal models. In humans the integrated intellectual nature of fear may be visualized as increases in amygdala activation in response not only to directly fearful stimuli such as a CS, but also to more ambiguous stimuli such as videos of another person being fear conditioned or being read a text describing instructions for the fear conditioning process [50, 51]. Importantly, increased amygdala activation is also observed in response to negatively valenced emotional stimuli, such as pictures of faces showing a fearful expression as well as positive emotional stimuli (Fig. 3.4) [52, 53]. These data suggest that the amygdala may be a nexus of emotional regulated responses not only for fear, but also more generally for emotionally salient stimuli [54, 55]. Studies like these highlight the complex intellectual and social elements involved in human fear and begin to suggest how circuit level dysregulation may result in varied perturbations to fear and other behaviors.

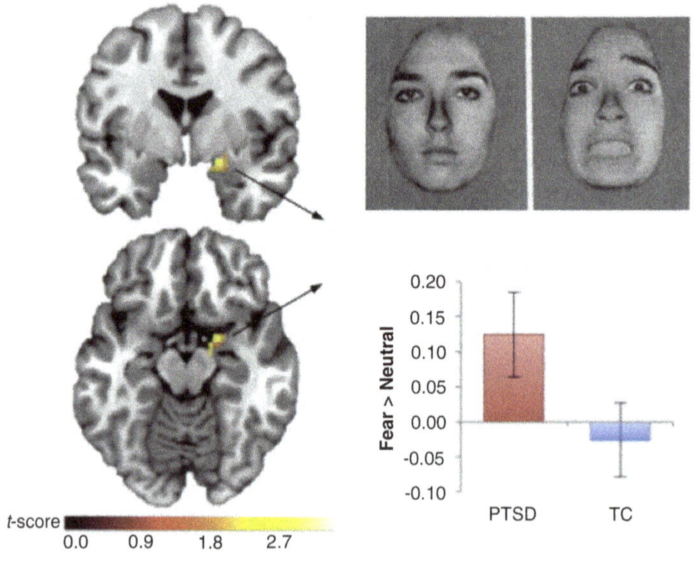

Fig. 3.4 Viewing images of fearful faces results in greater amygdala activation than viewing neutral faces. This effect is exacerbated in individuals with PTSD

Human functional brain regions involved in fear learning, processing and extinction correlate with those found in rodent models. The dorsal anterior cingulate cortex (dACC) and rostral ACC (rACC) in humans appear to correspond functionally to the PL described in rodents [56]. Activation in this area is correlated with fear expression as measured by increases in psychophysiological measures such as skin conductance [56–58]. Likewise, the ventromedial prefrontal cortex (vmPFC) in humans appears to correlate functionally with the IL in rodents [59, 60]. This region is activated during extinction learning and expression of extinction (meaning the successful suppression of fear responses to an extinguished CS) and activity in this region is inversely correlated with psychophysiological measures of fear [45, 59, 61]. Interestingly, activity in the amygdala is similarly modulated by the dACC and vmPFC where enhanced activity or thickness of the dACC is directly related to amygdala reactivity while activity or thickness of the vmPFC is inversely related to amygdala reactivity [45, 59]. In vivo imaging data suggests that the dACC and vmPFC represent crucial regions in the control of fear and fear extinction in humans.

Other important brain regions involved in the learning of fear and extinction are the insular cortex and the hippocampus. Increases in activation of both the insula and the hippocampus are found during fear conditioning [43, 57, 58, 62]. As the hippocampus is well known for its role in spatial learning and memory, it follows that it is involved in contextual fear learning as well as extinction of contextual fear where hippocampal activity is correlated with that of the vmPFC [61]. Many regions of the brain are intimately involved in the learning and extinction of fear and observing the interplay between these regions sheds light on the complex processing occurring in the humans brain.

Changes in Fear Circuitry and Behavior with PTSD

> But it was only for self-defense in that situation. But you can't just drop these behaviors once you get out of the situation. It becomes a part of who you are.

Processing of and responding to emotionally salient stimuli is foundational to an animal's ability to adapt to complex environments. The break-down of this adaptive learning process may result in pathological expression of fear and anxiety. One of the major findings from work with patients with PTSD is a deficit in extinction learning, which leads to over-active and over-generalized fear responses. These symptoms are accompanied by dramatic changes in the observed activity of fear-related neurocircuitries. Dysregulation of fear learning circuitries may underlie emotional learning deficits observed in patients with PTSD.

In PTSD patients the most dramatic changes in functional activity are found within limbic system areas mentioned above. Hyper-reactive emotional processing in PTSD patients may underlie the over-expression of fear behaviors. Work using fMRI confirms that the amygdala of PTSD patients is over-active at rest as well as in response to trauma-related stimuli such as images, odors, or sounds [63–66].

Likewise, the dACC, rACC, and insula, associated with fear expression, have been found to be hyper-reactive in PTSD patients while the vmPFC, associated with control of fearful behaviors and extinction, is hypo-reactive. The HPC, involved in regulating fear responses and identifying threatening stimuli, has aberrant activity in PTSD patients [67–69]. Smaller HPC and amygdala volumes provide several of the best-characterized risk factors for PTSD, and it has been suggested that chronic stress damages HPC, reducing its volume [70–75]. Both the ACC and PFC are also found to have reduced volumes in PTSD patients; twin studies suggest a causal relationship where trauma results in reductions in structure volume [76, 77]. Activity in a number of other regions such as orbitofrontal cortex (OFC) and parahippocampal gyrus is also dysregulated in PTSD patients [67, 78–80]. These observations together point towards an unbalancing of the fear controlling circuitry in PTSD where brain regions involved in production of fear (amygdala, dACC, rACC, and insula) are over-active while areas involved in fear suppression, emotional regulation, and extinction learning (HPC and vmPFC) are altered or under-reactive.

Strikingly, differences in network activity are accompanied by changes in response to threatening stimuli. In accordance with observed symptoms of PTSD, humans tend to over-generalize CS/US pairing in behavioral tasks [81]. When trained in fear conditioning tasks, veterans with PTSD who over-generalize the learned CS/US responses also have aberrant activation of fear controlling circuitries, such as in the vmPFC and insula [82]. This observation and many others establish the neurobiological basis for many of the behavioral alterations experienced by victims of PTSD.

Neuroimaging and psychophysiological markers of PTSD predict recovery as well. Investigations of changes in neural activation that predict recovery demonstrate that, as discussed, correlated activity between vmPFC and amydgala predicts current PTSD symptoms. Importantly, across time, changes in activity of HPC and ACC predict recovery [83]. Additionally, as smaller HPC volumes are a risk factor for current PTSD, larger HPC volumes actually predict recovery with treatment [84]. Likewise changes in psychophysiological measurements such as heart-rate variability and fear-potentiated startle correlate with recovery [85, 86]. These data demonstrate that neuroimaging and psychophysiological metrics closely track both the development of and recovery from PTSD.

Intersection of Fear and Addiction Circuitries

Neural circuitries involved in fear behaviors do not work in isolation and are instead involved in a vast array of other behaviors, most notably behavioral inhibition and emotional control. This is especially relevant in the context of the co-morbidity of PTSD with substance abuse and depression. Most notably, hypo-activity in the vmPFC is associated with drug abuse, pathological gambling, decision making, and emotional regulation [87–89]. Likewise, alterations in activity of the amygdala,

HPC, PFC, and ACC have been associated with negative affective states [90–92]. Widespread connectivity changes associated with PTSD affect many systems whose alteration may be associated with negative outcomes observed in PTSD patients.

Changes in the Stress Response System with PTSD

> But I wasn't crazy, I was tough, I was scared. And only I knew that. I was the only one who knew I was scared so what I'm gonna do is, … I'm going to do something really extreme

The neural circuitry responsible for direct execution of fear and anxiety behaviors is modulated by additional stress-responsive systems. Neurocircuitry for specific behaviors being under global control from stress response systems allows for adaptive (and maladaptive) modulation of behavioral states in response to the environment. The hypothalamic-pituitary-adrenal (HPA) axis (Fig. 3.5) [93] is one of the major systems for signaling stress that is recognized for playing a significant role in the psychopathology of TSRD. Very briefly, in response to stress the paraventricular nucleus of the hypothalamus synthesizes and releases corticotropin releasing factor (CRF). CRF binds to receptors on the pituitary gland, causing the release of adrenocorticotropic hormone (ACTH). ACTH binds to receptors in the adrenal cortex,

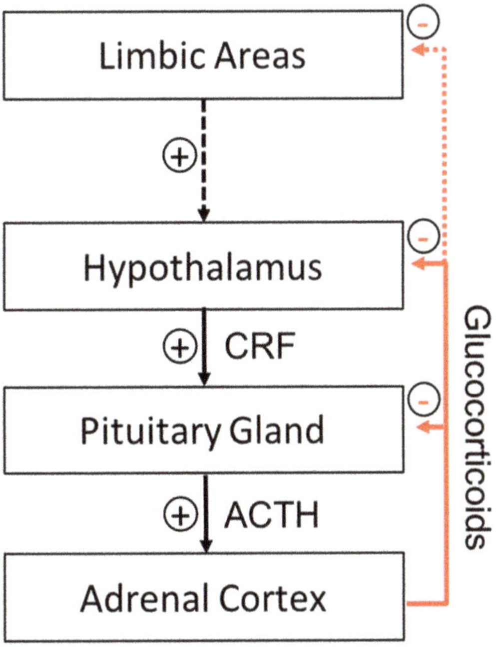

Fig. 3.5 The HPA axis affects and is affected by limbic regions including hippocampus and amygdala

which causes the release of glucocorticoids that negatively feed-back to hypothalamus and pituitary reducing the release of CRF and ACTH and suppressing further HPA activation [94–96]. Cortisol, a glucocorticoid, is the most widely studied stress hormone, as it is one of the most prominent effectors of HPA axis signaling. Another system with an important role in the stress response is the locus coeruleus-norepinephrine system. These stress-response systems are dysregulated in a variety of TSRD and other mood disorders [93].

While the precise causes and consequences of alterations in HPA-axis function are still being worked out, abnormalities in the stress response system are some of the most frequently reported with PTSD. The type and timing of trauma experienced have important consequences for how the HPA-axis is altered. The most common finding among veterans is that individuals with PTSD have decreased circulating cortisol and enhanced negative feedback to dexamethasone challenge [97]. These data suggest that enhanced sensitization of negative feedback in the HPA-axis may make the body hyper-responsive to stressors, thus potentiating anxiety and fear responses [97–99]. Alterations in stress response systems with PTSD increase psychological and psychological reactivity, further contributing to pathological symptomatology [100].

Interaction of PTSD with Community Dysfunction

Case Study

Colleen is a 7 year-old girl, presenting to regional diagnostic referral center with her father for question of autism. Father indicates that he is quite certain that Colleen has autism, but that she needs a medical diagnosis to access services.

At the start of the interview, Colleen is hiding behind the exam table. When asked what her preferred activities are, father explains that she is fixated on, obsessed with art. When some paper and crayons are placed on the desk and Colleen is invited to draw, she soon emerges from her hiding space, and spends the next 45 min of the interview, happily drawing. She draws houses, trees, flowers, clouds, birds, etc. She proudly and non-verbally shares her drawings and shares enjoyment in her drawings. She exhibits social smiles and liberally uses pointing, nodding, and other gestures, but says no words during the first half of the visit. By the end of the visit, she occasionally whispers a few words, directed only to her father.

While Colleen is drawing, father relates history. It is noted that Colleen has "always been aloof and disengaged," was never cuddly, never social, going back to infancy. During the social history, it is revealed that biological mother had history of substance addiction, but had been clean and sober through the

(continued)

pregnancy and until Colleen was 2 years of age. However, when Colleen was 2, mom began drinking again, escalating over the next several years, leading to parents' divorce when Colleen was 5. Father has been awarded sole custody, but Colleen has irregular visits with mom. Several months ago, mother was arrested for DUI while Colleen was in the car.

When diagnostic team relates their impression, that Colleen's presentation is most consistent with disrupted attachment and associated social anxiety and selective mutism, father expresses astonishment. He asks skeptically how such a young child could possibly have anxiety. When the DUI is pointed out as a possible trigger for anxiety in a small child, dad points out that Colleen has always been very emotionally disengaged, going back to infancy, to a time when mom was sober.

Several months later, the diagnostic team receives a call from father, inquiring about suggestions for treatment of Colleen's autism. He notes that they live in a small town. Father feels the town where they live has inadequate school and therapy services for children with autism. He wonders if there are better options for schooling and therapy for children with ASD in the city where the diagnostic referral center is located.

Diagnostic team points out that Colleen was not diagnosed with autism. Father informs the team that Colleen was seen by a local "neuro-psychologist" and diagnosed with autism with the use of an EEG. The psychologist informed dad that the EEG tracing was classic for autism. The diagnostic team objected that autism is a clinical diagnosis, based on interview and observational data, not on biomarkers, including EEG. Father simply insisted that Colleen had been diagnosed with autism and now he was turning to the team for suggestions about treatment. After all, aren't they an autism center?

Civilian PTSD

Symptoms of PTSD are debilitating and much has been done to understand its causes, treatments, and cures. Substantial research in this arena has been done in the context of service members returning from war. Much less recognized are the large numbers of civilians with PTSD and the costs to individual wellbeing, society, and infrastructure associated with these populations. An immediate example of the financial costs of PTSD to local infrastructure is that people with PTSD visit hospitals more frequently and have longer stays on average [101]. Likewise individuals who experience childhood abuse, itself a risk factor for later development of PTSD, have a high rate of poor physical and mental health leading to increased utilization of health care infrastructure [102]. PTSD among civilian populations is widespread and represents a significant mental health problem for local communities.

High profile situations that often result in PTSD include natural disasters such as hurricanes, earthquakes, or floods [8, 103–105]. Studies following Hurricane Katrina and Hurricane Hugo demonstrate that both acutely and long-term exposure to the physical and psychological stressors of these natural disasters greatly increased the rate of PTSD in the affected population especially among those who were children at the time of trauma [8, 105]. Man-made disasters such as the Oklahoma City bombing, Nairobi US Embassy bombing and World Trade Center attack of September 11th 2001, likewise result in increased rates of PTSD not only among victims and rescue workers, but also among neighborhood residents and witnesses to these tragedies [6, 7, 106–110]. In most cases, these events lead to large-scale and well-funded responses to provide financial and psychiatric assistance such that, in the case of 9/11 survivors, a majority of victims received at least some mental health treatment in the following years [109].

In contrast to survivors of natural and human-caused disasters, Americans living in metropolitan inner cities who are victims of high levels of chronic stress and violence receive remarkably little attention. Low-income residents of inner cities such as those living in Detroit, Chicago, Atlanta, Los Angeles, or Washington D.C. experience and witness violence at rates far higher than sub-urban residents. The youth living in these neighborhoods (generally 12–19 years of age) are especially at risk of exposure to violent assaults, mugging, rape, shootings, and death and are thus considered and referred to as being an at-risk population [109]. In Chicago, of this at-risk population 39% reported witnessing a shooting and 11% being shot at [111]. When examining urban youth in Philadelphia, 24% report witnessing a shooting compared to 4% of their sub-urban counterparts [112]. In Baltimore, of this at-risk population, 42% report witnessing a shooting versus 4% of middle and upper class youth [113]. While these rates of exposure to violence are very high, the rate of mental health assistance is concurrently very low; only 1% of Philadelphia respondents contacted a mental health professional [112]. By the time they have reached adulthood residents of these inner-city areas have accrued a high level of trauma. Nearly all of this population will have experienced or witnessed at least one trauma such as violent assault (especially high are rates of witnessing a murder when compared to sub-urban populations, 22–43% vs. 1–8% in some studies) and very few will have received mental health care [112–114]. Violence towards and witnessed by youth is especially important because trauma in this developmental time period dramatically affects developmental trajectories and risks of later development of mental illnesses such as PTSD.

Adult rates of PTSD largely reflect the high rates of trauma found in many low-income urban neighborhoods. Among residents of Atlanta, GA, interviewed at a primary care hospital (93% African American, low SES, men and women, $n = 1256$) 87.8% reported at least one lifetime traumatic event and 46.2% reached criteria for lifetime PTSD (36.7% reached criteria for lifetime MDD) [11]. Two very illuminating findings are discussed in this study and those like it. First, in terms of risk of development of PTSD, the sudden death of a loved one, one of the most common types of trauma experienced, is also one of the most likely to instigate PTSD [11, 115]. Such a result highlights that in communities with high

PTSD Symptoms (PSS) Mean±SE	Child Abuse None	Child Abuse 1 Type	Child Abuse 2 Types
Non-Child Abuse Trauma None	3.8±0.51	7.0±1.93	11.0±5.57
1 Type	5.6±0.73	11.3±2.43	10.7±2.59
2-3 Types	9.8±0.65	14.9±1.19	19.0±3.32
≥4 Types	14.5±0.95	18.5±1.14	23.4±1.86

Fig. 3.6 Childhood trauma potentiates and synergizes with adult trauma to increase risk for development of PTSD

rates of violence, not only are direct victims affected, but also their friends and family, who experience increases in trauma load. Second, childhood trauma followed by trauma exposure in adulthood, especially sexual abuse, are important interacting risk factors for lifetime development of PTSD [11, 116] (Fig. 3.6). In fact, the experience of three types of child abuse leads to a >20-fold increase in risk of developing PTSD, specifically in women [116]. These findings demonstrate that among civilian at-risk populations both childhood and adult trauma occur at high rates and that these are interacting risk factors for the development of PTSD [9, 11, 115, 117].

Civilian PTSD as Risk Factor for Interaction with Criminal Justice System

The United States criminal justice system has incarcerated 400% more people in the year 2005 than it did in the 1977 [118]. In 2005, the maintenance of correctional facilities required an outlay of $43 billion by the local and federal government. Although many explanations for these phenomena have been proposed, the most common and convincing is the initiation of the "War on Drugs" by the Nixon administration in 1971. This program resulted in exploding prison populations pushed by large increases in sentencing for drug related crimes; as evidenced by a 625% increase in California between 1982 and 1988, for example [119]. This enormous increase in the correctional population was disproportionately driven by the incarceration of Black and Latino (non-white minority) men [120]. Currently, high rates of trauma and community dysfunction, likely caused in part by mass incarceration, have created a "Cradle to Prison Pipeline" fed by cycles of trauma and incarceration exacerbated by epidemic rates of PTSD.

Social support and community cohesion are strong, but often under-appreciated, factors mediating mental health outcomes and, more specifically, risk for development of PTSD. Lack of social support is an important risk factor for development of a number of psychological disorders including major depressive disorder (MDD) and PTSD especially after a traumatic experience [121, 122]. Longitudinal studies

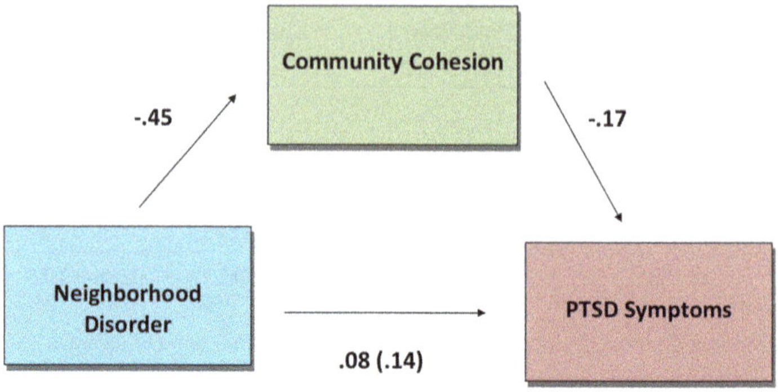

Fig. 3.7 Community cohesion buffers against increased risk of PTSD development caused by neighborhood disorder

demonstrate that high conflict and low support in an individual's social environment are very significant risk factors for development of PTSD and negatively impact recovery trajectories, suggesting that social support buffers an individual from development of PTSD and facilitates recovery [123–127]. On a community level, social support is often measured as perceived community cohesion referring to how individuals in a community relate to one another and provide support to each other [128, 129]. Low SES, low public services, high violence, and high stress communities such as those in urban centers discussed above have comparatively lower levels of social cohesion [130]. Perceived community cohesion is an important moderator of PTSD symptomology even when community disorder and trauma are accounted for, suggesting that strong communities may buffer individuals from PTSD even in at-risk neighborhoods (Fig. 3.7) [131, 132]. Areas with concentrated financial disadvantage and high rates of violence generally have concurrently low levels of community cohesion, which acts as an important risk factor for development of PTSD, exacerbating community problems and potentiating cycles of trauma.

PTSD and its co-morbidities strongly increase the frequency of risky behaviors that may involve individuals in the criminal justice system. Several of the cardinal symptoms of PTSD are increases in aggressive or violent behaviors and hyper-vigilance [133–135]. Increased violent behavior predisposes veterans and civilians with PTSD towards legal trouble resulting from violent encounters with civilians and police. Additionally, persons with PTSD are likely to also suffer from either a legal (alcohol) or illegal (marijuana, cocaine, heroin) substance abuse disorder (SUD). Long-term studies strongly support the hypothesis that increased rates of substance abuse is often attributable to individuals' self-medication of untreated symptoms of PTSD [136]. Research conducted among veteran populations finds that hyperarousal symptoms positively correlate with both aggression and problems with alcohol use [137, 138]. In a civilian population examined in the District of Colombia, the rate of PTSD among trauma-exposed individuals was 51%; the rate of SUD among trauma-exposed individuals was also 51% [115]. Likewise among individuals examined in Atlanta, GA, of people reaching criteria for PTSD, 40.3% also had a history of alcohol abuse or SUD compared to

22.2% of non-PTSD suffering individuals [139]. Importantly, consuming alcohol or illegal drugs independently increases rates of violent crime [140]. People suffering from PTSD are more likely to have substance abuse problems and be involved in violent altercations; these are the factors, which among others increase the likelihood that someone with PTSD will become involved in the criminal justice system.

Research has found that early life trauma increases the likelihood and severity of PTSD symptoms; likewise, early life trauma is associated with increased rates of substance abuse. Types of childhood abuse and trauma include neglect, physical abuse, emotional abuse, and sexual abuse. In an urban population from Atlanta, GA, childhood abuse and current PTSD symptoms correlate with rates of substance abuse in a trauma load dependent manner (Fig. 3.8) [141]. These results highlight that childhood abuse increases the risk for later development of both PTSD and substance abuse and this effect depends upon the severity of the early life abuse [102, 142, 143]. There is variability between sexes with regards to what type of child abuse was experienced and how trauma type influences the types of drugs of abuse used; however, as the number of types of child abuse experienced increases so does the risk of later substance use. Importantly, childhood abuse significantly increases risk of substance abuse, which in turn also increases risk for later

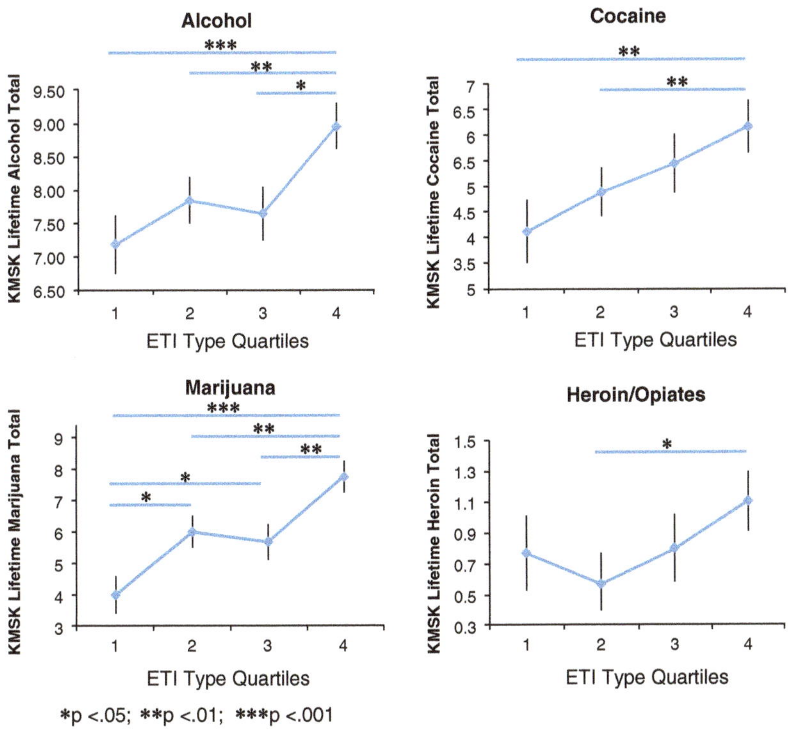

Fig. 3.8 Early life trauma load is a strong risk factor for later development of substance abuse disorders

experiencing of additional traumatic events and risky behavior, suggesting a causal chain between these events [144]. Early life trauma increases both rates of substance abuse and PTSD making it an important risk factor for later interaction with the criminal justice system.

The cycle of trauma perpetuated in part by PTSD may then be transferred between generations through the environment and from traumatized parents to their offspring. The biology of this process is complex; however, parents with PTSD are more likely to commit domestic violence, traumatizing their children. For example, veteran husbands and fathers who suffer from PTSD are more likely to commit domestic violence aimed at their spouse and children [145]. These instances of domestic violence are often discussed as traumas secondary to an initial trauma; however, from a child's perspective these represent primary traumas. Thus, risk for PTSD is behaviorally transferred from parent to child continuing cycles of trauma.

As discussed above, individuals suffering from PTSD are more likely to be imprisoned or incarcerated. In another population of urban Atlanta residents, individuals who met the criteria for PTSD were more likely to have been arrested (65.1% vs. 51.0%), jailed (61.6% vs. 47.7%), or imprisoned (16.7% vs. 11.2%). These results are even more remarkable when only males with PTSD are considered (88% arrested, 87% jailed, 36.3% imprisoned). Importantly, both trauma history and PTSD symptoms (when trauma history is controlled for) are significantly associated with charges relating to violence and incarceration [144]. In another study among incarcerated veterans, those that reach criteria for PTSD had both more history of substance abuse and problems with the legal system [146]. Finally, childhood trauma is one of the most significant variables associated with arrest and incarceration suggesting that, as this variable predates interaction with legal systems, there may be a direct relationship between childhood trauma and violent behavior resulting in arrest [139]. PTSD increases the likelihood that an individual will be arrested and incarcerated. Thus, from childhood residents of neighborhoods with high rates of violence and PTSD are often pushed towards entrance into the cradle to prison pipeline.

Prison sentences, ostensibly meant to increase public safety and remediate an individual's tendency towards criminal behavior, work against both goals and generally increase trauma load and violence in at-risk communities (*see above case study*). Meta-analyses of studies of rates of recidivism demonstrate that prison sentences should not be used as a method for reducing criminal behavior [147]. In fact when controlling for the criminal offense, individuals, especially adolescents, who are given a prison sentence are more likely to relapse than individuals given community-based sentences. Furthermore when given a prison sentence, those who are given longer sentences are more likely to commit additional crimes compared to individuals given a lesser sentence for the same offence [147, 148].

Prisoners are exposed to physical and sexual violence at high rates in prison putting them at further risk of development or worsening of PTSD [149–151]. Additionally, ex-prisoners returning to their communities have higher rates of negative health outcomes such as infectious diseases and hypertension [152, 153]. Increased rates of recidivism after incarceration may be due in part to cultural elements present in prisons; however, prison sentences are associated with increased exposure to traumatic events and negative health outcomes, which independently increase rates of PTSD and risk of illegal behavior.

While no one causal factor solely explains dramatic increases in rates of PTSD and incarceration over the last half century, many contributing factors contribute to the Cradle to the Prison pipeline operating in many of America's urban centers. Enormous increases in the rates of incarceration for drug offenses disproportionately negatively affect generations of minority men and women. Incarcerated people return to their communities with higher trauma loads and more negative health outcomes. Children living in these communities who experience trauma at home and in their neighborhood are more likely to develop substance abuse disorders and PTSD later in life putting them at further risk for interaction with the criminal justice system. Once an adolescent is sent to jail or prison they are more likely to reoffend further diminishing their chances of avoiding this cycle of trauma.

Risk and Resilience: Examples from Two Cases

Case Study

Ms X

"Ms. X is a 33 years old female. From the age of six, she has sustained severe physical and emotional abuse by her father and repeated sexual abuse by her step brother. She has significant symptoms of PTSD. She has 4 children. Her 8 years old stays with her mother, and the other children stay with her. She sounded annoyed by her own children ("my kids aggravate me") and is looking forward to having them stay with her mother for the summer. She described her relationship with her 15 years old daughter as "she can't stand me", her 16 years old son as "iffy", her 9 years old as "he loves me" and her 8 years old as "he doesn't know me". Having met her with her 9 years old son, I was surprised by her lack of warmth toward him."

Ms Y

"Ms. Y is a 25 years old female. Until the age of 7, she lived with her mother and father, who were addicted to crack cocaine. She witnessed a number of violent fights between her parents. At age 8 she moved in with her grandmother. But while still living with her parents, she was exposed to a lot of neighborhood violence. As a 7 years old, she survived a shootout between neighbors and dropped to the floor in the living room, trying to protect herself and her siblings from shots that came through the windows. She met current PTSD for this trauma. Ms. Y now has a 5 years old son and a 6 years old daughter. She was inspired by her daughter's strong interest in reading. She wants to be a role model for her children and is enrolled in a program to get her GED. Upon completing the GED program, Ms. Y hopes to do work in child advocacy."

In the excerpts above we find descriptions of two women; both of whom have experienced childhood trauma and meet criteria for PTSD. Ms. X exhibits many characteristics of a "risk" profile while Ms. Y demonstrates several "resilient" traits that set her on the path to recovery. Risk and resilience, often discussed as differential susceptibility, in the context of PTSD generally refers to the tendency of an individual to develop this disorder based upon the presence or absence of a number of resilience characteristics [154]. Risk and resilience are strongly influenced by a number of factors ranging from social and environmental factors to genetic factors that influence the way an individual's neurons react to the presence of stress hormones. Many of these factors most strongly play a role during development and influence a person's susceptibility for later development of PTSD. Below we will discuss individual, environmental, neurobiological and genetic risk factors for development of PTSD followed by a discussion of how these elements converge in so-called gene-by-environment (GxE) interactions.

Individual Risk and Resilience Characteristics in Parents and Children

On an individual level, personality traits that contribute to resilience can generally be considered to be those that support or encourage the development of successful coping strategies that result in success in important life domains such as work or relationships. Studies using self-report measures of individual traits such as durability, positivity, optimism, flexibility, and adaptive coping strategies have correlated these traits with resilience and tendency for recovery [155, 156]. Likewise external factors like strong community and social support as well as having meaningful goals and other fulfilling elements in life are major factor for resilience and recovery [156, 157]. Research measuring these attributes in an at-risk population demonstrates that resilience characteristics decrease lifetime alcohol and illicit drug abuse and lower rates of alcohol and illicit drug abuse disorders [158–160]. Risk and resilience towards developing PTSD are in part governed by individual personality traits that also protect against other negative life occurrences.

Examining the interview excerpts above Ms. X appears to have risk characteristics in that she lacks close personal relationships with her children, conversely Ms. Y demonstrates resilience traits through her goals of getting a GED, working in child advocacy and positive outlook inspired by her daughter. These interviews also clearly demonstrate another crucial element for development of resilience characteristics: supporting and nurturing environments during childhood development. As discussed above, childhood trauma such as neglect is one of the strongest risk factors for development of PTSD, SUD, and depression [161]. Thus, risk and resilience may be transferred intergenerationally from parents with PTSD to their children through child abuse or neglect.

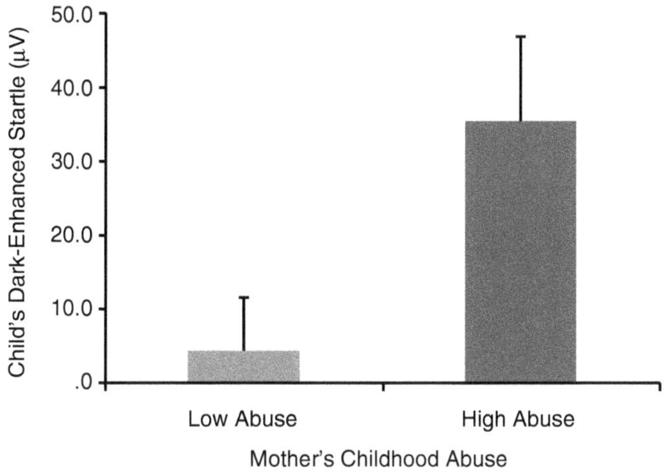

Fig. 3.9 The children of mothers who experienced high levels of child abuse have higher levels of dark-enhanced startle, a measure of anxiety

Intergenerational transmission of risk and resilience may take place on multiple levels from behavioral to genetic; however, psychophysiological measures demonstrate a strong link between the abuse history of a parent and the current behavior of children. Decades of evidence show that parental psychopathology can result in negative outcomes for children, specifically the presence of a parent with PTSD increases the likelihood of a child developing PTSD [162]. The most common measure for transgenerational transmission is the measurement of cortisol and of startle reflex, which are considered to be proxies for stress reactivity, anxiety, and hyper-vigilance [163, 164]. Startle reactivity is enhanced in adults who experienced high levels of childhood trauma [165]. In the study from which the interviews above were collected, mothers were queried for their and their children's trauma history then dark-enhanced startled was measured in their children [166]. The children of mothers who reported high levels of childhood abuse have significantly higher levels of dark-enhanced startle, which correlate with their own self-reported levels of anxiety (Fig. 3.9) [166]. This work suggests that childhood trauma in a parental generation increases both psychological and physiological measures of anxiety.

Using interviews with Ms. X and Ms. Y as case studies, we are able to examine the parental characteristics that may contribute to their own risk or resilience profiles as well as how these attributes will likely affect their children. Ms. X appears to behaviorally exhibit a risk profile while Ms. Y demonstrates an example of resilience traits. Examination of the dark-enhanced startle exhibited by these women's children anecdotally confirms this hypothesis. Ms. Y's child shows decreased enhancement in dark-enhanced startle while the child of Ms. X has an increased dark-enhanced startle, suggesting a higher level of anxiety (Fig. 3.10). Childhood

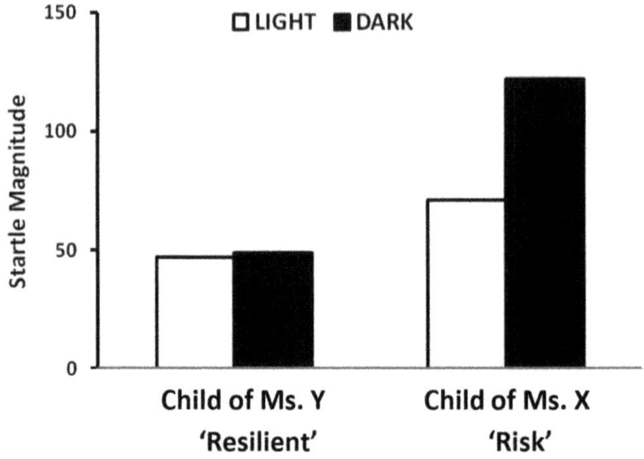

Fig. 3.10 The child of "resilient" Ms. Y has lower startle and anxiety than the child or "risk" Ms. X

trauma increases the risk of anxiety disorders and PTSD in not only the directly affected generation, but also in subsequent generations through transmission of transgenerational risk.

Genetic Mechanisms of Transgenerational Transmission of Trauma

Examination of behavioral and physiological correlates of intergenerational transmission of PTSD generates important evidence of this phenomenon; however, additional study into the mechanism of this transmission is necessary in order to both understand the underlying mechanism and prevent its transmission. While a large portion of transmission of risk and resilience appears to be environmental and behavioral, twin studies reveal that between 30% and 40% of risk for development of PTSD may be attributed to genetics [167, 168]. Although the heritability of risk for psychiatric disorders is well established, genome wide association studies (GWAS) have failed to identify significant numbers of loci that may be causing MDD or PTSD [169]. An interesting element that is particularly relevant to the study of the genetics of PTSD is the influence of both genetic and environmental factors on disease outcome. These gene by environment (G × E) relationships depend upon the presence of a genetic predisposition towards risk or resilience as well as a certain set of environmental factors such as trauma to predict disease outcomes. Here we will examine how childhood critical periods change developmental trajectories and also the gene FKBP5 as an example of a gene, whose G × E interaction with trauma during early critical periods may contribute to PTSD risk and resilience in adulthood.

Stress During Childhood Critical Periods

Critical developmental periods during childhood are times when environmental factors have large effects over developmental trajectories that set up an adult's state of risk or resilience. Depending on several factors, for humans this critical period is generally during early childhood. Quite a bit is known about critical periods for language and sensory system development; however, less is mechanistically known about how emotional learning in children modulates later susceptibility for psychiatric disorders [170, 171].

In rodent models, emotional learning and maternal care during critical periods dramatically alter behaviors in a cortisol dependent manner. When rats are older than postnatal day 12 (P12) and exposed to pairings of an odor and a shock they will later know to avoid that odor; however, if pups are exposed to the same odor shock pairings before P8, they will approach the aversively trained odor [172]. This critical period may be extended or closed by blocking or activating corticosterone receptors, respectively [173]. These findings suggest the presence of a critical transition period where noxious stimuli that may have been previously associated with maternal care become threat associated. That this critical period is modulated by corticosterone suggests that early life stress, which alters circulating corticosterone levels, may change trajectories of attachment and aversive learning. These results are translationally interesting because they suggest that infants become attached to parental stimuli regardless of their intrinsic positive or negative valence [174, 175]. This view is supported by data suggesting that maternal presence buffers young rats from stress and that rats that receive early life stress from low maternal care have altered attachment learning [176–178]. Taken together, rodent literature highlights the importance of maternal care for proper stress responses and suggests long lasting consequences of low-quality early-life care.

Non-human primate models have been critical for understanding the developmental trajectories and neural mechanisms of early life stress. Non-human primate models are also essential in that they bridge a phylogenetic gap between rodents and humans, thus providing enhanced translational relevance. Rhesus macaque monkeys have been particularly useful models to study the effects of early life stress due to their similarity in both behavioral and neural development to humans. Additionally, rhesus monkeys display complex maternal–offspring relationships, with monkeys having only single offspring that spend early life periods in close physical contact with the mother [179–183]. Monkeys reared without a mother and in social isolation displayed behavioral and social deficits along with increased fear and anxiety [184, 185]. Maternal separation across rodent and rhesus macaque models has been shown to increase acoustic startle reactivity and dysregulated HPA axis function, perhaps through chronic exposure to increased levels of stress hormones during early critical periods of development, as discussed above [186, 187].

In humans, institutional rearing, such as in orphanages abroad, followed by subsequent international adoption by families in the United States, has provided a special cohort of individual children and adolescents who have experienced maternal deprivation and early life stress during early developmental critical periods. The pre-adoption time period stands in stark contrast to the period following adoption, in which many children and adolescents receive high levels of care and support from their adopted families. Studies have found that these individuals have high rates of anxiety disorders and PTSD [188]. Additionally, individuals with a history of institutional care show increased amygdala volumes compared to "typically-raised" peers, and the length of stay in an institutional care setting is associated with increases in amygdala volume [188, 189]. In less extreme forms of early life stress, such as in children of clinically depressed mothers, such enhancements in amygdala volumes are also observed [190]. Children who experience moderate to severe early life stress have neurobiological changes that may predispose them towards anxiety disorders and PTSD [191].

FKBP5

The HPA axis is a crucial stress-response signaling system that allows the body, especially the brain, to rapidly and globally respond to stressful stimuli. As discussed above, alterations in this system are strongly associated with PTSD psychopathology [93]. FK506 Binding Protein-5 (FKBP5) is a crucial element of an ultra-short cortisol responsive negative feed-back loop (Fig. 3.11). Briefly, upon cortisol binding to the GR, the receptor complex is translocated to the nucleus where it initiates diverse changes in transcription, namely increasing transcription of the *FKBP5* gene. FKBP5 protein goes on to bind the GR receptor complex blocking

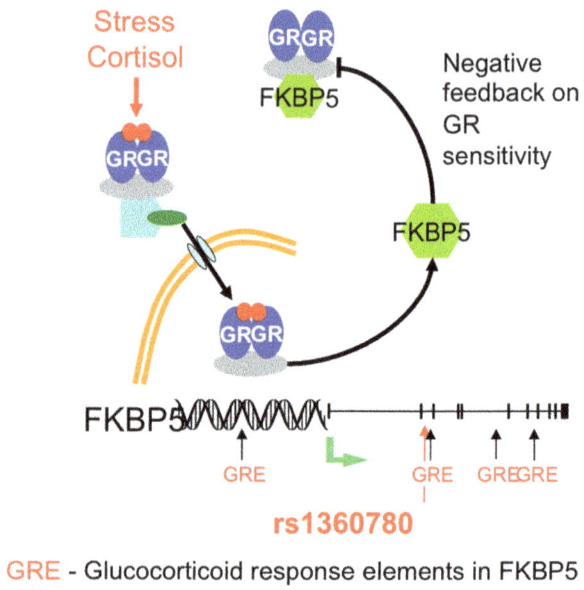

Fig. 3.11 The FKBP5 feed-back loop is a crucial brake on stress activated HPA activity

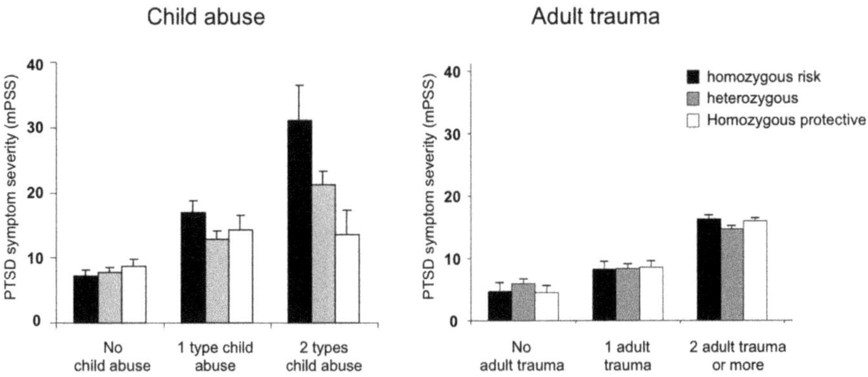

Fig. 3.12 Carrying the FKBP5 risk allele positively interacts with childhood trauma, but not adult trauma to increase risk of development of PTSD

further signal transduction [192–194]. This FKBP5 negative feed-back loop modulates stress response signaling, and changes in this signaling may alter the way a neuron (i.e., the brain) responds to stress.

Foundational work by Binder et al. demonstrated that a single nucleotide polymorphism (SNP) in *FPKB5* interacts with childhood trauma to predict PTSD symptoms [194]. Examination of this SNP found that the presence of the risk (A) allele predicts PTSD symptoms only in individuals highly traumatized as children (Fig. 3.12) [194]. Additionally, homozygous carriers of the risk allele (A/A) are at greater risk than heterozygous carriers (A/G) of developing PTSD. Importantly, this and subsequent studies have found no association with FKPB5, adult trauma, and PTSD demonstrating that this G × E interaction is specific for trauma during adolescence and early life [194, 195]. Polymorphisms in *FKBP5* interact with childhood trauma to predict severity of adult PTSD.

Examination of the mechanisms of this G × E interaction has revealed insight into the genetic and epigenetic control of stress responsiveness. In several follow-up studies researchers determined that the *FKBP5* risk allele changes the efficacy of a GR response element (GRE) activity in the *FKBP5* gene, leading to enhanced expression of *FKBP5* in response to GR binding, thus increasing the efficacy of this ultra-short cortisol response loop. Importantly, this effect is facilitated through an epigenetic mechanism that is genotype and trauma dependent [196–199]. Remarkably, the "risk" allele is also associated with decreases in lifetime PTSD when adults had not experienced childhood trauma, highlighting that "risk" and "resilience" factors may be entirely environmentally dependent (Fig. 3.13) [199]. Polymorphisms in *FKBP5* alter stress sensitivity through changes in stress responsive transcriptional regulation of FKBP5 during development; this correlates with adult outcomes towards risk and resilience in a G × E dependent manner.

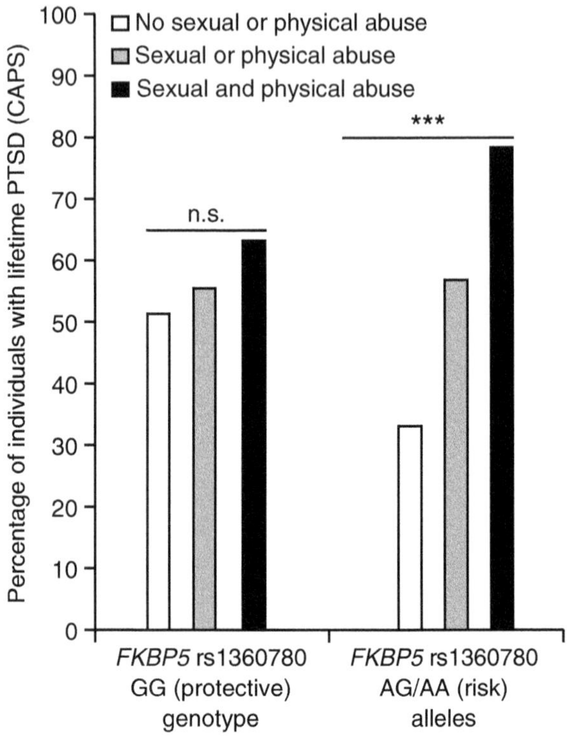

Fig. 3.13 The FKBP5 "Risk" allele is protective in the absence of childhood trauma, but deleterious in the presence of high trauma load

Summary

PTSD and other TSRDs have dramatic consequences for the lives of victims and the communities around them. Neurophysiologically, PTSD results in changes in the connectivity, activity, and in some cases size of brain regions involved in fear-related circuitry. These changes modify individuals' acute responses to fearful stimuli and may result in observed tendencies towards over-generalization of fear responses and deficits in extinction learning. Veterans returning from wars and individuals exposed to large-scale natural and man-made disasters suffer from high rates of PTSD. Historically underserved communities with high rates of violence and low rates of perceived community cohesion also exhibit increased rates of PTSD. PTSD may play a crucial role in the Cradle to the Prison pipeline by increasing rates of community trauma, substance abuse, and incarceration. Risk and Resilience traits are governed by multitude of interacting factors including personality characteristics, childhood trauma, and genetic risk factors, which may be transmitted intergenerationally. An example of two important and interacting risk factors are childhood trauma and FKBP5 polymorphisms, which may transfer risk and resilience through a G × E interaction. Decreasing rates of PTSD presents a difficult challenge; however, by addressing social and biological challenges in conjunction, palpable progress may be made.

Acknowledgements and Disclosures The authors declare no competing financial interests. Support was provided by NIH (R01MH096764) and by an NIH/NCRR base grant (P51RR000165) to Yerkes National Primate Research Center.

References

1. Association, A. P. Diagnostic and statistical manual of mental disorders (DSM-5®). 5th ed. Washington, DC: American Psychiatric Association; 2013.
2. Kessler RC, et al. LIfetime prevalence and age-of-onset distributions of dsm-iv disorders in the national comorbidity survey replication. Arch Gen Psychiatry. 2005;62:593–602. https://doi.org/10.1001/archpsyc.62.6.593.
3. Kessler RC, Sonnega A, Bromet E, Hughes M, Nelson CB. POsttraumatic stress disorder in the national comorbidity survey. Arch Gen Psychiatry. 1995;52:1048–60. https://doi.org/10.1001/archpsyc.1995.03950240066012.
4. Tanielian TL, Jaycox L. Invisible wounds of war: psychological and cognitive injuries, their consequences, and services to assist recovery, vol. 1. Santa Monica: Rand Corporation; 2008.
5. Schlenger WE, et al. The prevalence of post-traumatic stress disorder in the Vietnam generation: a multimethod, multisource assessment of psychiatric disorder. J Trauma Stress. 1992;5:333–63. https://doi.org/10.1002/jts.2490050303.
6. Galea S, et al. Trends of probable post-traumatic stress disorder in New York City after the September 11 terrorist attacks. Am J Epidemiol. 2003;158:514–24.
7. Grieger TA, Fullerton CS, Ursano RJ. Posttraumatic stress disorder, alcohol use, and perceived safety after the terrorist attack on the pentagon. Psychiatr Serv. 2003;54:1380.
8. Galea S, et al. Exposure to hurricane-related stressors and mental illness after Hurricane Katrina. Arch Gen Psychiatry. 2007;64:1427–34. https://doi.org/10.1001/archpsyc.64.12.1427.
9. Singer MI, Anglin TM, Song LY, Lunghofer L. Adolescents' exposure to violence and associated symptoms of psychological trauma. JAMA. 1995;273:477–82.
10. Schwartz AC, Bradley RL, Sexton M, Sherry A, Ressler KJ. Posttraumatic stress disorder among African Americans in an inner city mental health clinic. Psychiatr Serv. 2005;56:212.
11. Gillespie CF, et al. Trauma exposure and stress-related disorders in inner city primary care patients. Gen Hosp Psychiatry. 2009;31:505–14.
12. Davidson JR, Stein DJ, Shalev AY, Yehuda R. Posttraumatic stress disorder: acquisition, recognition, course, and treatment. J Neuropsychiatry Clin Neurosci. 2004;16:135–47. https://doi.org/10.1176/jnp.16.2.135.
13. Breslau N. The epidemiology of posttraumatic stress disorder: what is the extent of the problem? J Clin Psychiatry. 2001;62(Suppl 17):16–22.
14. Jovanovic T, Ressler KJ. How the neurocircuitry and genetics of fear inhibition may inform our understanding of PTSD. Am J Psychiatry. 2010;167:648–62.
15. Rothbaum BO, et al. A pilot study of an exposure-based intervention in the ED designed to prevent posttraumatic stress disorder. Am J Emerg Med. 2008;26:326–30. https://doi.org/10.1016/j.ajem.2007.07.006.
16. LeDoux J. Emotional networks and motor control: a fearful view. Prog Brain Res. 1996;107:437–46.
17. Gross CT, Canteras NS. The many paths to fear. Nat Rev Neurosci. 2012;13:651–8.
18. Morrison FG, Ressler KJ. From the neurobiology of extinction to improved clinical treatments. Depress Anxiety. 2013;31:279. https://doi.org/10.1002/da.22214.
19. Fanselow MS. Conditioned and unconditional components of post-shock freezing. Pavlov J Biol Sci. 1980;15:177–82.
20. Blanchard RJ, Blanchard DC. Crouching as an index of fear. J Comp Physiol Psychol. 1969;67:370–5. https://doi.org/10.1037/h0026779.

21. Myers KM, Davis M. Mechanisms of fear extinction. Mol Psychiatry. 2007;12:120–50. https://doi.org/10.1038/sj.mp.4001939.
22. Andero R, Dias BG, Ressler KJ. A role for Tac2, NkB, and Nk3 receptor in normal and dysregulated fear memory consolidation. Neuron. 2014;83:444. https://doi.org/10.1016/j.neuron.2014.05.028.
23. Maren S, Holmes A. Stress and fear extinction. Neuropsychopharmacology. 2016;41:58–79. https://doi.org/10.1038/npp.2015.180.
24. Pare D, Quirk GJ, Ledoux JE. New vistas on amygdala networks in conditioned fear. J Neurophysiol. 2004;92:1–9. https://doi.org/10.1152/jn.00153.2004.
25. LeDoux J. The amygdala. Curr Biol. 2007;17:R868–74. https://doi.org/10.1016/j.cub.2007.08.005.
26. LeDoux JE. Coming to terms with fear. Proc Natl Acad Sci U S A. 2014;111:2871–8. https://doi.org/10.1073/pnas.1400335111.
27. Pape HC, Pare D. Plastic synaptic networks of the amygdala for the acquisition, expression, and extinction of conditioned fear. Physiol Rev. 2010;90:419–63. https://doi.org/10.1152/physrev.00037.2009.
28. Campeau S, Davis M. Involvement of the central nucleus and basolateral complex of the amygdala in fear conditioning measured with fear-potentiated startle in rats trained concurrently with auditory and visual conditioned stimuli. J Neurosci. 1995;15:2301–11.
29. Repa JC, et al. Two different lateral amygdala cell populations contribute to the initiation and storage of memory. Nat Neurosci. 2001;4:724–31. https://doi.org/10.1038/89512.
30. Pitkanen A, Savander V, LeDoux JE. Organization of intra-amygdaloid circuitries in the rat: an emerging framework for understanding functions of the amygdala. Trends Neurosci. 1997;20:517–23.
31. Gentile CG, Jarrell TW, Teich A, McCabe PM, Schneiderman N. The role of amygdaloid central nucleus in the retention of differential pavlovian conditioning of bradycardia in rabbits. Behav Brain Res. 1986;20:263–73.
32. LeDoux JE, Iwata J, Cicchetti P, Reis DJ. Different projections of the central amygdaloid nucleus mediate autonomic and behavioral correlates of conditioned fear. J Neurosci. 1988;8:2517–29.
33. Pikkarainen M, Ronkko S, Savander V, Insausti R, Pitkanen A. Projections from the lateral, basal, and accessory basal nuclei of the amygdala to the hippocampal formation in rat. J Comp Neurol. 1999;403:229–60.
34. McDonald AJ, Mott DD. Functional neuroanatomy of amygdalohippocampal interconnections and their role in learning and memory. J Neurosci Res. 2016;95:797. https://doi.org/10.1002/jnr.23709.
35. Sierra-Mercado D, Padilla-Coreano N, Quirk GJ. Dissociable roles of prelimbic and infralimbic cortices, ventral hippocampus, and basolateral amygdala in the expression and extinction of conditioned fear. Neuropsychopharmacology. 2011;36:529–38. https://doi.org/10.1038/npp.2010.184.
36. Davis M. Neural systems involved in fear and anxiety measured with fear-potentiated startle. Am Psychol. 2006;61:741–56. https://doi.org/10.1037/0003-066x.61.8.741.
37. Stuber GD, et al. Excitatory transmission from the amygdala to nucleus accumbens facilitates reward seeking. Nature. 2011;475:377–80. https://doi.org/10.1038/nature10194.
38. Ambroggi F, Ishikawa A, Fields HL, Nicola SM. Basolateral amygdala neurons facilitate reward-seeking behavior by exciting nucleus accumbens neurons. Neuron. 2008;59:648–61. https://doi.org/10.1016/j.neuron.2008.07.004.
39. Di Ciano P, Everitt BJ. Direct interactions between the basolateral amygdala and nucleus accumbens core underlie cocaine-seeking behavior by rats. J Neurosci. 2004;24:7167–73. https://doi.org/10.1523/jneurosci.1581-04.2004.
40. Fox MD, Raichle ME. Spontaneous fluctuations in brain activity observed with functional magnetic resonance imaging. Neuroscience. 2007;8:700–11. https://doi.org/10.1038/nrn2201.

41. Logothetis NK, Wandell BA. Interpreting the BOLD signal. Annu Rev Physiol. 2004;66:735–69. https://doi.org/10.1146/annurev.physiol.66.082602.092845.
42. Mahan AL, Ressler KJ. Fear conditioning, synaptic plasticity and the amygdala: implications for posttraumatic stress disorder. Trends Neurosci. 2012;35:24–35. https://doi.org/10.1016/j.tins.2011.06.007.
43. Alvarez RP, Biggs A, Chen G, Pine DS, Grillon C. Contextual fear conditioning in humans: cortical-hippocampal and amygdala contributions. J Neurosci. 2008;28:6211–9. https://doi.org/10.1523/jneurosci.1246-08.2008.
44. Barrett J, Armony JL. Influence of trait anxiety on brain activity during the acquisition and extinction of aversive conditioning. Psychol Med. 2009;39:255–65. https://doi.org/10.1017/s0033291708003516.
45. Milad MR, et al. Recall of fear extinction in humans activates the ventromedial prefrontal cortex and hippocampus in concert. Biol Psychiatry. 2007;62:446–54. https://doi.org/10.1016/j.biopsych.2006.10.011.
46. Knight DC, Smith CN, Cheng DT, Stein EA, Helmstetter FJ. Amygdala and hippocampal activity during acquisition and extinction of human fear conditioning. Cogn Affect Behav Neurosci. 2004;4:317–25.
47. Critchley HD, Mathias CJ, Dolan RJ. Fear conditioning in humans: the influence of awareness and autonomic arousal on functional neuroanatomy. Neuron. 2002;33:653–63.
48. Norrholm SD, et al. Baseline psychophysiological and cortisol reactivity as a predictor of PTSD treatment outcome in virtual reality exposure therapy. Behav Res Ther. 2016;82:28–37. https://doi.org/10.1016/j.brat.2016.05.002.
49. van Well S, Visser RM, Scholte HS, Kindt M. Neural substrates of individual differences in human fear learning: evidence from concurrent fMRI, fear-potentiated startle, and US-expectancy data. Cogn Affect Behav Neurosci. 2012;12:499–512. https://doi.org/10.3758/s13415-012-0089-7.
50. Ma Q, Huang Y, Wang L. Left prefrontal activity reflects the ability of vicarious fear learning: a functional near-infrared spectroscopy study. Sci World J. 2013;2013:652542. https://doi.org/10.1155/2013/652542.
51. Olsson A, Nearing KI, Phelps EA. Learning fears by observing others: the neural systems of social fear transmission. Soc Cogn Affect Neurosci. 2007;2:3–11. https://doi.org/10.1093/scan/nsm005.
52. Thomas KM, et al. Amygdala response to fearful faces in anxious and depressed children. Arch Gen Psychiatry. 2001;58:1057–63.
53. Stevens JS, et al. Disrupted amygdala-prefrontal functional connectivity in civilian women with posttraumatic stress disorder. J Psychiatr Res. 2013;47:1469–78. https://doi.org/10.1016/j.jpsychires.2013.05.031.
54. Phan KL, et al. Activation of the medial prefrontal cortex and extended amygdala by individual ratings of emotional arousal: a fMRI study. Biol Psychiatry. 2003;53:211–5.
55. Phillips ML, et al. Differential neural responses to overt and covert presentations of facial expressions of fear and disgust. NeuroImage. 2004;21:1484–96. https://doi.org/10.1016/j.neuroimage.2003.12.013.
56. Milad MR, et al. A role for the human dorsal anterior cingulate cortex in fear expression. Biol Psychiatry. 2007;62:1191–4. https://doi.org/10.1016/j.biopsych.2007.04.032.
57. Buchel C, Morris J, Dolan RJ, Friston KJ. Brain systems mediating aversive conditioning: an event-related fMRI study. Neuron. 1998;20:947–57.
58. Marschner A, Kalisch R, Vervliet B, Vansteenwegen D, Buchel C. Dissociable roles for the hippocampus and the amygdala in human cued versus context fear conditioning. J Neurosci. 2008;28:9030–6. https://doi.org/10.1523/jneurosci.1651-08.2008.
59. Phelps EA, Delgado MR, Nearing KI, LeDoux JE. Extinction learning in humans: role of the amygdala and vmPFC. Neuron. 2004;43:897–905. https://doi.org/10.1016/j.neuron.2004.08.042.
60. Milad MR, Quirk GJ. Fear extinction as a model for translational neuroscience: ten years of progress. Annu Rev Psychol. 2012;63:129–51. https://doi.org/10.1146/annurev.psych.121208.131631.

61. Kalisch R, et al. Context-dependent human extinction memory is mediated by a ventromedial prefrontal and hippocampal network. J Neurosci. 2006;26:9503–11. https://doi.org/10.1523/jneurosci.2021-06.2006.
62. Lang S, et al. Context conditioning and extinction in humans: differential contribution of the hippocampus, amygdala and prefrontal cortex. Eur J Neurosci. 2009;29:823–32.
63. Shin LM, et al. Regional cerebral blood flow in the amygdala and medial prefrontal cortex during traumatic imagery in male and female Vietnam veterans with PTSD. Arch Gen Psychiatry. 2004;61:168–76. https://doi.org/10.1001/archpsyc.61.2.168.
64. Morey RA, et al. The role of trauma-related distractors on neural systems for working memory and emotion processing in posttraumatic stress disorder. J Psychiatr Res. 2009;43:809–17. https://doi.org/10.1016/j.jpsychires.2008.10.014.
65. Bryant RA, et al. Neural networks of information processing in posttraumatic stress disorder: a functional magnetic resonance imaging study. Biol Psychiatry. 2005;58:111–8. https://doi.org/10.1016/j.biopsych.2005.03.021.
66. Bryant RA, et al. Enhanced amygdala and medial prefrontal activation during nonconscious processing of fear in posttraumatic stress disorder: an fMRI study. Hum Brain Mapp. 2008;29:517–23. https://doi.org/10.1002/hbm.20415.
67. Etkin A, Wager TD. Functional neuroimaging of anxiety: a meta-analysis of emotional processing in PTSD, social anxiety disorder, and specific phobia. Am J Psychiatry. 2007;164:1476–88. https://doi.org/10.1176/appi.ajp.2007.07030504.
68. Bremner JD, et al. MRI and PET study of deficits in hippocampal structure and function in women with childhood sexual abuse and posttraumatic stress disorder. Am J Psychiatry. 2003;160:924–32. https://doi.org/10.1176/appi.ajp.160.5.924.
69. Shin LM, Liberzon I. The neurocircuitry of fear, stress, and anxiety disorders. Neuropsychopharmacology. 2010;35:169–91. https://doi.org/10.1038/npp.2009.83.
70. Kitayama N, Vaccarino V, Kutner M, Weiss P, Bremner JD. Magnetic resonance imaging (MRI) measurement of hippocampal volume in posttraumatic stress disorder: a meta-analysis. J Affect Disord. 2005;88:79–86. https://doi.org/10.1016/j.jad.2005.05.014.
71. Sapolsky RM, Uno H, Rebert CS, Finch CE. Hippocampal damage associated with prolonged glucocorticoid exposure in primates. J Neurosci. 1990;10:2897–902.
72. O'Doherty DC, Chitty KM, Saddiqui S, Bennett MR, Lagopoulos J. A systematic review and meta-analysis of magnetic resonance imaging measurement of structural volumes in posttraumatic stress disorder. Psychiatry Res. 2015;232:1–33. https://doi.org/10.1016/j.pscychresns.2015.01.002.
73. Pare D, Duvarci S. Amygdala microcircuits mediating fear expression and extinction. Curr Opin Neurobiol. 2012;22:717–23. https://doi.org/10.1016/j.conb.2012.02.014.
74. Kim EJ, Pellman B, Kim JJ. Stress effects on the hippocampus: a critical review. Learn Mem. 2015;22:411–6. https://doi.org/10.1101/lm.037291.114.
75. van Rooij SJ, et al. Smaller hippocampal volume as a vulnerability factor for the persistence of post-traumatic stress disorder. Psychol Med. 2015;45:2737–46. https://doi.org/10.1017/s0033291715000707.
76. Kasai K, et al. Evidence for acquired pregenual anterior cingulate gray matter loss from a twin study of combat-related posttraumatic stress disorder. Biol Psychiatry. 2008;63:550–6. https://doi.org/10.1016/j.biopsych.2007.06.022.
77. Carrion VG, Weems CF, Richert K, Hoffman BC, Reiss AL. Decreased prefrontal cortical volume associated with increased bedtime cortisol in traumatized youth. Biol Psychiatry. 2010;68:491–3. https://doi.org/10.1016/j.biopsych.2010.05.010.
78. Abe O, et al. Voxel-based diffusion tensor analysis reveals aberrant anterior cingulum integrity in posttraumatic stress disorder due to terrorism. Psychiatry Res. 2006;146:231–42. https://doi.org/10.1016/j.pscychresns.2006.01.004.
79. Thomaes K, et al. Reduced anterior cingulate and orbitofrontal volumes in child abuse-related complex PTSD. J Clin Psychiatry. 2010;71:1636–44. https://doi.org/10.4088/JCP.08m04754blu.

80. Rogers MA, et al. Smaller amygdala volume and reduced anterior cingulate gray matter density associated with history of post-traumatic stress disorder. Psychiatry Res. 2009;174:210–6. https://doi.org/10.1016/j.pscychresns.2009.06.001.
81. Pole N, et al. Prospective prediction of posttraumatic stress disorder symptoms using fear potentiated auditory startle responses. Biol Psychiatry. 2009;65:235–40. https://doi.org/10.1016/j.biopsych.2008.07.015.
82. Morey RA, et al. Fear learning circuitry is biased toward generalization of fear associations in posttraumatic stress disorder. Transl Psychiatry. 2015;5:e700. https://doi.org/10.1038/tp.2015.196.
83. Dickie EW, Brunet A, Akerib V, Armony JL. Neural correlates of recovery from post-traumatic stress disorder: a longitudinal fMRI investigation of memory encoding. Neuropsychologia. 2011;49:1771–8. https://doi.org/10.1016/j.neuropsychologia.2011.02.055.
84. Rubin M, et al. Greater hippocampal volume is associated with PTSD treatment response. Psychiatry Res. 2016;252:36–9. https://doi.org/10.1016/j.pscychresns.2016.05.001.
85. Norte CE, et al. They know their trauma by heart: an assessment of psychophysiological failure to recover in PTSD. J Affect Disord. 2013;150:136–41. https://doi.org/10.1016/j.jad.2012.11.039.
86. Robison-Andrew EJ, et al. Changes in trauma-potentiated startle with treatment of post-traumatic stress disorder in combat Veterans. J Anxiety Disord. 2014;28:358–62. https://doi.org/10.1016/j.janxdis.2014.04.002.
87. Bechara A. Risky business: emotion, decision-making, and addiction. J Gambl Stud. 2003;19:23–51.
88. Reuter J, et al. Pathological gambling is linked to reduced activation of the mesolimbic reward system. Nat Neurosci. 2005;8:147–8. https://doi.org/10.1038/nn1378.
89. Verdejo-Garcia A, Bechara A. A somatic marker theory of addiction. Neuropharmacology. 2009;56(Suppl 1):48–62. https://doi.org/10.1016/j.neuropharm.2008.07.035.
90. Mayberg HS. Targeted electrode-based modulation of neural circuits for depression. J Clin Invest. 2009;119:717–25. https://doi.org/10.1172/JCI38454.
91. Drevets WC, Price JL, Furey ML. Brain structural and functional abnormalities in mood disorders: implications for neurocircuitry models of depression. Brain Struct Funct. 2008;213:93–118. https://doi.org/10.1007/s00429-008-0189-x.
92. Mayberg HS. Limbic-cortical dysregulation: a proposed model of depression. J Neuropsychiatry Clin Neurosci. 1997;9:471–81. https://doi.org/10.1176/jnp.9.3.471.
93. de Kloet CS, et al. Assessment of HPA-axis function in posttraumatic stress disorder: pharmacological and non-pharmacological challenge tests, a review. J Psychiatr Res. 2006;40:550–67. https://doi.org/10.1016/j.jpsychires.2005.08.002.
94. Smith SM, Vale WW. The role of the hypothalamic-pituitary-adrenal axis in neuroendocrine responses to stress. Dialogues Clin Neurosci. 2006;8:383–95.
95. Munck A, Guyre PM, Holbrook NJ. Physiological functions of glucocorticoids in stress and their relation to pharmacological actions. Endocr Rev. 1984;5:25–44. https://doi.org/10.1210/edrv-5-1-25.
96. Bamberger CM, Schulte HM, Chrousos GP. Molecular determinants of glucocorticoid receptor function and tissue sensitivity to glucocorticoids. Endocr Rev. 1996;17:245–61. https://doi.org/10.1210/edrv-17-3-245.
97. Yehuda R. Advances in understanding neuroendocrine alterations in PTSD and their therapeutic implications. Ann N Y Acad Sci. 2006;1071:137–66. https://doi.org/10.1196/annals.1364.012.
98. de Quervain DJ, Margraf J. Glucocorticoids for the treatment of post-traumatic stress disorder and phobias: a novel therapeutic approach. Eur J Pharmacol. 2008;583:365–71. https://doi.org/10.1016/j.ejphar.2007.11.068.
99. Meewisse ML, Reitsma JB, de Vries GJ, Gersons BP, Olff M. Cortisol and post-traumatic stress disorder in adults: systematic review and meta-analysis. Br J Psychiatry. 2007;191:387–92. https://doi.org/10.1192/bjp.bp.106.024877.

100. Sherin JE, Nemeroff CB. Post-traumatic stress disorder: the neurobiological impact of psychological trauma. Dialogues Clin Neurosci. 2011;13:263–78.
101. Kartha A, et al. The impact of trauma exposure and post-traumatic stress disorder on healthcare utilization among primary care patients. Med Care. 2008;46:388–93. https://doi.org/10.1097/MLR.0b013e31815dc5d2.
102. Arnow BA. Relationships between childhood maltreatment, adult health and psychiatric outcomes, and medical utilization. J Clin Psychiatry. 2004;65(Suppl 12):10–5.
103. Madakasira S, O'Brien KF. Acute posttraumatic stress disorder in victims of a natural disaster. J Nerv Ment Dis. 1987;175:286–90.
104. Cao H, McFarlane CA, Klimidis S. Prevalence of psychiatric disorder following the 1988 Yun Nan (China) earthquake. Soc Psychiatry Psychiatr Epidemiol. 2003;38:204–12. https://doi.org/10.1007/s00127-003-0619-2.
105. Thompson MP, Norris FH, Hanacek B. Age differences in the psychological consequences of Hurricane Hugo. Psychol Aging. 1993;8:606–16.
106. North CS, et al. Psychiatric disorders among survivors of the Oklahoma City bombing. JAMA. 1999;282:755–62.
107. North CS, et al. The postdisaster prevalence of major depression relative to PTSD in survivors of the 9/11 attacks on the World Trade Center selected from affected workplaces. Compr Psychiatry. 2015;60:119–25. https://doi.org/10.1016/j.comppsych.2015.02.009.
108. Zhang G, et al. Psychiatric disorders after terrorist bombings among rescue workers and bombing survivors in Nairobi and rescue workers in Oklahoma City. Ann Clin Psychiatry. 2016;28:22–30.
109. Grieger TA, Waldrep DA, Lovasz MM, Ursano RJ. Follow-up of Pentagon employees two years after the terrorist attack of September 11, 2001. Psychiatr Serv. 2005;56:1374–8. https://doi.org/10.1176/appi.ps.56.11.1374.
110. Liu B, Tarigan LH, Bromet EJ, Kim H. World Trade Center disaster exposure-related probable posttraumatic stress disorder among responders and civilians: a meta-analysis. PLoS One. 2014;9:e101491. https://doi.org/10.1371/journal.pone.0101491.
111. Bell CC, Jenkins EJ. Community violence and children on Chicago's southside. Psychiatry. 1993;56:46–54.
112. Campbell C, Schwarz DF. Prevalence and impact of exposure to interpersonal violence among suburban and urban middle school students. Pediatrics. 1996;98:396–402.
113. Gladstein J, Rusonis EJ, Heald FP. A comparison of inner-city and upper-middle class youths' exposure to violence. J Adolesc Health. 1992;13:275–80.
114. Fitzpatrick KM, Boldizar JP. The prevalence and consequences of exposure to violence among African-American youth. J Am Acad Child Adolesc Psychiatry. 1993;32:424–30. https://doi.org/10.1097/00004583-199303000-00026.
115. Alim TN, et al. Trauma exposure, posttraumatic stress disorder and depression in an African-American primary care population. J Natl Med Assoc. 2006;98:1630–6.
116. Schneider R, Baumrind N, Kimerling R. Exposure to child abuse and risk for mental health problems in women. Violence Vict. 2007;22:620–31.
117. Breslau N, et al. Trauma and posttraumatic stress disorder in the community: the 1996 detroit area survey of trauma. Arch Gen Psychiatry. 1998;55:626–32. https://doi.org/10.1001/archpsyc.55.7.626.
118. Pfaff JF. The empirics of prison growth: a critical review and path forward. J Crim Law Criminol. 2008;98:547–619.
119. Austin J, McVey AD. The impact of the war on drugs. 1989.
120. Greenberg DF, West V. State prison populations and their growth, 1971–1991. Criminology. 2001;39:615–54.
121. Gillespie CF, Phifer J, Bradley B, Ressler KJ. Risk and resilience: genetic and environmental influences on development of the stress response. Depress Anxiety. 2009;26:984–92. https://doi.org/10.1002/da.20605.

122. Dean G, Kilpatrick PD, et al. The serotonin transporter genotype and social support and moderation of posttraumatic stress disorder and depression in hurricane-exposed adults. Am J Psychiatr. 2007;164:1693–9. https://doi.org/10.1176/appi.ajp.2007.06122007.
123. Robinaugh DJ, et al. Understanding the relationship of perceived social support to post-trauma cognitions and posttraumatic stress disorder. J Anxiety Disord. 2011;25:1072–8.
124. Dai W, et al. Association between social support and recovery from post-traumatic stress disorder after flood: a 13–14 year follow-up study in Hunan, China. BMC Public Health. 2016;16:194.
125. Coker AL, et al. Social support protects against the negative effects of partner violence on mental health. J Womens Health Gend Based Med. 2002;11:465–76. https://doi.org/10.1089/15246090260137644.
126. Brewin CR, Andrews B, Valentine JD. Meta-analysis of risk factors for posttraumatic stress disorder in trauma-exposed adults. J Consult Clin Psychol. 2000;68:748–66.
127. Ozer EJ, Best SR, Lipsey TL, Weiss DS. Predictors of posttraumatic stress disorder and symptoms in adults: a meta-analysis. Psychol Bull. 2003;129:52–73.
128. Cutrona CE, Russell DW, Hessling RM, Brown PA, Murry V. Direct and moderating effects of community context on the psychological well-being of African American women. J Pers Soc Psychol. 2000;79:1088–101.
129. Obasaju MA, Palin FL, Jacobs C, Anderson P, Kaslow NJ. Won't you be my neighbor? Using an ecological approach to examine the impact of community on revictimization. J Interpers Violence. 2009;24:38–53. https://doi.org/10.1177/0886260508314933.
130. Sampson RJ, Raudenbush SW, Earls F. Neighborhoods and violent crime: a multilevel study of collective efficacy. Science. 1997;277:918–24.
131. Gapen M, et al. Perceived neighborhood disorder, community cohesion, and PTSD symptoms among low-income African Americans in an urban health setting. Am J Orthopsychiatry. 2011;81:31–7. https://doi.org/10.1111/j.1939-0025.2010.01069.x.
132. Johns LE, et al. Neighborhood social cohesion and posttraumatic stress disorder in a community-based sample: findings from the Detroit Neighborhood Health Study. Soc Psychiatry Psychiatr Epidemiol. 2012;47:1899–906. https://doi.org/10.1007/s00127-012-0506-9.
133. McFall M, Fontana A, Raskind M, Rosenheck R. Analysis of violent behavior in Vietnam combat veteran psychiatric inpatients with posttraumatic stress disorder. J Trauma Stress. 1999;12:501–17. https://doi.org/10.1023/a:1024771121189.
134. Elbogen EB, Beckham JC, Butterfield MI, Swartz M, Swanson J. Assessing risk of violent behavior among veterans with severe mental illness. J Trauma Stress. 2008;21:113–7. https://doi.org/10.1002/jts.20283.
135. Glenn DM, et al. Violence and hostility among families of Vietnam veterans with combat-related posttraumatic stress disorder. Violence Vict. 2002;17:473–89.
136. Haller M, Chassin L. Risk pathways among traumatic stress, posttraumatic stress disorder symptoms, and alcohol and drug problems: a test of four hypotheses. Psychol Addict Behav. 2014;28:841–51. https://doi.org/10.1037/a0035878.
137. Fetzner MG, Abrams MP, Asmundson GJ. Symptoms of posttraumatic stress disorder and depression in relation to alcohol-use and alcohol-related problems among Canadian forces veterans. Can J Psychiatr. 2013;58:417–25.
138. Taft CT, et al. Posttraumatic stress disorder symptoms, physiological reactivity, alcohol problems, and aggression among military veterans. J Abnorm Psychol. 2007;116:498–507. https://doi.org/10.1037/0021-843x.116.3.498.
139. Donley S, et al. Civilian PTSD symptoms and risk for involvement in the criminal justice system. J Am Acad Psychiatry Law. 2012;40:522–9.
140. Lundholm L, Haggard U, Moller J, Hallqvist J, Thiblin I. The triggering effect of alcohol and illicit drugs on violent crime in a remand prison population: a case crossover study. Drug Alcohol Depend. 2013;129:110–5. https://doi.org/10.1016/j.drugalcdep.2012.09.019.

141. Khoury L, Tang YL, Bradley B, Cubells JF, Ressler KJ. Substance use, childhood traumatic experience, and posttraumatic stress disorder in an urban civilian population. Depress Anxiety. 2010;27:1077–86. https://doi.org/10.1002/da.20751.
142. Dube SR, Anda RF, Felitti VJ, Edwards VJ, Croft JB. Adverse childhood experiences and personal alcohol abuse as an adult. Addict Behav. 2002;27:713–25.
143. Neigh GN, Gillespie CF, Nemeroff CB. The neurobiological toll of child abuse and neglect. Trauma Violence Abuse. 2009;10:389–410. https://doi.org/10.1177/1524838009339758.
144. Kingston S, Raghavan C. The relationship of sexual abuse, early initiation of substance use, and adolescent trauma to PTSD. J Trauma Stress. 2009;22:65–8. https://doi.org/10.1002/jts.20381.
145. Galovski T, Lyons JA. Psychological sequelae of combat violence: a review of the impact of PTSD on the veteran's family and possible interventions. Aggress Violent Behav. 2004;9:477–501.
146. Saxon AJ, et al. Trauma, symptoms of posttraumatic stress disorder, and associated problems among incarcerated veterans. Psychiatr Serv. 2001;52:959–64. https://doi.org/10.1176/appi.ps.52.7.959.
147. Gendreau P, Goggin C, Smith P. Generating rational correctional policies: an introduction to advances in cumulating knowledge. Correct Manag Q. 2000;4:52–60.
148. Gendreau P, Cullen FT, Goggin C. The effects of prison sentences on recidivism. Solicitor General Canada Ottawa, 1999.
149. Wolff N, Blitz CL, Shi J, Bachman R, Siegel JA. Sexual violence inside prisons: rates of victimization. J Urban Health. 2006;83:835–48.
150. Blitz CL, Wolff N, Shi J. Physical victimization in prison: the role of mental illness. Int J Law Psychiatry. 2008;31:385–93.
151. Wooldredge JD. Inmate crime and victimization in a southwestern correctional facility. J Crim Just. 1994;22:367–81.
152. Golembeski C, Fullilove R. Criminal (in)justice in the city and its associated health consequences. Am J Public Health. 2005;95:1701–6.
153. Wang EA, et al. Incarceration, incident hypertension, and access to healthcare: findings from the coronary artery risk development in young adults (CARDIA) study. Arch Intern Med. 2009;169:687–93.
154. Parsons RG, Ressler KJ. Implications of memory modulation for post-traumatic stress and fear disorders. Nat Neurosci. 2013;16:146–53. https://doi.org/10.1038/nn.3296.
155. Feder A, Nestler EJ, Charney DS. Psychobiology and molecular genetics of resilience. Nat Rev Neurosci. 2009;10:446–57. https://doi.org/10.1038/nrn2649.
156. Southwick SM, Vythilingam M, Charney DS. The psychobiology of depression and resilience to stress: implications for prevention and treatment. Annu Rev Clin Psychol. 2005;1:255–91. https://doi.org/10.1146/annurev.clinpsy.1.102803.143948.
157. Alim TN, et al. Trauma, resilience, and recovery in a high-risk African-American population. Am J Psychiatry. 2008;165:1566–75. https://doi.org/10.1176/appi.ajp.2008.07121939.
158. Wingo AP, Ressler KJ, Bradley B. Resilience characteristics mitigate tendency for harmful alcohol and illicit drug use in adults with a history of childhood abuse: a cross-sectional study of 2024 inner-city men and women. J Psychiatr Res. 2014;51:93–9.
159. Campbell-Sills L, Stein MB. Psychometric analysis and refinement of the Connor-Davidson resilience scale (CD-RISC): validation of a 10-item measure of resilience. J Trauma Stress. 2007;20:1019–28. https://doi.org/10.1002/jts.20271.
160. Connor KM, Davidson JR. Development of a new resilience scale: the Connor-Davidson resilience scale (CD-RISC). Depress Anxiety. 2003;18:76–82. https://doi.org/10.1002/da.10113.
161. Heim C, Shugart M, Craighead WE, Nemeroff CB. Neurobiological and psychiatric consequences of child abuse and neglect. Dev Psychobiol. 2010;52:671–90. https://doi.org/10.1002/dev.20494.
162. Yehuda R, Halligan SL, Bierer LM. Relationship of parental trauma exposure and PTSD to PTSD, depressive and anxiety disorders in offspring. J Psychiatr Res. 2001;35:261–70.

163. Grillon C, et al. Families at high and low risk for depression: a three-generation startle study. Biol Psychiatry. 2005;57:953–60. https://doi.org/10.1016/j.biopsych.2005.01.045.
164. Yehuda R, Bierer LM. Transgenerational transmission of cortisol and PTSD risk. Prog Brain Res. 2008;167:121–35. https://doi.org/10.1016/s0079-6123(07)67009-5.
165. Jovanovic T, et al. Childhood abuse is associated with increased startle reactivity in adulthood. Depress Anxiety. 2009;26:1018–26.
166. Jovanovic T, et al. Physiological markers of anxiety are increased in children of abused mothers. J Child Psychol Psychiatry. 2011;52:844–52. https://doi.org/10.1111/j.1469-7610.2011.02410.x.
167. Stein MB, Jang KL, Taylor S, Vernon PA, Livesley WJ. Genetic and environmental influences on trauma exposure and posttraumatic stress disorder symptoms: a twin study. Am J Psychiatry. 2002;159:1675–81. https://doi.org/10.1176/appi.ajp.159.10.1675.
168. True WR, et al. A twin study of genetic and environmental contributions to liability for posttraumatic stress symptoms. Arch Gen Psychiatry. 1993;50:257–64.
169. Sharma S, Powers A, Bradley B, Ressler KJ. Gene x environment determinants of stress- and anxiety-related disorders. Annu Rev Psychol. 2016;67:239–61. https://doi.org/10.1146/annurev-psych-122414-033408.
170. Antonini A, Stryker MP. Rapid remodeling of axonal arbors in the visual cortex. Science. 1993;260:1819–21.
171. Werker JF, Hensch TK. Critical periods in speech perception: new directions. Annu Rev Psychol. 2015;66:173–96. https://doi.org/10.1146/annurev-psych-010814-015104.
172. Sullivan RM, Landers M, Yeaman B, Wilson DA. Neurophysiology: good memories of bad events in infancy. Nature. 2000;407:38–9.
173. Moriceau S, Wilson DA, Levine S, Sullivan RM. Dual circuitry for odor-shock conditioning during infancy: corticosterone switches between fear and attraction via amygdala. J Neurosci. 2006;26:6737–48. https://doi.org/10.1523/jneurosci.0499-06.2006.
174. Sullivan R, The M. Neurobiology of attachment to nurturing and abusive caregivers. Hastings Law J. 2012;63:1553–70.
175. Roth TL, et al. Neurobiology of secure infant attachment and attachment despite adversity: a mouse model. Genes Brain Behav. 2013;12:673–80. https://doi.org/10.1111/gbb.12067.
176. Moriceau S, Shionoya K, Jakubs K, Sullivan RM. Early-life stress disrupts attachment learning: the role of amygdala corticosterone, locus ceruleus corticotropin releasing hormone, and olfactory bulb norepinephrine. J Neurosci. 2009;29:15745–55. https://doi.org/10.1523/jneurosci.4106-09.2009.
177. Moriceau S, Roth TL, Sullivan RM. Rodent model of infant attachment learning and stress. Dev Psychobiol. 2010;52:651–60. https://doi.org/10.1002/dev.20482.
178. Sarro EC, Wilson DA, Sullivan RM. Maternal regulation of infant brain state. Curr Biol. 2014;24:1664–9. https://doi.org/10.1016/j.cub.2014.06.017.
179. Barbas H. Connections underlying the synthesis of cognition, memory, and emotion in primate prefrontal cortices. Brain Res Bull. 2000;52:319–30.
180. Croxson PL, et al. Quantitative investigation of connections of the prefrontal cortex in the human and macaque using probabilistic diffusion tractography. J Neurosci. 2005;25:8854–66. https://doi.org/10.1523/jneurosci.1311-05.2005.
181. Preuss TM, Goldman-Rakic PS. Ipsilateral cortical connections of granular frontal cortex in the strepsirhine primate Galago, with comparative comments on anthropoid primates. J Comp Neurol. 1991;310:507–49. https://doi.org/10.1002/cne.903100404.
182. Preuss TM. Do rats have prefrontal cortex? The rose-Woolsey-Akert program reconsidered. J Cogn Neurosci. 1995;7:1–24. https://doi.org/10.1162/jocn.1995.7.1.1.
183. Ongur D, Price JL. The organization of networks within the orbital and medial prefrontal cortex of rats, monkeys and humans. Cereb Cortex. 2000;10:206–19.
184. Seay B, Gottfried NW. A phylogenetic perspective for social behavior in primates. J Gen Psychol. 1975;92:5–17. https://doi.org/10.1080/00221309.1975.9711323.

185. Suomi SJ, Harlow HF, Kimball SD. Behavioral effects of prolonged partial social isolation in the rhesus monkey. Psychol Rep. 1971;29:1171–7. https://doi.org/10.2466/pr0.1971.29.3f.1171.
186. Sanchez MM, et al. Alterations in diurnal cortisol rhythm and acoustic startle response in nonhuman primates with adverse rearing. Biol Psychiatry. 2005;57:373–81. https://doi.org/10.1016/j.biopsych.2004.11.032.
187. Sanchez MM, Ladd CO, Plotsky PM. Early adverse experience as a developmental risk factor for later psychopathology: evidence from rodent and primate models. Dev Psychopathol. 2001;13:419–49.
188. Tottenham N, et al. Prolonged institutional rearing is associated with atypically large amygdala volume and difficulties in emotion regulation. Dev Sci. 2010;13:46–61. https://doi.org/10.1111/j.1467-7687.2009.00852.x.
189. Fareri DS, Tottenham N. Effects of early life stress on amygdala and striatal development. Dev Cogn Neurosci. 2016;19:233–47. https://doi.org/10.1016/j.dcn.2016.04.005.
190. Lupien SJ, et al. Larger amygdala but no change in hippocampal volume in 10-year-old children exposed to maternal depressive symptomatology since birth. Proc Natl Acad Sci U S A. 2011;108:14324–9. https://doi.org/10.1073/pnas.1105371108.
191. Callaghan BL, Sullivan RM, Howell B, Tottenham N. The international society for developmental psychobiology Sackler symposium: early adversity and the maturation of emotion circuits--a cross-species analysis. Dev Psychobiol. 2014;56:1635–50. https://doi.org/10.1002/dev.21260.
192. Davies TH, Ning YM, Sanchez ER. A new first step in activation of steroid receptors: hormone-induced switching of FKBP51 and FKBP52 immunophilins. J Biol Chem. 2002;277:4597–600. https://doi.org/10.1074/jbc.C100531200.
193. Wochnik GM, et al. FK506-binding proteins 51 and 52 differentially regulate dynein interaction and nuclear translocation of the glucocorticoid receptor in mammalian cells. J Biol Chem. 2005;280:4609–16. https://doi.org/10.1074/jbc.M407498200.
194. Binder EB, et al. Association of FKBP5 polymorphisms and childhood abuse with risk of posttraumatic stress disorder symptoms in adults. JAMA. 2008;299:1291–305.
195. Xie P, et al. Interaction of FKBP5 with childhood adversity on risk for post-traumatic stress disorder. Neuropsychopharmacology. 2010;35:1684–92.
196. Klengel T, Binder EB. FKBP5 allele-specific epigenetic modification in gene by environment interaction. Neuropsychopharmacology. 2015;40:244–6.
197. Klengel T, Binder EB. Epigenetics of stress-related psychiatric disorders and gene X environment interactions. Neuron. 2015;86:1343–57. https://doi.org/10.1016/j.neuron.2015.05.036.
198. Sabbagh JJ, et al. Age-associated epigenetic upregulation of the FKBP5 gene selectively impairs stress resiliency. PLoS One. 2014;9:e107241. https://doi.org/10.1371/journal.pone.0107241.
199. Klengel T, et al. Allele-specific FKBP5 DNA demethylation mediates gene-childhood trauma interactions. Nat Neurosci. 2013;16:33–41.

Chapter 4
Trauma and Neurodevelopmental Disorder: Assessment, Treatment, and Triage

Lisa Prock and Jason M. Fogler

> *Based on a careful evaluation of neurocognitive and personality factors, the neuropsychologist can offer an objective view of the patient's experience and adaptive resources or limitations. Such a perspective may indeed be objective without sacrificing empathy.*
>
> —*L. Seidman (1994) [1]*

Vignettes

Vignette #1: Marianne: "Marianne," age 7½, was adopted from a Russian orphanage at 4 years of age and has been in a stable adoptive home since her adoption. Her birth parents were characterized as "unstable," and her early history is significant for reported neglect, failure to thrive, malnutrition, and developmental delays with many additional details unknown. Presenting difficulties for this clinical visit included marked inattention, possible learning disability/disabilities, frequent (often violent) nightmares, and recently, "hearing voices." Marianne's parents have had a longstanding concern that Marianne would "talk to and go off with anybody," and this has not appreciably improved in the 3 years that Marianne has been living with her parents.

Marianne's neurocognitive testing performance was salient for asking questions about the examiner and team members, frequent time checks/checking in with her adoptive parents, and saying that she is having "so much fun" and "wants to stay here forever." (Despite her expressed wish to check in

L. Prock
Division of Developmental Medicine, Boston Children's Hospital, Boston, MA, USA

Harvard Medical School, Boston, MA, USA
e-mail: Lisa.Prock@childrens.harvard.edu

J. M. Fogler (✉)
Developmental Medical Center, Boston Children's Hospital, Boston, MA, USA
e-mail: Jason.Fogler@childrens.harvard.edu

J. M. Fogler, R. A. Phelps (eds.), *Trauma, Autism, and Neurodevelopmental Disorders*, https://doi.org/10.1007/978-3-030-00503-0_4

frequently with her adoptive parents during the testing, she asks if she can spend breaks with the examiner). It often seems as if Marianne is attending to the examiner's tone of voice and facial expressions rather than the test items and she benefits from consistent redirection from chatting back to task in order to demonstrate her true abilities. Her behavior abruptly shifts to hyperactive and silly upon being told that the assessment was ending and that she would be going home soon.

Vignette #2: Ken: "Ken" is a now 7-year-old who joined his family via adoption from South Korea at 18 months of age. He is the second child in his family with a history of international adoption and cleft lip/palate; and his parents felt very prepared prior to his adoption to support his medical needs. Ken's adoptive parents were aware that he would need to have surgical repairs of his cleft lip/palate shortly after arriving home. Although his parents were prepared for his expected surgeries and speech and language therapy related to his known cleft lip and palate—they are now more concerned about his behavioral and emotional concerns than they expected to be prior to his adoption. Ken's local therapist (who describes her area of expertise to include "attachment therapy") is working with the family based on the assumption that he has a diagnosis of reactive attachment disorder. Comprehensive psychological assessment in our center suggested a diagnosis of autism spectrum disorder based on his performance during the ADOS in conjunction with history provided by his mother during his assessment. Specifically, testing was notable for decreased social responsiveness (reduced eye contact; limited use of nonverbal communication) and play that was immature for his age—leading to an autism diagnosis. Ken's mother is now quite confused—as she does not see him as on the autism spectrum, has noted positive behavioral challenges with attachment-focused interventions, and reports she is confused regarding where to go with next steps with Ken in terms of school-based and other services. She is also concerned that no "tests" have considered his "trauma history"—including his pre-adoptive life and multiple interventions/surgery post-adoption.

These two cases raise a host of different diagnostic issues and treatment challenges related to diagnostic categories that may arise with children with a history of traumatic experiences including presenting with symptoms of inattention and hyperactivity, learning disability, disinhibited social engagement/reactive attachment, autism spectrum disorders, and the question of traumatic dissociation versus (or plus) auditory hallucinations. These overlapping symptoms are the norm rather than the exception when children have experienced a combination of neglect, trauma, and toxic stress given the pervasive effects of adverse childhood experiences on neurodevelopment and brain architecture [2]. We can no longer draw arbitrary distinctions between "mind" (psychiatric)- and "brain" (neurodevelopmental)-related challenges, because a chronically stressed brain will not only be at risk for a hyperaroused "fight or flight" system but also impaired learning and executive functioning. One's level of regulation (or dysregulation) also significantly impacts the ability to learn, regulate interpersonal relationships, and regulate mood and reactions to others.

The correlation between negative experiences in childhood and later health and mental health concerns in adulthood has been well documented. The Adverse Childhood Experiences Study (ACES) [3] describes the self-reports and medical records of more than 17,000 Kaiser Permanente HMO health insurance members longitudinally considering both childhood exposures and adult outcomes. Participants were asked about childhood experiences including psychological, physical, and sexual abuse and neglect as well as exposure to caretakers and other adults with substance abuse, mental illness, domestic violence, and criminal behavior. An increased number of adverse childhood events contributed to an increased adult risk of both mental health concerns (generalized anxiety disorder, major depressive disorder) and chronic medical concerns (hypertension, cardiac disease, and diabetes) [3].

Complicating matters further, children with neurodevelopmental disorders are at increased risk for bullying and maltreatment [4], particularly if they also have intellectual disability and communication disorders [5]. A recent systematic review of studies of youth at clinical high risk (CHR) for developing psychosis has rates of trauma and extreme stress in their histories as high as 80% [6]. The National Child Traumatic Stress Network provides guidelines for assessing traumatic stress in developmentally disordered children [7], highlighting that children with developmental delays or disabilities may internalize blame for their victimization and apply magical thinking to make sense of what happened to them. These guidelines underscore the importance of watching for *deviations* from usual patterns of self-soothing, sensory seeking, selective attention, and idiosyncratic speech or behavior. In addition, it is critical to carefully monitor children's symptoms over time as emotional and behavioral reactions to one or more stressors may manifest immediately or quite some time after traumatic exposure.

In the absence of clear biological markers, or a thorough history (inclusive of psychological trauma), the majority of healthcare providers—primary, subspecialty, or allied—may understandably interpret emotionally dysregulated behavior, distractibility, restlessness, social withdrawal, and so on according to their specific set of cognitive biases and clinical heuristics. One audiologist's auditory processing disorder is another occupational therapist's sensory processing disorder or another developmental-behavioral pediatrician's "rule out for ADHD or autism spectrum disorder." These labels are neither necessarily "wrong," nor are they mutually exclusive from trauma- and stressor-related disorder (TSRD); but each diagnostic label alone may not sufficiently capture the scope of the child's difficulties—or, more importantly, point present and future clinicians toward the most parsimonious or efficacious treatments to address the underlying primary challenges that hamper a child's development.

That said, "treating the symptom" will sometimes benefit the child regardless of diagnosis, especially in the case of behavioral strategies that promote self-care and healthy parenting. Many of our broadband wellness-oriented treatments that promote relaxation, exercise, healthy diet, better sleep, and positive, consistent parenting are truly transdiagnostic [8–10]. Although helpful for most, these treatments may need to be *adapted* for children who don't like to be touched (whether due to autism-related sensory sensitivities or TSRD-related hyperarousal), have levels of impulsivity that preclude the use of certain kinds of exercise equipment, or have food allergies or sensory aversions. On the other hand, when TSRD is the main driver of a child's difficulties and if that child is in a state of acute distress as a direct consequence of posttraumatic symptoms, symptom-focused treatments like psychostimulants, behavioral exposure, or refuting automatic negative thoughts are not helpful—as they are both likely to fail and risk alienating or, in the case of side effects, harming the child. When a child has already experienced the worst-case scenario, the well-meaning cognitive therapist's "What's the worst that can happen?"—meant in the motivating spirit of trying a new healthy behavior—can feel like the cruelest of insults and may prevent future progress.

What Is a Clinician to Do?

Many parents and professionals referring a child for a psychological/neuropsychological assessment are seeking a definitive diagnosis and treatment plan for a child. However, the diagnostic/treatment picture is typically far more complicated for children with a trauma history than simply arriving at "the diagnosis," which easily maps onto a treatment plan for a specific individual. Diagnostic conundrums stem from both the considerable overlap between features of these disorders and the inadequacy of appropriate DSM-5 diagnostic categories (Table 4.1). These diagnostic conundrums are often compounded by absence of a child's key history within the context of foster care, adoption, and/or non-parental care. When assessing children with a history of known or suspected trauma, it is critical to appreciate that all history that could be helpful may simply not be available to the clinician and that each child's presentation may best be viewed as a "snapshot in time" with additional important clues observed outside of the usual observations documented during psychological assessments. This chapter will identify key considerations with respect to history gathering, assessment, and treatment recommendations when working with children and adolescents with a history of trauma.

Components of a comprehensive psychological assessment for a child with a history of trauma will at a minimum include (1) gathering a history, (2) formal cognitive and academic assessment, and (3) a review of formal and informal reports and measures of executive functioning and emotional functioning. The evaluator (s) will review all components of the assessment and previous evaluations in order to formulate the best summary of an individual's current functioning, identify diagnoses if appropriate, and formulate a treatment plan to provide families with a road map for recommended interventions and monitoring.

The various symptom domains of trauma- and stressor-related disorders (TSRD) span a wide range of phenomena that can mirror symptoms also seen in other neurodevelopmental and psychiatric conditions (Table 4.1). Rates of co-occurring diagnoses are exceedingly high in cases of TSRD—which makes the

Table 4.1 Symptom overlap between trauma- and stressor-related disorders and other conditions[a]

DSM-5 PTSD criterion symptoms	Comparable features in other neurodevelopmental disorders
Criterion A: traumatic event criterion A Event"	*N/A*
Criterion B: re-experiencing (flashbacks, nightmares, and intrusive thoughts)	Hallucinations in the schizophrenia spectrum and other psychotic disorders Perseverations in autism spectrum disorder, intellectual disability, and obsessive-compulsive disorder Rumination and catastrophizing in generalized anxiety disorder
Criterion C: avoidance of internal and external reminders ("emotional numbing")	Social disconnection in autism spectrum disorder Emotional constriction in anxiety disorders Rituals in obsessive-compulsive disorder
Criterion D: negative cognitions and mood (sense of foreshortened future)	Depressive disorder, flat affect in autism spectrum disorder
Criterion E: alterations in arousal and reactivity (hyperarousal and hypervigilance)	Hyperactive/impulsive symptoms in ADHD Panic attacks Other anxiety disorders (especially if manifesting as irritability)
Associated features: attachment problems and dissociation	Social pragmatic problems and disconnection in autism spectrum disorder Problems with personal space and boundaries in ADHD Inattention and "spacing out" in ADHD and schizophrenia spectrum and other psychotic disorder

[a]PTSD was chosen as the "prototypical" TSRD in that its criteria are observed among the other TSRDs in different combinations and levels of severity

task of determining which diagnosis should be the "leading foot" in a clinician's conceptualization and treatment planning especially difficult. Recognition of trauma(s) as the etiology for symptom onset, or traumatic reminders as the consistent trigger of seemingly isolated or random incidents, can assist with the differential diagnosis. Broadly speaking, the symptoms of TSRD will seem more *reactive* than the symptoms of other neuropsychiatric disorders, even if what "set off" the reaction initially seems unclear. For example, whereas children with ADHD will usually be inattentive, hyperactive (or both) at baseline and throughout an assessment, children with TSRD will seem *selectively* inattentive and hyperactive and usually under emotionally charged conditions by history and during an assessment. Similarly, "social withdrawal" will present very differently, especially in regard to affective quality, in children with a primary autism spectrum disorder (ASD) vs. TSRD. For example, a child with ASD will be consistently (and often euthymically) disconnected from other people, be they caregivers or clinicians; but the child with TSRDs disconnection is more likely to stem from hypervigilance and trust issues—and therefore apt to fluctuate with the child's comfort level with the clinician that she/he is working with.

History Gathering: Considering the Role of Trauma in the Story

History gathering is fundamental to generating an appropriate differential diagnosis, identifying an appropriate diagnosis/es and developing an appropriate treatment plan in any child's situation. All available history should be gathered and gaps noted. However, children and young adults with a history of trauma and their parents/caretakers may or may not be fully aware of the details of a child's history. Children with TSRDs and their parents—who may be victims or perpetrators of violence themselves—may also not be especially forthcoming in discussing their trauma history, and/or some of this history may be out of their awareness in whole or part due to the defensive mechanism of dissociation [11–13]. As Judith Herman describes so eloquently in her widely influential book *Trauma and Recovery*, survivors of trauma are often caught between the dynamics of desperately wanting to reveal and unburden themselves of what has happened to them and hiding what for them are deeply shameful experiences of their victimhood and internalized sense of having "deserved" their traumas. (For why else would God or a parent allow such terrible things to happen to me?) [14].

In addition to general details shared about a child's history—the working narrative that caregivers use to understand their child/ren as vulnerable or resilient—*the trajectory of change* with respect to a child's affect and behaviors over time and the multiple reasons or triggers for specific behaviors should also be appreciated. For children who have had multiple transitions and caretakers, creating a "timeline" of events may be helpful with respect to both a clinician's understanding a child's history and a child personally understanding his/her own history (see Sidebar, Table 4.2). Key historical events may include a child's entering child protective custody, a move to a new/foster/pre-adoptive home, significant trauma/abuse, loss of meaningful adults and children via death, transition, and exposure to potentially re-traumatizing events (e.g., visits with birth family members including siblings with whom they may have a positive or negative relationship). Observations about how a child's regulation abilities (e.g., activity level, mood, interpersonal relationships) change over time and in relation to key events are helpful [15].

For example, in Ken's case—his local therapist worked specifically with Ken and his mother and noted the challenges he had with relating to his mother and interacting with her in a positive manner. As she started working with him prior to repair of

Table 4.2 Sample historical events in the assessment and treatment of TSRD

• Entering child protective custody
• Move to a new/foster/pre-adoptive home, significant trauma/abuse
• Loss of meaningful adults and children via death, incarceration/institutionalization, move or other transitions
• Exposure to potentially re-traumatizing events (e.g., visits with birth family members including siblings with whom they may have a very positive relationship; return to country of origin)

his cleft lip and palate—and she appreciated that English was not his first language—she took his nonverbal communication challenges and lack of routine response to his mother as consistent with an "attachment disorder." In contrast, a later evaluation in a new setting with a psychologist was notable for decreased social responsiveness (reduced eye contact; limited use of nonverbal communication) and play that was quite immature for his age—leading to an autism diagnosis. Ultimately, Ken's family and treating providers agreed that he had features of many different developmental disorders; but that treatment needed to prioritize his emotional connections with his family as well as help him cultivate better social skills. This was a case in which the team felt strongly that appreciating the role of Ken's history was more critical than addressing the autistic symptoms in isolation from their emotional content. Over time, Ken appeared "less autistic" and more socially related, albeit still with some social pragmatic vulnerabilities—which gradually improved with treatment.

The Effects of Trauma on Neurocognitive Functioning: A Psychometric Perspective

Whereas history helps to contextualize children's difficulties within certain temporal parameters (i.e., dates of onset/offset; sequence relative to hypothesized causal factors and triggers; behavioral "chaining"), psychometric testing helps to provide a here-and-now snapshot of the scope and severity of these difficulties. Psychometric testing is predicated on the assumption that neurocognitive abilities are normally distributed in the population and can be normed to reference groups based on age and developmental level. As a result, a population of typically developing children has a roughly even distribution of cognitive abilities established by the "set point" of their genetic potential, which is subsequently moderated by the (positive or negative) effects of environmental factors. Potential moderating and mediating factors include prenatal substance exposure, pre- and postnatal nutrition, quality of language exposure and educational instruction, socioeconomic status, and multiple environmental stressors. Psychometric tests are thought to provide a reference normed, performance-based proxy for different neurocognitive abilities. When there are large, statistically significant discrepancies between test performances, the pattern of disparities may suggest different clinical syndromes. For example, a significant weakness on tests of reading in comparison with the rest of a child's neurocognitive profile, especially in conjunction with family history, would support a diagnosis of dyslexia.

The effects of traumatic stress on neuropsychological functions have been well documented. Chronic stress particularly contributes to diminished prefrontal and hippocampal functioning, with corresponding performance problems on test of working memory, anterograde memory/learning process, sustained attention, and behavioral inhibition [16]. Notably these neuropsychological deficits can also be observed in routine disorders of learning and executive dysfunction.

In our experience, a key difference between children presenting with predominantly uncomplicated learning disorders and those presenting with primarily trauma- and stressor-related disorders is how they *approach the testing experience*. A child with learning disorders might resist being evaluated in the areas in which they struggle but otherwise be well regulated during the administration of other measures and during the physical examination. In contrast, the child with a history of traumatic stress will approach the examiner or setting with general wariness and, as many survivors do, may take refuge in the structured cognitive tasks but become more dysregulated with less structured and more emotionally laden tasks. Similarly, whereas the child with primary ASD will be consistently socially disconnected during a play-based evaluation like the Autism Diagnostic Observation Schedule-2 and euthymic as long as she/he is left to pursue his/her self-directed interests, the child with primary TSRD will likely have wide fluctuations in social response and affect regulation depending on whether or not she/he has been triggered. We would make a similar observation about the difference between inattention and hyperactivity that is primarily due to ADHD vs. TSRD. In contrast to the relatively consistent and euthymic hyperactivity and distractibility observed in children with ADHD, children with TSRD might become highly dysregulated at specific triggering events during the testing but may seem highly controlled and focused during nonthreatening tasks.

There are a wide range of questionnaire measures and semi-structured interviews targeted at the assessment of traumatic stress symptoms and potentially traumatic

Table 4.3 Commonly used measures in the assessment of traumatic stress symptoms

Content type	Measure	Age (years)	# items	Respondent	Languages	Psychometrics
Traumatic stress symptoms	TSCYC	3–12	90	Caregiver	English, Spanish	+++
	TSS	8–16	54	Caregiver	English, Spanish	+++
	PTSD-RI Modified	6–17 (3–5)	20 (22)	Child Child	English English	++ (+)
	PTSD-PAC	3–5	18	Caregiver	English	+
	PT-SIC	4–8	30	Child	English	+++
PTE/violence exposure	TESI-PR	3–18	24	Caregiver	English, Spanish	+
	TESI-PRR	0–6	15	Caregiver	English, Spanish	0
	VEX-PV	4+	25	Child	English, Spanish, Hebrew	++
	VEX-PR	4–6	22	Caregiver	English	++
	DOSE	n.s.	50	Caregiver	English	0

+ internal consistency or test-retest reliability, ++ two dimensions, including interrater reliability or convergent validity, +++ three dimensions, including predictive validity, *0* non-normed, *n.s.* not specified events [17, 18]. The purpose of this chapter is not to provide an exhaustive review of these measures—although we have provided a table listing some of the better supported ones in the empirical literature (see Table 4.3)—but rather to highlight two key points. The first is that *children and caregivers may be reluctant to disclose the full extent of their symptoms*, and thus we advise following up on any endorsed item even if responses do not aggregate to a clinically significant standard score or clinical cutoff. The second is that it is more often the norm than the exception for children and caregivers to *provide the most salient or extreme potentially traumatic experience* rather than recognizing the everyday chaos in their lives as being of equal importance or impact.

The Science and Craft of Assessment

From a psychometric testing perspective, one needs to "read between the scores" to begin to differentiate symptoms and clarify diagnosis (es) as appropriate. For example, a symptom such as inattention that is primarily due to a neurodevelopmental disorder (or full or prodromal psychotic and schizophrenia spectrum disorder) vs. similar symptoms primarily related to trauma- and stressor-related disorders (including dissociation) vs. symptoms that may suggest other psychiatric conditions (including primary anxiety disorder) should be continually considered throughout the assessment. Direct questioning using our standard questionnaire measures may not yield very much if the child is reluctant to disclose. And it is not uncommon for children to underreport their symptoms on a questionnaire, while their observed or reported behavior tells a very different story [19]. Edith Kaplan's Boston Process Approach—which emphasizes the behavioral observations (e.g., error patterns) underlying how an examinee arrived at a particular test score—can be especially helpful in this regard [20]. For example, the child who "times out" of a Block Design due to obsessive checking and rechecking of her work may benefit from quite different interventions provided to the child who playfully assembles houses and walls and never engages with the item at hand. With disorders that impact cognition and concentration, children will develop all manner of compensatory strategies and strong feelings about the tasks we put in front of them. The pattern of an individual's behavioral and emotional shifts, and which tasks do or do not activate them, will be incredibly helpful to us in interpreting the standard scores. Embedded in traumatic stress symptoms is often a sense of "when the other shoe is going to drop" in relationships with adults; and that feeling may drive desperate needs to be "the best" in order to "keep the adult happy" or avoid tasks altogether. The testing of relationships with overly aggressive play or pointed comments described by our colleagues in the preceding chapter (Chapter "Posttraumatic Stress Disorder: From Neurobiology to Cycles of Violence": Van Scoyoc et al.) is a very common scenario when testing children with TSRDs; and professionals need to be prepared to manage them decisively without overreacting. Sometimes the child can be (literally and figuratively) disarmed with a request to see a toy that she/he has just struck you with (and even better when you model a constructive or relational purpose for that same toy), a question about who taught him or her that particular game, or a simple statement about how "we don't hit each other here." For the child who is accustomed to being hit for transgressions, this kind of statement is more than the rote reiteration of a classroom rule; it may be a corrective emotional experience. Of course, emergency precautions need to be taken if a child is in danger of hurting herself or others, but a calm and caring manner, coupled with selective attention to constructive behavior and transparency about the order of events during your evaluation, can have surprising power to redirect and diffuse dysregulated behavior.

Because our assessments can "raise the emotional stakes" for our examinees, it is critical to establish trust and safety—in all cases and especially so in cases of TSRD. "Safety" can be achieved in a variety of ways, ranging from giving the examinee his/her choice of the order of subtest or test administration to letting the child know that she/he is "in the driver's seat" in terms of taking breaks or how much or little to disclose when asked questions about feelings or family. A clinician's leading question or opening remark to a potentially traumatized child is critical to building a sense of trust: *Confirming that a child has permission to engage and disclose (or not engage and disclose) at her pace is crucial.* There are many traces and clues that can guide the attuned and experienced clinician toward this opening question, but there is much to be said for being kind, motivated, and well-intentioned at any level of training. My (JF) personal assessment approach when working with a child with a known or possible history of trauma is part algorithm and part intuition and includes elements of Eriksonian psychosocial stage theory, Piaget's model of cognitive development, the skip logic of structured clinical interviews like the SCID and K-SADS, and the guiding principle of wanting the child in front of me to know, when the time is right, and when she is ready, she can tell someone her story and she will be believed and supported in her grieving.

For example, school-aged children, in the psychosocial phase of industry vs. inferiority, might prefer to start the conversation about their favorite video game, how many levels they have achieved, and when they started noticing when the game started becoming less fun (and did they also notice whether they felt more tired, achy, and hopeless around this time too). Younger children, many of whom are in the phase of "magical thinking," need reassurance that what happened to them is not their fault and compassion when they desperately try to hold onto a positive image of their abuser (yet are experiencing symptoms that directly run counter to that positive belief). Readers will likely not say anything explicitly about a child's metacognitive processes or developmental stage to the child in front of them; but wondering this to oneself will make it easier to maintain one's equilibrium when the child balks at drawing a picture of his "family doing something together" or perseveratively asks if he or she is "doing a good job" with different subtests.

Although data gathering is important during an assessment, providing corrective and even therapeutic feedback for children with a history of trauma is also critical. I (JF) have become very fond of the phrase, "Some kids we see..." to start a discussion about symptoms or problematic behavior without making children feel like they are "under the microscope." It simultaneously lets children know that they are not alone in their experiences while giving them the option of saying that the experience does not apply to them. If trauma is an overwhelming loss of control, we want our assessments to provide the corrective emotional experience of titrated control under safe and structured conditions. Yes, the *primary purpose* of assessment is gathering data, but I feel equally strongly about the therapeutic function of assessment: imparting the idea throughout an assessment that the child can find refuge in the helping relationship now or at some point in the future. I take comfort in the fact that there can be another assessment in this child's life, and if I have done my job well, she will have an easier time participating in that assessment the next time around.

Once we have acquired some data, both objective and observational, several heuristics can guide the assessor in describing a child's underlying profile; I highlight two of the more common ones below:

1. The *dichotomy of "cold" and "hot" executive functioning (EF)*—"cold" EF referring to the tests of sequencing, switching, and behavioral inhibition commonly administered as part of neuropsychological test batteries and "hot" EF referring to our ability to stay focused and organized under emotionally charged conditions [21]. Our field is vastly better at assessing cold than hot executive functioning in a standardized manner, but variability in test performance can be a helpful way to make the differential. Whereas "pure" ADHD without additional negative affect will tend to translate into a baseline level of disinhibition and hyperactivity during the entire battery, it is not uncommon to observe the child struggling with traumatic stress perform well on "cold" tests of cognitive functioning and become disorganized and disinhibited during projective testing or conversation about his or her family (where more "hot" EF is required).
2. Quite specific to the profile of a trauma survivor is the *reenactment of victim-perpetrator-rescuer*. Whether one puts stock in mirror neurons [22] or the psychoanalytic idea of *reverie* [23], our survivor patients and examinees get us to "tune in" to their hypervigilant tests of trust and safety. Mirror neurons often feel more accessible to the scientifically minded practitioner: If the person in front of us appears to be scared, angry, or frowning, mirror neurons will subtly activate those same facial expressions, shoulder tension, and autonomic arousal in us as well. For fleeting moments, we are "sitting in the other person's shoes"—at least neuromuscularly—and this interoceptive input can guide hypotheses about how the person in front of us may be feeling and what triggered those shifts.

Reverie is a more fantastical idea from psychoanalysis that is probably based on similar neuronal mechanisms. Essentially, the attuned therapist is able to play out a daydream or movie in her mind based on what the patient or examinee is saying, and this vivid narrative can provide clues about the examinee's history or emotional state. I believe that I have experienced reverie when a working narrative comes to mind about the examinee's history and the examinee assents to the correctness of it when I introduce it in displacement: "Some kids we see..."

Mirror neurons and reverie are likely at work when we feel unconsciously compelled to punish or rescue the child for their cries for help or dysregulated behavior and perhaps act accordingly out of character. This is what we mean by the *trauma dynamic*. When we feel ourselves pulled into playing out a trauma dynamic [11, 12], we have to "trust our gut" as much as the standard scores and be sensitive to the closely related dynamics of constriction and hyperarousal [12]. Simultaneously, it is critical to realize a child's equally desperate but conflicting wishes to disclose their traumas and keep them secret. Put more simply, children are often terrified of what has happened to them and what may still be happening to them; but they may also have learned or internalized an equally strong fear of what will or might happen to them if they try to escape. One might conceptualize the examiner's victim-perpetrator-rescuer dynamic as being driven, directly or indirectly, by the survivor's constriction/hyperarousal dynamic. These dynamics will naturally override, or at least strongly influence, the survivor's motivation to engage with the assessment process. We may not get all possible data, but the most important gift we can share is to make that possibility "ok" for the examinee.

In the absence of a traumatic history, notwithstanding the unconscionably high rates of maltreatment that many children with developmental disabilities experience, it is highly unlikely that we would feel the same kinds of emotional pulls while evaluating a child with intellectual disability or autism spectrum disorder alone. More often than not, these children's wants, needs, and habits are on the surface: "What you see is what you get." There is no sense of hidden agenda or having stumbled into another's nightmare. Children with autism spectrum disorder will spin the wheels of toy cars near the corners of their eyes whether we are in the room or not. Our attempts at engagement are momentary distractions from their perseverative interests. Higher-functioning autistic children might attempt to engage us in one-sided conversation about the finer points of architecture, *Pokemon*, or *Thomas the Tank Engine*—and it will quickly become clear that it is "their show."

Disclosure Is Rarely Convenient

The "doorknob comment," the archetypal disclosure of a major clinical issue as the patient is leaving the room—presumably in order to unburden him or herself while avoiding having to dwell on it further—creates a dilemma for the caring clinician. Do I act on this information, "strike while the iron is hot," and possibly move the patient to a higher level of consciousness and understanding? Do I make myself complicit in the avoidance, either in the name of "not pushing the patient away" or out of a sense of obligation to the next patient waiting for my services—or colleagues, students, or family waiting for me outside the clinic? What do I do if the disclosure pertains to safety (of if I *suspect* that it pertains to safety) and requires me to act in my role as a mandated reporter?

Neither we nor the child in front of us *want* a long evening in the emergency room, a potentially long and unsatisfying process of filing a report of possible abuse/neglect and anticipating the call to get screened out or an uncomfortable conversation with a guardian who has been accused of harming his/her child. The child wants the pain to stop, broadly defined, and we as therapists want to feel helpful and useful. The dynamics of trauma directly play into a sense of learned helplessness: What's the use of disclosing/intervening if our actions could potentially make the situation worse? Nonetheless, we feel the pang of conscience: Who else could get hurt if I remain silent?

I encourage readers and colleagues to view these exquisitely inconvenient "doorknob comments," especially when they pertain to disclosures of trauma and abuse, as similar to a desperate prisoner tapping morse code through prison walls. Even if there is nothing we can do immediately and in the moment, letting that child know that their message was received can be powerfully therapeutic in itself.

Real-Life Strategies Regarding History Gathering, Assessment, and Treatment

We have hopefully communicated our impression that it is incredibly difficult and probably undesirable, to separate the functions of assessment and therapy when working with a potentially traumatized child. However challenging her behaviors may be, the traumatized child is, at her core, a terrified child, and she needs a corrective emotional experience to begin to feel safe before she can grow, learn, and even begin to comply with the assessment process. For our purposes, safety means a sense of "I can be myself here, and I will not be judged, and no one is going to get hurt—by me or anyone else." When children feel stable and steady, we can better trust their performances on psychometric tests and answers to our questions. We describe practical tips and strategies for maintaining this delicate balance during history gathering, assessment, and therapy below:

History Gathering Tips (LP)

1. All children presenting with any developmental, behavioral, and emotional concerns benefit from treating professionals viewing their history of presenting concerns within an environmental and dynamic context. However, this approach is especially important for children, young adults, and adults with a history of trauma exposure. As available, a *chronologic history should be gathered highlighting periods of significant stress/trauma and transition* (e.g., child entering child protective custody, move to a new/foster/pre-adoptive home, significant trauma/abuse, loss of meaningful adults via death, transition, exposure to potentially re-traumatizing events such as visits with birth family members including siblings with whom they may have a very positive relationship); and correlations between ongoing behavioral observations and other life events should be noted.

2. Gathering additional information about a *child's behavioral "trajectory of change"* within the context of being in a stable or chaotic setting is especially important in providing guidance with respect to treatment and later expectations. For example, "excellent behavior" for a preschool or school-aged child within the first few weeks/months of joining a new family may reflect a "honeymoon period" which may be expected following transition to a new setting—and subsequent increased behavioral challenges as one becomes more comfortable in a new home setting is quite common. In addition, changes in behavior with exposure to birth family members or previous foster parents (whether the relationship/interaction is a positive or negative one) is to be expected.

Assessment Tips (JF)

1. *Heed the "cry for help" in whatever form it takes.* People suffering from traumatic stress symptoms—especially in combination with other mental health conditions—are likely to be experiencing and reporting unusual levels of distress and symptomatology compared to a "typical" child presenting with a simple phobia or adjustment reaction to a recent stressor. These heightened levels might trigger a "validity scale" on a psychometric measure, indicating that a child or caregiver is "exaggerating" or "faking bad." David Tolin and colleagues of the National Center for Posttraumatic Stress Disorder write cogently about how the *F*-scale, also known as the "fake bad" scale, is routinely elevated in the MMPI-2 profiles of combat veterans with PTSD [24]. This phenomenon has come to be understood as a declaration of global distress that needs to be taken seriously. We encourage examiners to consider elevated validity scales on questionnaires (e.g., Trauma Symptom Checklist for Children/Young Children) and computer administered tests of clinical prototype matching like the Millon Inventories in a similar light.
2. Convey a simultaneous *attitude of willingness to listen and respect for reticence.* Many survivors downplay their distress. I (JF) conduct trauma symptom checklists as clinical interviews, expressing interest in any item endorsed, at no matter how low a level. I let examinees know that "they're in the driver's seat" and can tell me "as much or as little as they feel comfortable talking about." I speak in the abstract to normalize survivors' experiences: "Some kids we see sometimes feel like X." My goal is to create a safe environment for survivors to disclose as much or as little as they wish, setting the stage for disclosure as a current or future therapeutic activity.
3. Appreciate that you will need to *shift fluidly between modes of assessment and treatment/stabilization.* Traumatic re-experiencing, whether or not events are actually disclosed, can be highly unmooring and often require grounding techniques from the mindfulness-based school of cognitive-behavioral therapy to restore psychological homeostasis [11, 12, 15]. I do discourage disclosure if I know I do not have enough time to help the examinee return to baseline, opting

instead for psychoeducation about the importance of self-care and "putting memories away" until they can be addressed at a therapeutic pace. Judith Herman established clear guidelines in trauma-focused work for the progression through phases of safety, mourning, and recovery. Ideally, and notwithstanding our earlier guidance about managing "doorknob comments," a survivor should not begin to reprocess traumatic material until she/he has developed some degree of mastery over the emotional reactions that it engenders.

4. When working with *children with co-occurring developmental delays/disabilities and traumatic stress, follow the recommended guidelines of the National Child Traumatic Stress Network* [7]. For example, calibrate expectations for emotional regulation and ability to verbalize past experiences to the child's cognitive-developmental level (rather than chronological age). Lower-functioning children with younger cognitive-developmental presentations will process events more concretely than their typically developing peers and may even apply magical thinking to potentially traumatic events—ascribing unusual levels of power to perpetrators and unfortunate levels of blame to themselves.
5. "*Collaborate, collaborate, collaborate*": Given multiple and competing needs, work with children with co-occurring neurodevelopmental disorders and traumatic stress necessitates thoughtful conversations about transfer of care to subspecialists vs. consulting to local providers vs. true co-management. One should endeavor to cultivate a rich professional support network of psychologists, psychiatrists, developmental-behavioral pediatricians, social workers, and other helping professions as collaborators and co-managers.

Treatment Tips

1. Especially if treatment needs are complex—we suggest that it is important to *prioritize treatment needs* for each child/adolescent with family/caretakers. Addressing overwhelming anxiety and/or safety concerns is critical to support any child's improved connections with caretakers and to allow him or her to be available for both emotional and academic learning. We have found that addressing anxiety and safety concerns in all settings (home, school, extracurricular activities) is critical prior to being able to address learning or attentional concerns. It is worth noting that children may not feel comfortable describing their emotional distress in the school setting; but this does not mean that they feel comfortable and are available to learn in that setting. The core treatment goals for any traumatized child are distress tolerance, grounding, and self-care. Offering hope and normalizing a child's experience are the key ingredients to gaining the child's assent to this undertaking [25].
2. Diagnostic and treatment decisions for children shortly after experiencing a significant trauma or joining a new family can be viewed as "current profile" and "current (Band-Aid?) treatment"—with an expectation that treatment will continue to be modified over time. Consider each assessment as "one snapshot in

time"—appreciating that years may pass before a child's full potential is realized. For example, initial treatment of symptoms of inattention and anxiety from a behavioral and/or pharmacologic perspective may be warranted following trauma exposure. But acute treatment to achieve improved regulation may not indicate a need for long-term treatment of these symptoms. Ongoing monitoring is required to determine evolving long-term treatment needs.

3. Although children with a history of trauma may benefit from working with an experienced clinician with an array of skills including trauma-informed cognitive-behavioral therapy, mindfulness, executive function coaching and family therapy, and an understanding of the development of healthy attachment relationships and identity development—this is a very long and perhaps unattainable wish list for any single provider. Collaboration and co-management are essential. We have found *that prioritizing treatment needs based on a child/family's greatest area of need and considering local resources* is an important place to start.

We want to stress, in closing, that one need not be an expert in trauma-focused assessment and therapy to be able to comfort and appropriately triage a traumatized child. We hope that familiarity with common themes and dynamics as described above will help the clinician to steer clear from the pitfalls of "symptom chasing" that can delay time to a desired outcome. More important than gathering every ounce of data is creating a safe space for a child to unburden oneself of haunting memories or the somatic experience of relived terror—now or in the future. This need is especially true for our vulnerable patients with neurodevelopmental disabilities and their caregivers, who may themselves be battling with their own traumas, stresses, and health conditions.

References

1. Seidman L. Listening, meaning, and empathy in neuropsychological disorders: case examples of assessment and treatment. In: Ellison JM, Weinstein CS, Hodel-Malinofsky T, editors. The psychotherapist's guide to neuropsychiatry. Washington, DC: American Psychiatric Press; 1994. p. 1–22.
2. Center on the Developing Child at Harvard University. Key concepts; brain architecture. http://developingchild.harvard.edu/science/key-concepts/brain-architecture/.
3. Felitti VJ, Anda RF, Nordenberg D, Williamson DF, Spitz AM, Edwards V, Koss MP, Marks JS. Relationship of childhood abuse and household dysfunction to many of the leading causes of death in adults: the Adverse Childhood Experiences (ACE) Study. Am J Prev Med. 1998;14(4):245–58. https://doi.org/10.1016/S0749-3797(98)00017-8.
4. Goldson E. Maltreatment among children with disabilities. In 14th international congress on child abuse and neglect. Denver, Colorado; 2002.
5. Sullivan PM, Knutson JF. The association between child maltreatment and disabilities in a hospital-based epidemiological study. Child Abuse Negl. 1998;22:271–88.
6. Mayo D, Corey S, Kelly LH, Yohannes S, Youngquist AL, Stuart BK, Niendam TA, Loewy RL. The role of trauma and stressful life events among individuals at clinical high risk for psychosis: a review. Front Psychiatry. 2017;8:55. https://doi.org/10.3389/fpsyt.2017.00055.

7. National Child Traumatic Stress Network Adapted Trauma Treatment Standards Work Group (Subgroup on Developmental Disabilities). Facts on traumatic stress and children with developmental disabilities. 2004. http://www.nctsn.org/sites/default/files/assets/pdfs/traumatic_stress_developmental_disabilities_final.pdf.
8. Weisz JR, Chorpita BF, Palinkas LA, Schoenwald SK, Miranda J, Bearman SK, et al. Testing standard and modular designs for psychotherapy treating depression, anxiety, and conduct problems in youth: a randomized effectiveness trial. Arch Gen Psychiatry. 2012;69(3):274–82.
9. Chorpita BF, Weisz JR, Daleiden EL, Schoenwald SK, Palinkas LA, Miranda J, et al. Long-term outcomes for the Child STEPs randomized effectiveness trial: a comparison of modular and standard treatment designs with usual care. J Consult Clin Psychol. 2013;81(6):999–1009.
10. Sanders MR. Triple P-Positive Parenting Program: towards an empirically validated multilevel parenting and family support strategy for the prevention of behavior and emotional problems in children. Clin Child Fam Psychol Rev. 1999;2(2):71–90.
11. Chu JA. Rebuilding shattered lives: responsible treatment of complex post-traumatic and dissociative disorders. New York: Wiley; 1998.
12. Herman JL. Trauma and recovery: the aftermath of violence—from domestic abuse to political terror. New York: Basic Books; 1992.
13. Terr LC. Childhood traumas: an outline and overview. Am J Psychiatry. 1991;148:10–20. https://doi.org/10.1176/ajp.148.1.10.
14. McMackin RA, Keane TM, Kline PM, editors. Understanding the impact of clergy sexual abuse: betrayal and recovery. London: Routledge, a division of Taylor & Francis; 2009.
15. Saxe GN, Ellis BH, Kaplow JB. Collaborative treatment of traumatized children and teens: the trauma systems therapy approach. 1st ed. New York: Guilford Press; 2007.
16. MacDonald HZ, Franz MR, Vasterling JJ. Assessment and treatment of neuropsychological deficits in posttraumatic stress disorder. In: McMackin RA, Newman E, Fogler JM, Keane TA, editors. Trauma therapy in context: the science and craft of evidence-based practice. Washington, DC: American Psychiatric Press; 2012. p. 331–52.
17. National Child Traumatic Stress Network. Measures review database. http://www.nctsnet.org/resources/online-research/measures-review.
18. National Center for PTSD. Child measures of trauma and PTSD. https://www.ptsd.va.gov/professional/assessment/child/index.asp.
19. Newman E, Briere J, Kirlic N. Clinical assessment as a form of listening and intervention. In: McMackin RA, Newman E, Fogler JM, Keane TA, editors. Trauma therapy in context: the science and craft of evidence-based practice. Washington, DC: American Psychiatric Press; 2012.
20. Ashendorf L, Swenson R, Libon DJ. The Boston process approach to neuropsychological assessment: a practitioner's guide. New York: Oxford University Press; 2013.
21. Anderson V, Anderson PJ, Jacobs R, Smith MS. Development and assessment of executive function: from preschool to adolescence. In: Anderson V, Jacobs R, Anderson PJ, editors. Executive functions and the frontal lobes: a lifespan perspective. Philadelphia, PA: Taylor & Francis; 2008. p. 123–54.
22. Gallese V, Eagle MN, Migone P. Intentional attunement: mirror neurons and the neural underpinnings of interpersonal relations. J Am Psychoanal Assoc. 2007;55(1):131.
23. Ogden T. Reverie and metaphor. Some thoughts on how I work as a psychoanalyst. Int J Psychoanal. 1997;78(4):719–32.
24. Tolin DF, Maltby N, Weathers FW, Litz BT, Knight J, Keane TM. The use of the MMPI-2 infrequency–psychopathology scale in the assessment of posttraumatic stress disorder in male veterans. J Psychopathol Behav Assess. 2004;26(1):23–9.
25. Yohani SC, Larsen DJ. The cultivation of hope in trauma-focused counseling. In: McMackin RA, Newman E, Fogler JM, Keane TA, editors. Trauma therapy in context: the science and craft of evidence-based practice. Washington, DC: American Psychiatric Press; 2012.

Chapter 5
The Challenge and Importance of Differentiating Trauma and Stress-Related Disorders from Autism Spectrum Disorders

Amanda Van Scoyoc, Melissa B. Marquardt, and Randall A. Phelps

Vignette

History: Jayden is a 4-year 7-month-old boy, brought in by his mother for comprehensive diagnostic assessment. Mom's primary concerns are that Jayden doesn't "mind" her, i.e., that he is consistently defiant. Mom notes that Jayden's first response to her is "always" to be negative and that their relationship is "constantly" adversarial: "He says 'no' even when he does mean yes." When asked what Jayden likes to do, mom replies, "being a pain in my butt."

Mom reports that she is never able to just relax and enjoy being with Jayden. He says the same thing over and over, for example, constantly asking to go to the park to play or wanting to watch the same videos over and over. He sits on his bed and rocks his body back and forth, often for hours before falling asleep at night. Jayden resists cuddling with her and seems to avoid eye

A. Van Scoyoc (✉)
University of Oregon, Eugene, OR, USA

Oregon Health and Sciences University, Portland, OR, USA

Yale School of Medicine, Yale Child Study Center, New Haven, CT, USA
e-mail: Amanda.vanscoyoc@yale.edu

M. B. Marquardt
University of Oregon, Eugene, OR, USA

Oregon Health and Sciences University, Portland, OR, USA

Department of Psychiatry, University of New Mexico, Health Sciences Center, Albuquerque, NM, USA
e-mail: mbmarquardt@salud.unm.edu

R. A. Phelps
Oregon Health & Sciences University, Eugene, OR, USA
e-mail: phelpsr@ohsu.edu

J. M. Fogler, R. A. Phelps (eds.), *Trauma, Autism, and Neurodevelopmental Disorders*, https://doi.org/10.1007/978-3-030-00503-0_5

contact. He often fails to respond to her, "almost like he's deaf," yet is hypersensitive to sound. Loud, unpredictable noises provoke agitation and sometimes even rage and aggression. He hits his mother when he hears a loud noise, even if it came from a neighboring apartment or from outside, and there was no way that she could have been responsible for making the sound.

Mom also reports that Jayden frequently "lies" sometimes to avoid punishment, but sometimes for no purpose at all, even when it is obvious that he is lying. Mom gives the example of refusing to use the bathroom even when it is obvious that he needs to, and then continuing to deny that he had an accident after urinating and defecating in his pants. It especially distresses her when Jayden puts his hands in his pants and smears feces around the house.

In contrast with Jayden's behavior toward her, Mom reports that Jayden is overly friendly with strangers, striking up conversations and sharing personal details with random people in stores. She reports being concerned that he will "walk off with strangers." Jayden attends preschool. He participates in structured activities and is very eager for the attention of his teachers. However, he either ignores his classmates or tries to control their play.

Social History: Based on an interview with Jayden's mother and on a review of records provided by Child Protective Services, social history is significant for the fact that mother drank alcohol throughout the pregnancy and then continued to drink daily, to excess, for the first 3 years of Jayden's life. During this time, she had several partners, one of whom raped Jayden. Multiple calls from teachers and neighbors over the first 3 years of Jayden's life led to the involvement of Child Protective Services.

Jayden was removed from mother's custody at age 3 and placed in nonrelative foster care. In his first foster placement, where there were seven other foster children, Jayden frequently raged, smeared feces, and repeatedly physically attacked an infant also in foster care in the home. It was noted that these behaviors were exacerbated following weekly supervised visits with mom. Due to these behaviors, he was removed from this first placement and placed in a second home after just 2 months. Weekly visits with mom continued. Similar behaviors ensued in the second home, in which there were three other high-need foster children. He was removed from this home after 3 months. Next, he was placed in a "therapeutic" foster home, with just one other foster child, a teenage girl with cerebral palsy. He continued to have regular supervised visits with mom. He remained in this home for 10 months, where his behavior stabilized somewhat, until he was reunited with his mother, 13 months after his removal from her custody. At this point, mom now has had physical custody for 6 months, though Child Welfare retains legal custody, thus retaining the right to make decisions impacting Jayden's welfare.

Mom's Diagnostic Concerns: Mom wonders whether Jayden might have "fetal alcohol syndrome," acknowledging that she drank heavily throughout the pregnancy. She wonders if this might account for his challenging and bizarre behaviors. Mom also offers that Jayden may have post-traumatic stress disorder, acknowledging that Jayden was raped and generally exposed to abuse, neglect, and domestic violence. However, mom reports that she most suspects that Jayden has autism. She thinks he has autism because of his poor eye contact, the way he ignores her, that he is sensitive to loud sounds, that he rocks his body, and because he doesn't get along well with his peers. Mom reports that Jayden's pediatrician, his preschool teachers, and the caseworker through Child Protective Services have all suggested that Jayden might have autism. She notes that Jayden's cousin is just like Jayden, and he has been diagnosed with autism. Also, a neighbor is very similar to Jayden and also has autism. Both of these other children have greatly benefitted from the autism diagnosis. They have accessed more help at school, applied behavior analysis therapy at home, respite and personal support worker hours through the county office of developmental disabilities services, and supplemental income through Social Security.

Observations and Formal Assessments: At the start of the visit, Jayden turns to the examiner, makes good eye contact, smiles, and spontaneously starts a conversation about the toy barn in the room. He brings toy animals to the examiner and makes animal noises. During the interview, Jayden plays contentedly and appropriately with various toys, often engaging the examiner in play. During the examination, Jayden pretends to examine the examiner with stethoscope, otoscope, etc. He hits the examiner a little too hard with the reflex hammer and pronounces with a sly smile that the examiner is "very sick, very sick."

On formal assessments by an interdisciplinary team, including developmental-behavioral pediatrician, psychologist, speech language pathologist, and occupational therapist, it is found that cognitive skills, language, and motor skills are average. Structured observations, on the Autism Diagnostic Observation Schedule, are not consistent with autism spectrum disorders. Structured interview of autism symptoms, based on the DSM-5, is equivocal, given mom's description of such concerns, for example, "poor eye contact, the way he ignores her, that he is sensitive to loud sounds, that he rocks his body, and because he doesn't get along well with his peers." Adaptive skills, per mom's report, are impaired. Jayden has normal growth, weight, head circumference, and non-dysmorphic facial features.

Diagnostic Formulation: Jayden's presentation does not meet criteria for a diagnosis of autism spectrum disorder, although it is understandable that his constellation of symptoms including social difficulties and repetitive behaviors has led his mom and others to contemplate this diagnosis. Prenatal alcohol exposure is acknowledged, and behavioral challenges might be attributable, at least in part, to this prenatal exposure. Past medical history, review of systems, and examination do not indicate any of the birth defects that may be associated with FASD, but these findings are not always present even with clinically significant prenatal alcohol exposure.

Post-traumatic stress disorder is in the differential diagnosis given Jayden's history of potentially traumatic events, hypersensitivity, and severe associated agitation to loud sounds and self-soothing behaviors. After thorough evaluation, our team determined that the most appropriate diagnosis was a trauma- and stressor-related disorder, more specifically disinhibited social engagement disorder. This diagnosis fits the available data given Jayden's history of inconsistent and unavailable caregivers and his tendency toward indiscriminately friendly behavior with strangers. Beyond the symptoms that characterize disinhibited social engagement disorder, Jayden's presentation more broadly suggests the impact of his experiences of abuse and social neglect during early childhood. For example, many children who experience abuse and neglect in early childhood struggle with toileting, self-soothe through repetitive behaviors, engage in oppositional behaviors, and have impoverished relationships with their primary caregiver. The constellation of Jayden's difficulties can best be understood by considering the impact of early inconsistent caregiving on Jayden's ability to understand reciprocal social interactions, as well as Jayden's ability to learn how to self-regulate his emotions.

Giving Feedback: In an attempt at a strength-based and compassionate approach to feedback, the team member giving the feedback starts with the good news that Jayden's presentation is not really suggestive of fetal alcohol spectrum disorder. Next, the "good news" is given that Jayden doesn't have ASD, either. Before the clinician can go on, to explain the diagnosis of disinhibited social engagement disorder and the rule-out diagnosis of post-traumatic stress disorder, mom explodes, "You're telling me my kid is normal! You're not listening to me! I'm telling you, this kid is severely disabled! This kid is not normal!" The clinician explains to the mom that not having fetal alcohol spectrum disorder or autism does not mean that the clinician or team are being dismissive of mom's concerns or suggesting that there are no problems with Jayden's behavior, merely that the source of the behavior problems does not seem to be either fetal alcohol exposure or autism. Mom calms slightly, enough to inquire what the recommendations are.

The clinician suggests that before giving the recommendations for treatment, it would be helpful for mom to understand the diagnosis. Mom again flies into a rage, takes out her cell phone, calls her boyfriend, and stalks into the hall, where she can be overheard, saying, "They won't help me! They won't tell me how to treat Jayden!" Again, the clinician helps mom to calm down and explains the diagnosis of disinhibited social engagement disorder. Mom asks how it is treated. The clinician recommends placement in a therapeutic preschool program, which includes family therapy and intensive parent education programming. Mom leaves in a huff, clearly unconvinced and dissatisfied.

Epilogue: The team contacts the child welfare caseworker, who expresses disappointment in the diagnosis of disinhibited social engagement disorder, noting that she had hoped to access respite supports through the Developmental Disability system and applied behavior analysis through the mental health system for the family with the help of an autism diagnosis. The team contacts the preschool teacher, who also expresses disappointment with the diagnosis noting that "more services" would be available with an autism diagnosis. The pediatrician refers Jayden to a neurologist, to work up the lack of response to mom, questioning absence seizures. Jayden was very agitated in the neurologist's office; he hid under the table, rocked, and screamed throughout the neurologist's consultation. The neurologist confers a diagnosis autism, further confusing mom. However, we were able to work with the child welfare caseworker and public health nurse to arrange referral to a therapeutic preschool for children who have experienced abuse/neglect and to arrange for enrollment of Jayden and mom in family therapy through that program.

Differential Diagnosis of Autism Spectrum Disorders and Trauma- and Stressor-Related Disorders

As Jayden's case study demonstrates, children who have experienced early environmental stress and trauma often have a complex array of difficulties across many domains of functioning. These difficulties often seemingly map onto the broad categories of symptoms that are diagnostic of autism spectrum disorders (ASD) including the areas of social communication/social interaction and repetitive patterns of behavior. This overlap in the broad areas of functioning can lead to confusion and even misdiagnosis. Children with ASD and children with trauma- and stressor-related disorders (TSRDs) tend to exhibit difficulties interpreting and responding to social cues, communicating effectively, and regulating their emotional state. In addition, both children who are diagnosed on the autism spectrum and children who have experienced stress and trauma often have difficulties with repetitive behaviors, eating, sleeping, and gastrointestinal functioning.

Although there is an overlap in these broad areas of functioning that are impacted by ASD and TSRD, specific symptoms differ. For example, although both children with ASD and TSRDs have difficulties with social interactions, these difficulties are notably different. For children with ASD, difficulties with social interactions often include a lack of normal reciprocal interactions, reduced nonverbal communication including eye contact and gestures, and a general lack of peer relationships. In contrast, children with trauma and stressor-related disorders can have quite varied presentations in terms of social interactions. For example, children who have such TSRDs as reactive attachment disorder (RAD) and disinhibited social engagement disorder (DSED) often have impoverished or explosive interactions with their primary caregiver. They may have difficulties with social interactions due to social distancing, social disinhibition, and diminished positive affect. While they may demonstrate these impoverished interactions with their primary caregiver or other close adults, they may also intermittently demonstrate more reciprocal and typical (if overly familiar) social interactions with relative strangers or acquaintances. Additionally, the core features of ASD, including having difficulty expressing oneself through gestures or understanding others' intentions during reciprocal interactions (i.e., "theory of mind" deficits), are not generally considered symptoms of these TSRDs.

Given this overlap in symptomatology, the *Diagnostic and Statistical Manual*, 5th Edition (DSM-5), acknowledges the importance of differentiating TSRDs and ASD. For example, in the differential diagnosis section on RAD, it is identified that, "Aberrant social behaviors manifest in young children with reactive attachment disorder, but they also are key features of autism spectrum disorder. Specifically, young children with either condition can manifest dampened expression of positive emotions, cognitive and language delays, and impairments in social reciprocity" [1].

Despite acknowledgement of difficulties in differential diagnosis, currently very little research has considered this similarity of symptoms for children with ASD and TSRD. One study identified that children with RAD and children with ASD who have normative intellectual abilities often have similarly impoverished aspects of pragmatic language skills. Sixty percent of children in the sample who had RAD had clinically significant language problems, and 20% exhibited clinically significant difficulties with repetitive movement, when evaluated using the Autism Diagnostic Interview-Revised [2]. This study suggests that some children with RAD have language and behavioral difficulties that are similar to children with ASD or meet diagnostic criteria for specific symptoms of ASD. Notably, this research identifies symptoms in children with RAD that may lead to diagnostic confusion, as repetitive movement as well as language problems map onto a diagnosis of ASD and are not diagnostic of RAD.

There is evidence from the research literature that children who have severe attachment problems, related to early experiences of prolonged neglect, can manifest with *autism-like* symptoms. In particular, studies with children who were adopted from Romanian orphanages in the 1990s are well-suited to the examination of the effects of severe neglect. Children who spent their first few years of life in Romanian orphanages were deprived of normative caregiving experiences. Rather than living with a family, their care was institutionalized. In this setting, caregivers prioritized meeting children's physical needs by providing them with a crib, food, toileting needs, etc. However, children's need for safe, stable, and responsive caregiving was generally not met. In these institutionalized settings, infants' bids for attention were often left unattended. Rather than being held, talked to, and fed by caregivers, infants spent their days isolated in a crib, often automatically fed through propped bottles. Thus, these children most often had very limited experiences engaging in reciprocal and rewarding interactions with their caregivers.

Research with children who have this background of severe neglect indicates that many of these children have persistent difficulties resulting from these early-life experiences. Sir Michael Rutter et al. [3] identified that for children who were adopted from Romanian orphanages by families in the UK, a subset of this population exhibited symptoms of autism. Specifically, 6% of these children, when assessed at the ages of 4 and 6, had overall patterns of behavior that looked like autism, and an additional 6% had features of autism including stereotyped repetitive movements and difficulties in understanding social boundaries. Rutter et al. refer to these children's repertoire of autism-like behaviors as "quasi-autistic patterns" noting that although these children exhibit symptoms that look similar to ASD, there are key differences. First, in comparison with ASD, which is generally accepted to be a neurodevelopmental disorder present at birth, these quasi-autistic patterns were related to early experiences of deprivation. In their sample, children who exhibited quasi-autistic patterns of behaviors had experienced a longer duration of neglect within an orphanage setting. There were other notable differences between children with these quasi-autistic patterns and children with ASD. Whereas boys are more likely than girls to be diagnosed with ASD, there was no difference in gender prevalence for children with autism-like symptoms resulting from early neglect. In addition, at the age of 6, children with quasi-autistic patterns had greater improvement in ASD-like symptoms, demonstrating differences in long-term outcomes for children with ASD and children with trauma-related symptoms that parallel ASD. In another study of school-aged children who were adopted from Romanian orphanages (Mean Age = 8 years), one third exhibited stereotypic behaviors as well as communication and language disorders common to ASD. In addition, 16% of the sample met criteria for ASD, with boys and girls being equally likely to meet criteria [4].

Given this overlap in symptoms, as well as current difficulties in differential diagnosis between attachment problems and ASD, Dr. Heather Moran has created a clinical tool to help clarify differences in the clinical presentations of high-functioning children with ASD and children with significant attachment problems [5]. The tool was developed after noticing difficulties in differential diagnosis for children with significant trauma histories and caregiver instability and for children with ASD as both groups of children had difficulties with "social use of language, emotional regulation, social skills and repetitive and routinized behaviors."

This tool, called the Coventry Grid, identifies eight key symptoms of ASD and describes shared aspects of these symptoms for children with both ASD and attachment problems, while also describing the typical presentation of these symptoms for ASD and the typical presentation for children with attachment problems. For example, both children with ASD and children with attachment problems can have sensory integration problems and, in particular, can have difficulty integrating information about physical cues. The Coventry Grid notes that this difficulty is shared with the two diagnoses, but then provides a description of differences in typical presentation. Specifically, children with ASD often are either notably overly or under-sensitive to some stimuli and may have difficulty communicating what is causing them distress. In contrast, children with attachment difficulties typically have a strong reaction to discomfort and may become angry or blame the caregiver. The Coventry Grid provides a starting place for clinical conversations and research around difficulties in diagnosis; however currently it is developed based upon clinical impressions rather than data-driven research.

There is a strong need for clinical diagnostic tools to better differentiate these two diagnoses. Without these tools, differential diagnosis is perhaps too strongly impacted by clinician interpretation of symptomology and too likely to be impacted by knowledge of children's early experiences of adversity. Many clinicians, who are frequently differentially assessing ASD in comparison with attachment disorders, have likely developed differential diagnosis grids in their own minds to help with diagnoses, identifying which behaviors lend evidence to attachment disorders and which behaviors lend evidence to ASD. Greater consideration of the challenges of differential diagnosis and development of assessment tools will help to align diagnostic efforts and enable more children to access treatments that are well-matched to their clinical needs.

A Neurobiological Basis of Impairment for Trauma- and Stressor-Related Disorders

When considering why TSRD may manifest with symptoms that in some ways parallel ASD, it is important to consider the neurobiological basis of impairment for these two diagnoses. Numerous researchers have identified that the failure to have expected caregiving experiences, the basis of TSRDs, undermines normative human development. For example, considering children who spent their first years in orphanages, their need for comfort, initially demonstrated through infant crying, is oftentimes ignored. In addition to the large evidence base supporting the psychological sequelae of these critical events, there is increasing evidence of a *neurological* basis of impairment related to negative early-life experiences.

Shonkoff et al. writing on "toxic stress" considers the ways in which early experiences impact long-term health outcomes [6]. "Toxic stress" refers to the frequent and lasting activation of the body's stress-response system in childhood. Their work suggests that experiences within the first few years of life, including early caregiving experiences, have a lasting impact on brain development. Whereas supportive caregiving sets the stage for emotional regulation and optimal learning under calm conditions, frequent and prolonged stress responses can lead to changes in the brain during the sensitive developmental period of early childhood, impacting trajectories for both poor physical health and mental health throughout the lifespan [7]. For children who have supportive caregivers, the caregiver's response to children's need for comfort alleviates the negative impact of activating this stress-response system, by helping the child learn to calm himself/herself. However, children who have caregivers who either inconsistently meet their needs or who are unavailable or abusive do not experience the same support to learn how to calm themselves and thereby become vulnerable to a host of poor health and psychosocial outcomes. As Dr. Anne Masten describes in an article about human resilience, "The great threats to human development are those that jeopardize the systems underlying these adaptive processes, including brain development and cognition, caregiver-child relationships, regulation of emotion and behavior, and motivation for learning and engaging in the environment" [8].

Children who do not experience nurturing caregiver-child interactions during their first years of life are at risk for a host of negative outcomes, as their development is altered by absence of expected caregiving. Increasingly, research indicates that reciprocal and responsive caregiving experiences are a key ingredient for typical development.

Children who experience social neglect and other forms of adversity in early childhood are at increased risk for affective disorders (anxiety, depression), substance abuse, increased stress, and poor health (e.g., severe obesity, sleep problems). The widespread impact on different aspects of health and mental health suggests an effect on underlying body regulatory systems, with researchers hypothesizing that a neurobiological impact on the developing brain during early childhood underlies the widespread negative outcomes [9].

Although research on the neurobiology underlying trajectories of health and mental health is still gaining momentum, this accumulation of evidence thus far suggests that early stressful experiences that deviate from expected infant-caregiver relationships can have a lasting impact on neurobiology, underlying persistent impairments in health and mental health. In this way, early adversity and prolonged trauma-related diagnoses can be conceptualized as being related to alterations in early brain development, leading to difficulties that can be similar to ASD—a diagnosis that is neurodevelopmental in nature. Future research may reveal that the overlap in TSRD and ASD symptoms may stem from a common disruption or defect in underlying brain architecture and/or function—one that is presumably inherited or activated in the case of ASD and acquired in the case of TSRD.

The Increased Prevalence of ASD

Until advances in our technology permit us to diagnose neurodevelopmental and psychiatric disorders with a "blood test" in the way we do for common medical conditions, we are limited in our ability to diagnose beyond what we see and learn through clinical interview and data from psychometric tests. It is therefore especially challenging to discuss diagnoses of ASD and particularly to discuss differential diagnosis with TSRD or any other condition, without acknowledging the increased prevalence of ASD. In March of 2014, the CDC identified that 1 in 68 American Children were diagnosed as having an autism spectrum disorder. This marks more than tenfold increase in the diagnosis of ASD in the last 40 years. In California since the early 1990s, the prevalence of ASD in children aged 3–6 years has increased drastically, shifting from approximately 17.5 in 10,000 to 43.5 in a thousand [10]. Families, researchers, and clinicians alike are discussing what may be contributing to this increase in prevalence. While many factors have been posited such as environmental toxins and the increasing age of parents, some factors that stand out in the literature include changes in the diagnostic criteria of ASD itself; changes in diagnostic standards, practice, and procedure; greater public and pediatric knowledge of the symptoms of ASD; and diagnostic substitution, the renaming of clinical phenomena under new names based on new research findings or popular trends [10–12].

Chakrabarti and Fombonne [11] propose that changes in both how ASD is diagnosed and its core diagnostic criteria account for much of the increase in prevalence. An ASD diagnosis is conferred based on interpreting behavioral signs of the disorder and is thusly a *qualitative* decision based largely on observation and interviewing. Symptoms of ASD have widened in breadth. In fact, this is clearly demonstrated in the switch in terminology in the DSM-5 to "autism spectrum disorder" rather than the previously used terms of autistic disorder, Asperger's disorder, or the especially problematic Pervasive Developmental Disorder-Not Otherwise Specified (PDD-NOS). Research supports a conceptualization of ASD in which symptoms fluctuate in intensity and severity along a continuum over the course of the lifespan rather than clustering into discrete categories, making the "autism spectrum" diagnosis seem more appropriate and empirically grounded than the subcategories that preceded it. However, when we consider the characteristic symptoms along a spectrum, we may also be more likely to include and label typical variation in symptoms as clinically relevant. In support of this proposed explanation, Chakrabarti and Fombonne identified that when using the same diagnostic criteria that were used 15 years ago to identify the presence of pervasive developmental disorders in a sample of individuals in the UK, they find a similar incidence as to those reported 15 years ago.

It is also possible that social influence or diffusion of information is responsible for contributing to this increased prevalence. Living within close proximity to children with ASD increases the likelihood of a diagnosis of ASD [10]. Parents are more aware of ASD and what potential symptoms look like. For example, spending time with other children diagnosed with ASD or speaking to parents who have children with an ASD can make individuals more aware and knowledgeable of potential symptoms and can provide information on how to access clinicians who may be able to provide assistance through diagnosis or providing services. Thus, it is possible that an increase in prevalence is in part due to parents identifying symptoms that previously may not have seemed concerning or contact physicians with specific questions regarding an ASD diagnosis [13]. In the case of Jayden, other care providers and preschool teachers suggested to his mother that he may have ASD. Additionally, his mother compared his behavior to his cousin and a neighbor, both of whom have existing diagnoses of ASD. In this case, it appears that this social influence contributed to Jayden's mother specifically *seeking* a diagnosis of ASD.

In addition to the knowledge of ASD and related symptoms being more dispersed to parents, there has also been an increase in professional education on ASD in both early childhood and pediatric settings which result in more referrals and diagnosis. For example, the American Academy of Pediatrics' policy on early identification and referral calls for developmental screening at 9, 18, and 20 or 24 months. Additionally, ASD-specific screening is recommended at 18 and 24 months [14].

An additional factor contributing to the increased number of children diagnosed with ASD may be that that populations of children with disabilities may have been previously diagnosed under a different category [15]. The increase in ASD as a diagnosis is also associated with a decline in diagnoses of intellectual disability and other developmental disabilities. Previously, these conditions were considered rare for children and clearly identified as discrete categories. However, currently, as several childhood disorders have expanded their criteria (such as ASD), the number of children being diagnosed with intellectual disability has decreased, and there is more overlap between existing disorders than ever before. ASD, for example, now includes an added descriptor for "with/without cognitive impairment," thus increasing its overlap with intellectual disability [1]. With greater appreciation of the overlap and co-occurrence of psychiatric and neurodevelopmental disorders, children today are less likely to fall into discrete diagnostic categories.

Challenges for Assessing Trauma- and Stressor-Related Disorders

Diagnosing TSRD is complicated both by the nature of the diagnoses and by the lack of assessment tools related to these diagnoses. Currently there is not a gold standard assessment protocol for identifying problems related to early environmental stress including reactive attachment disorder and disinhibited social engagement disorder. Without validated and widely used tools for assessing these diagnoses, clinicians' assessments and recommendations for treatment are often inconsistent.

The first challenge in assessing TSRD is identifying that a child has had the types of experience in early childhood that underlie these diagnoses. For a child to be diagnosed with reactive attachment disorder or disinhibited social engagement disorder, the clinician first must identify that the child experienced impoverished early caregiving such that they were not able to develop a selective attachment. Although this criterion may be easily established for some children (e.g., children reared in an institutional setting, children with a documented history of early maltreatment), for children who do not have a documented history, it can be difficult to ascertain this information.

Caregivers may be reluctant to discuss their own difficulties providing adequate care for their children. For example, caregivers often struggle to provide consistent and sensitive caregiving when they have mental health issues including substance addiction or postpartum depression. For caregivers, recounting difficulties providing adequate care for infants and young children can be shameful, embarrassing, and distressing. These conversations inherently suggest that the caregiver plays a strong role in the etiology of the diagnosis. Despite clinicians' best efforts to remain positive and supportive of both the caregiver and the child, this conversation can lead caregivers to feel attacked and blamed. Additionally, in some instances, caregivers may also not want to discuss this information due to concerns about child welfare involvement.

An additional challenge is that often by the time the caretaker is seeking an assessment for their child, they may already have strong beliefs about the etiology of their child's difficulties. In some instances, pediatricians, daycare providers, other professionals, and even friends may have suggested the possibility of a neurodevelopmental etiology of the child's behavior. Parents, who expect that their child may be on the autism spectrum, may not have considered the possibility of early environmental trauma as the etiology of the child's behavior. Thus, discussing this pertinent history can seem to some parents to be unrelated to their reason for referral.

As we saw in the case of Jayden, although his mother was willing to openly discuss Jayden's history of prenatal substance exposure, abuse, and being reared while she struggled with addiction, she entered the clinic with a strong belief about Jayden's symptoms being rooted in autism. This belief had been clearly shaped by conversations with other individuals who interacted with Jayden. His pediatrician, preschool teacher, and child welfare caseworker all had brought up this possibility, lending credibility to this possible diagnosis. As is often the case, by the time Mom brought Jayden in for an assessment, she already had a clear explanation in her mind for Jayden's behaviors. This explanation balances acknowledgment of her struggle during his early childhood while also relieving some of the burden for being responsible for his current symptoms.

Once a history of early environmental stress is established, there are further challenges in diagnosing TSRDs. As O'Connor and Zeanah identified in their 2003 comprehensive article on the state of assessment and treatment approaches for attachment disorders, there are no existing observational protocols designed to assess attachment disorders, including reactive attachment disorder and disinhibited social engagement disorder [16]. The Strange Situation [17] is a widely used assessment tool, particularly in research studies, for identifying the *quality* of attachment between a child and caregiver, not specific diagnoses. Given its utility in diagnosing disturbances of attachment, it may be assumed to help with diagnosis of a TSRD. However, as O'Connor and Zeanah note, this tool specifically considers attachment behaviors within relationships in which there is an existing and selective attachment. It was not designed to identify instances in which a selective attachment is in question. Furthermore, research has demonstrated that children can exhibit both disinhibited behavior with strangers alongside more normative and detached behaviors with their primary caregiver. This combination of behaviors complicates the use of the Strange Situation as an assessment tool because this tool is primarily focused on identifying reactions to the primary caregiver and may miss significant aspects of the child engaging with a stranger.

There are also drawbacks to using a questionnaire-based assessment. First off, parents may not understand the questions asked, and it may be difficult to identify, based on questionnaires, when a behavior is clinically significant. For example, the

Early Childhood Inventory-4 is a questionnaire that measures the behavioral symptoms of DSM-IV diagnoses relevant to preschool-aged children including diagnostic symptoms of attachment disorders. The specific symptoms for attachment disorders include asking a parent if their child "seeks affection from people, even strangers," and is "afraid, distrustful with people" [18]. Given the normal range of child introversion and extroversion, it is easy to imagine that many parents would highly endorse these types of questions for children whose behavior is not problematic. Thus, the nuances of social interactions may be difficult to identify through these types of child behavioral checklists. It is also possible that some caregivers might not know if certain behaviors are present or how their children respond in certain situations. In this event there is the risk that parents may choose to record responses that are more socially desirable.

Semi-structured interviews hold promise for identifying whether children have disinhibited and inhibited behaviors across situations and across time. In addition, a semi-structured interview is often necessary to understand children's early-life history of insufficient care for diagnosis. However, currently there are no widely used interviews for assessing these difficulties. Research on interview procedures suggest that interviews have a tendency to overdiagnose RAD [19]. This may be in part due to the symptom overlap with other diagnoses (e.g., PTSD, social anxiety disorder), as well as the tendency for some children to have personality characteristics that reflect reactive attachment disorder or disinhibited social engagement disorder [20].

As considered above, children who are particularly socially inhibited or socially extroverted may be incorrectly diagnosed with reactive attachment disorder and disinhibited social engagement disorder, respectively. Symptoms that hold less clinical relevance in the general public may seem particularly clinically relevant in children who are known to have experienced significant early adversity. Children who have spent their early years with insufficient care may also be particularly likely to exhibit idiosyncratic or odd behaviors, which may or may not relate to an attachment disorder—or, as described previously, an autism spectrum disorder.

Given this reported lack of clear assessment tools and tendency toward overdiagnosis, numerous researchers have written about the importance of careful differential diagnosis by qualified mental health professionals [16, 20, 21]. Diagnosis of attachment disorder typically occurs through a convergence of data based upon behavioral observation and clinical interview, and in the absence of validated protocols, there is much clinician interpretation of behavioral- and interview-based information during differential diagnosis, and this interpretation can be easily biased by the clinician's worldview and dominant paradigm. Autism specialists tend to have selective attention for symptoms of ASD, trauma-focused clinicians tend to be selectively attuned to indicators of traumatic stress, and so on. It is critically important for professionals to carefully consider alternative possible diagnoses and consult specialists in areas outside their expertise when they are in doubt or "on the fence."

Important Considerations for Providing Diagnostic Feedback to Families

Feedback sessions can be particularly challenging when identifying a new TSRD diagnosis. In particular, if parents are anticipating that their child will meet the criteria for ASD, feedback identifying that symptoms are instead related to early environmental stress can pose a number of challenges.

First, if the caregivers are the same caregivers who were parenting the child during infancy, this diagnosis identifies that the caregivers likely hold some responsibility for the child's current difficulties. If a caregiver was not thinking in these terms before the assessment, feedback must be presented carefully to both clearly convey the etiology while preventing a rupture in communication. Despite the difficulty of relaying information about the impact of caregiving on current symptomatology, it is essential that this information is conveyed. Explaining that the child's symptoms are impacted by caregiving environment is necessary for the caregiver to clearly understand the diagnosis, and this information sets the stage for treatment recommendations that focus on the caregiver-child relationship.

As we see with Jayden's case, conveying this information can also be complicated because a diagnosis of ASD often is associated with greater access to resources and social support than a diagnosis related to trauma. In Jayden's case we see that the parent, preschool teacher, and the child welfare caseworker are each aware that an ASD diagnosis would lead to greater access to resources that could provide helpful support to this family. Although differential diagnosis should not be impacted by (real or perceived) differential ease of access to services, it is important for clinicians to be aware that a trauma-related diagnosis often does not garner the same level of support. In addition to differential access to mental health services, ASD also garners greater social support. For caregivers of children with this diagnosis, it is easy to find local support groups, to access helpful information online, or even to join fundraising efforts to "cure" ASD. There are many ways for caregivers to access social support following a diagnosis and to feel a connection to a greater cause.

A diagnosis of ASD also can provide a basis for explaining children's challenging behaviors in everyday social situations. For example, imagine being a parent trying to explain to a new teacher why Jayden may have challenging behaviors in a preschool classroom. A diagnosis of ASD provides a shorthand way of explaining the basis of these behaviors without imputing blame to any particular family member. Like diabetes and asthma, ASD is a condition that many "take at face value." On the other hand, explaining that a child's current behaviors are related to early environment infers parental blame and may bring up aspects of the family history that a caregiver may wish not to have to discuss. A diagnosis related to early trauma is not associated with the same social support network and does not provide an acceptable way of explaining children's challenging behaviors.

It is within this context that clinicians can understand a parent's strongly aversive reactions during feedback sessions. As we see with Jayden's case, Jayden's caregiver is reacting to the clinician based upon her prior knowledge of these two different diagnoses. Expecting a diagnosis of ASD, she is upset by learning that her child is not given that diagnosis. She seems to have come into the assessment with the strong belief that this diagnosis would be helpful for her son and for her family. In contrast, a trauma-related diagnosis is likely less familiar and includes the implication of parental impact, highlighting past difficulties in establishing a stable and consistent caregiving environment for Jayden.

Why Does "Getting It Right" Matter?

Thus far we have spent a considerable amount of time discussing the differential diagnosis between ASD and TSRD. We have considered the overlapping symptomology as well as the key factors to consider for an accurate differential diagnosis that include differences in how the symptoms manifest themselves. It is now critical for us to understand the importance of correctly differentiating those children who have ASD from those who have TSRD. In other words, why does getting it right matter? Why is it imperative to identify and name the correct diagnosis when there is such overlap in symptomology?

Treatment for ASD and TSRDs varies significantly. Extensive research has identified that direct teaching of social skills through behavioral methods is most effective for treating children with autism and improving their ability to successfully integrate with neuro-typical children [22, 23]. Intervention methods often include teaching children to recognize facial expressions; using social stories to teach behavioral and communicative repertoires for how to react in various situations; recognizing, monitoring, and managing their emotions; and teaching pragmatic language skills such as taking turns in a conversation and using gestures to augment one's communications. Commonly, and in what is considered best practice, children who have ASD are provided behavioral supports and intervention such as an applied behavior therapist who works with the child in their own home [24]. The behavioral therapists teach important skills to successfully negotiate inclusive settings such as school or community locations including parks, libraries, and stores. Effective behavior therapists also provide parent education and provide family members with resources to help maintain and practice these skills at home and in the community while they work directly with the child.

A diagnostic label of ASD also qualifies children for extensive resources at school that are explicitly designed to extend their direct social skills training, functional language, and academic performance that is more commensurate with their assessed cognitive potential. As was identified earlier in the referral information for Jayden, a label of ASD can also provide access to Developmental Disabilities Services, which in turn can yield some financial supports to families as well as funding for Personal Support Workers that can both further extend social skills training and provide respite for tired caregivers.

Treatment for TSRD, on the other hand, must often take a different approach in order to best address the cause of the behaviors. Therapy and intervention for TSRDs and attachment-based disorders are much less researched, and the majority of available research targets adoption and supportive foster care as effective treatment approaches [25]. The assumption in these cases is that the adoptive or foster families provide higher quality caregiving. In general, the extant research suggests that effective treatment for an attachment disorder focuses on improving the relationship with the primary caregiver while establishing supportive caregiving behaviors [25, 26]. They tend to focus on the attachment between the child and their primary caregiver. With the support of a therapist, families increase activities that are designed to strengthen positive interactions and emotional attachments [27, 28]. Family therapy is also utilized to improve communication with the child and to establish effective behavior management strategies that do not jeopardize the quality of the relationship [29]. In some instances, children engage in individual therapy to help process the trauma that contributed to their diagnosis or reduce behavioral symptoms [30]. However, as has been discussed, in TSRDs such as reactive attachment disorder or disinhibited social engagement disorder, the disrupted parent-child relationship serves an integral etiological role in symptomology. Current research suggests that the best predictor for improving behavioral and mental health outcomes stems from improving this disrupted relationship. Thus, treatment for TSRDs should prioritize the child and caregiver working together.

Therapeutic preschools, or in some cases behavior plans at school, are also important for children with TSRDs but serve a different purpose than for children with ASD. A benefit of such therapeutic programs, as was suggested in the recommendations for Jayden, is to provide a supportive environment with well-trained and sensitive staff members who have experience working with children with behavioral symptoms. This will provide an environment for children to continue to be supported in learning social, pragmatic language, and self-regulation skills. While these structured programs and supports may be helpful for children diagnosed with a TSRD, they tend to have minimal impact in the absence of a therapeutic program targeting the relationship between the child and a primary caregiver. It is important to note that a diagnosis of a TSRD alone does not qualify families to receive social security support or other supports for developmental disability. This may be assumed to be one of the factors that made feedback so challenging for Jayden's mother. Jayden's mother came to her assessment with existing knowledge about services and supports appropriate for a child with an ASD, and a particular challenge for clinicians is finding ways to clearly communicate why these same resources may not be available or helpful for their child.

The supports that are available for children with a diagnosis of ASD are often designed to help families access therapeutic skill builders or support workers that can help teach social skills and pragmatic language skills. Furthermore, resources are offered to provide respite for families. As has been discussed, children with a TSRD will benefit most from being engaged in therapy *with* their primary caregiver, thus making outside skill builders and respite care providers less effective for achieving long-term goals. A personal support worker may reduce the amount of time that a child has to build a predictable and secure relationship with their caregiver. The challenge is that parents with a child with a TSRD may be similarly tired as parents of a child with ASD from managing behaviors and would themselves benefit from respite.

Circling back to the question, why does getting it right matter? If we solely focus on treating the symptoms, children with a TSRD or attachment-based disorder will have limited opportunities to establish a healthy relationship with their primary caregiver. In the absence of establishing or working toward establishing this relationship, behavior problems are likely to persist, further straining the quality of that relationship. Additionally, getting inappropriately labeled as ASD can significantly determine classroom placement and services that may be inappropriate for the child. In summary, the goal when considering treatment for ASD is often to develop compensatory behaviors to make up for a lack of aptitude for empathy. In these instances, early intervention is most successful. The goal of treating RAD, on the other hand, is to increase empathy by creating a healthy attachment to caregivers. This highlights the difference between a lack of ability to develop empathy due to a fundamental deficit in social cognition and unlearned empathy due to chronic activation of fear mechanisms and survival strategies. Treatment for ASD helps children to identify skills and strategies to navigate life without empathy, whereas children with a TSRD should be provided with appropriate opportunities to learn empathy, starting within their relationship with their primary caregiver.

Let's consider the effect of "getting it right" for Jayden. While his mother may benefit from monetary support and respite, the interventions that he would have received with a diagnosis of ASD would not appropriately emphasize building a healthy attachment with his mother and as a result would not work to help him learn empathy. Although some social skills and language supports may benefit him—without directly targeting his relationship with his mother—he would likely to continue struggling within that relationship. However, both Jayden's mother and caseworker were not pleased with this outcome and were seeking additional services.

Situations such as this often set up a struggle for clinicians who strive to provide an accurate diagnostic label in order to provide the most appropriate services and the impression that more services mean better services. In the case of Jayden, it is understandable to see why his neurologist ultimately provided a diagnosis of ASD. By providing this label, Jayden's family would be able to access the most services that seemingly would provide a high level of support. Many professionals conclude that in these situations, it is best to obtain the most services for high-need families. While this temptation is understandable, especially with pressure from both a primary caregiver and caseworker, in the long run, this decision may be detrimental to children diagnosed with a TSRD for many of the reasons cited above. The "most services" that Jayden may receive are not the "most appropriate" services for his diagnosis. By not being provided supports to build a secure relationship with his mother, Jayden risks not being provided with the necessary supports and opportunities to develop his capacity for empathy. One is tempted to speculate that if Jayden's mother had been engaged in the feedback conversation for longer, her clinician may have suggested that she pursue supports through her local Developmental Disability Services Department on the basis of his prenatal alcohol exposure, which can be argued to have caused his functional impairments (see Chap. 5, this volume).

References

1. American Psychiatric Association. Diagnostic and statistical manual of mental disorders: DSM-5. Washington, DC: American Psychiatric Association; 2013.
2. Sadiq FA, Slator L, Skuse D, Law J, Gillberg C, Minnis H. Social use of language in children with reactive attachment disorder and autism spectrum disorders. Eur Child Adolesc Psychiatry. 2012;21(5):267–76.
3. Rutter M, Andersen-Wood L, Beckett C, Bredenkamp D, Castle J, Groothues C, et al. Quasi-autistic patterns following severe early global privation. J Child Psychol Psychiatry. 1999;40(4):537–49.
4. Hoksbergen R, ter Laak J, Rijk K, van Dijkum C, Stoutjesdijk F. Post-institutional autistic syndrome in Romanian adoptees. J Autism Dev Disord. 2005;35(5):615–23.
5. Moran H. Clinical observations of the differences between children on the autism spectrum and those with attachment problems: The Coventry Grid. Good Autism Practice. 2010;11(2):46–59.
6. Shonkoff JP, Garner AS, Section on Developmental and Behavioral Pediatrics. The lifelong effects of early childhood adversity and toxic stress. Pediatrics. 2012;129(1):e232–46.
7. Shonkoff JP, Callister G, Oberklaid F. The science of early childhood development: closing the gap between what we know and what we do. Victoria: Department of Human Services; 2006.
8. Masten AS. Ordinary magic. Resilience processes in development. Am Psychol. 2001;56(3):227–38.
9. Anda RF, Felitti VJ, Bremner JD, Walker JD, Whitfield C, Perry BD, et al. The enduring effects of abuse and related adverse experiences in childhood. A convergence of evidence from neurobiology and epidemiology. Eur Arch Psychiatry Clin Neurosci. 2006;256(3):174–86.
10. Liu KY, King M, Bearman PS. Social influence and the autism epidemic. Am J Sociol. 2010;115(5):1387–434.
11. Chakrabarti S, Fombonne E. Pervasive developmental disorders in preschool children: confirmation of high prevalence. Am J Psychiatr. 2005;162(6):1133–41.
12. Rice CE, Rosanoff M, Dawson G, Durkin MS, Croen LA, Singer A, Yeargin-Allsopp M. Evaluating changes in the prevalence of the autism spectrum disorders (ASDs). Public Health Rev. 2012;34(2):1–22.
13. Keyes KM, Susser E, Cheslack-Postava K, Fountain C, Liu K, Bearman PS. Cohort effects explain the increase in autism diagnosis among children born from 1992 to 2003 in California. Int J Epidemiol. 2012;41:495–503.
14. American Academy of Pediatrics. Recommendations for preventive pediatric health care. 2015. https://www.aap.org/en-us/Documents/periodicity_schedule_oral_health.pdf.
15. Shattuck PT. The contribution of diagnostic substitution to the growing administrative prevalence of autism in US special education. Pediatrics. 2006;117(4):1028–37.
16. O'Connor TG, Zeanah CH. Attachment disorders: assessment strategies and treatment approaches. Attach Hum Dev. 2003;5(3):223–44.
17. Ainsworth MDS, Blehar MC, Waters E, Wall S. Patterns of attachment: a psychological study of the strange situation. Hillsdale: Erlbaum; 1978.
18. Sprafkin J, Volpe RJ, Gadow KD, Nolan EE, Kelly K. A DSM-IV–referenced screening instrument for preschool children: the Early Childhood Inventory-4. J Am Acad Child Adolesc Psychiatry. 2002;41(5):604–12.
19. O'Connor TG, Rutter M, Beckett C, Keaveney L, Kreppner JM. The effects of global severe privation on cognitive competence: extension and longitudinal follow-up. Child Dev. 2000;71(2):376–90.
20. Chaffin M, Hanson R, Saunders BE, Nichols T, Barnett D, Zeanah C, et al. Report of the APSAC task force on attachment therapy, reactive attachment disorder, and attachment problems. Child Maltreat. 2006;11(1):76–89.
21. Hanson RF, Spratt EG. Reactive attachment disorder: what we know about the disorder and implications for treatment. Child Maltreat. 2000;5(2):137–45.

22. Dawson G, Jones EJ, Merkle K, Venema K, Lowy R, Faja S, et al. Early behavioral intervention is associated with normalized brain activity in young children with autism. J Am Acad Child Adolesc Psychiatry. 2012;51(11):1150–9.
23. Virués-Ortega J. Applied behavior analytic intervention for autism in early childhood: meta-analysis, meta-regression and dose–response meta-analysis of multiple outcomes. Clin Psychol Rev. 2010;30(4):387–99.
24. Volkmar F, Siegel M, Woodbury-Smith M, King B, McCracken J, State M, The American Academy of Child and Adolescent Psychiatry (AACAP) Committee on Quality Issues (CQI). Practice parameter for the assessment and treatment of children and adolescents with autism spectrum disorder. J Am Acad Child Adolesc Psychiatry. 2014;53(2):237–57.
25. Zeanah CH, Gleason MM. Annual research review: attachment disorders in early childhood–clinical presentation, causes, correlates, and treatment. J Child Psychol Psychiatry. 2015;56(3):207–22.
26. McGoron L, Gleason MM, Smyke AT, Drury SS, Nelson CA, Gregas MC, Zeanah CH. Recovering from early deprivation: attachment mediates effects of caregiving on psychopathology. J Am Acad Child Adolesc Psychiatry. 2012;51(7):683–93.
27. Allen B, Timmer SG, Urquiza AJ. Parent–Child Interaction Therapy as an attachment-based intervention: theoretical rationale and pilot data with adopted children. Child Youth Serv Rev. 2014;47:334–41.
28. Batzer S, Berg T, Godinet MT, Stotzer RL. Efficacy or chaos? Parent–child interaction therapy in maltreating populations: a review of research. Trauma Violence Abuse. 2018;19(1):3–19. https://doi.org/10.1177/1524838015620819.
29. Thomas R, Zimmer-Gembeck MJ. Parent-child interaction therapy: an evidence-based treatment for child maltreatment. Child Maltreat. 2012;17(3):1–14. https://doi.org/10.1177/1077559512459555.
30. Garland AF, Landsverk JL, Hough RL, Ellis-MacLeod E. Type of maltreatment as a predictor of mental health service use for children in foster care. Child Abuse Negl. 1996;20(8):675–88.

Chapter 6
Fetal Alcohol Spectrum Disorders: Diagnostic Considerations for Children with a History of Trauma

Prachi E. Shah, Danielle Shapiro, Tedi Milgrom, and H. Eugene Hoyme

Case Presentation

Edward is a 16-year-old boy in residential care who was adopted from a Ukrainian orphanage at 6 years of age. He is here with his caseworker for a diagnostic evaluation to determine whether he meets diagnostic criteria for a fetal alcohol spectrum disorder diagnosis.

Adoption records indicate that his mother had a history of schizophrenia, depression, and a learning disability, and she completed school to the ninth grade. His biological mother was also an alcoholic who drank heavily when she was pregnant with him. Pregnancy was notable for no prenatal care. He was in the care of his biological mother until 3 years of age, at which time there was a fire in their home, and Edward and his sister were found tied up in the basement of his home. Edward was placed in foster care and parental rights were terminated. Edward had a history of significant externalizing behavior problems, resulting in multiple foster care placements over the next 2 years. In foster care, he experienced physical abuse and neglect, resulting in placement in a Ukrainian orphanage at age 4. Records indicate that at the time of his placement, he demonstrated failure to thrive, with his height and weight less than the fifth percentile. He also had a history of microcephaly and had third degree burns over his body at the time of placement in the orphanage. When he was adopted by an American couple at 6 years of age, he was noted to have a history of significant disruptive behaviors. He had a history of hoarding and stealing and began starting fires in the fifth grade. He developed an interest in pornography in the sixth grade and began engaging in voyeuristic behaviors toward his

P. E. Shah (✉) · D. Shapiro · T. Milgrom
University of Michigan, Ann Arbor, MI, USA
e-mail: prachis@umich.edu; dnshap@med.umich.edu

H. Eugene Hoyme
University of Arizona, Tucson, AZ, USA
e-mail: Gene.Hoyme@sanfordhealth.org

J. M. Fogler, R. A. Phelps (eds.), *Trauma, Autism, and Neurodevelopmental Disorders*, https://doi.org/10.1007/978-3-030-00503-0_6

adopted sister. He was diagnosed with reactive attachment disorder, autism spectrum disorder, conduct disorder, ADHD, and a learning disability. He was placed on an IEP under the qualification of "emotional impairment" and was started on numerous psychotropic medications. Due to his sexual predatory behavior toward his adopted sister, and history of impulse control disorder, the adoption was terminated. He was removed from the adopted home and placed into a foster home. This foster placement was terminated due to his aggression and pathological behaviors including lying and stealing, and he was placed briefly in two other foster homes before he was placed in a residential treatment facility at age 14.

Edward underwent comprehensive neuropsychological testing at age 16 which revealed highly variable abilities, including impairments in expressive language, reading, attention, foundational and complex executive functions, learning and memory for visually presented information, fine motor skills, and adaptive and behavioral functioning. He demonstrated low-average verbal reasoning skills, average visual-perceptual reasoning abilities, mildly impaired expressive language, and impaired graphomotor visuo-construction. Assessment of his academic abilities revealed moderately impaired reading, phonemic awareness, and phonetic decoding. He displayed remarkable deficits in his adaptive functioning, and assessment of attention and executive function demonstrated impairments in processing speed, working memory, and sustained attention. Assessments of learning and memory corroborated significant deficits in visuo-constructional and picture memory. Broadband assessment of emotional and adaptive functioning revealed clinically significant concerns in the domains of attention, social withdrawal, aggression, atypical social behavior, and adaptive functioning. He presents with his caseworker for a diagnostic evaluation to determine whether he meets diagnostic criteria for a fetal alcohol spectrum disorder.

Introduction

Edward's history illustrates the diagnostic complexity and challenge of identifying a unifying diagnosis for the origins of his pathological behaviors. The etiology of Edward's symptoms is likely multifactorial, related to both individual and situational risk factors in the biopsychosocial ecology [1–3], including a history of early prenatal exposure to alcohol, genetic history of psychiatric disorders, learning problems, history of ASD, and history of early trauma, early pathogenic care, and caregiving inconsistency. However, given Edward's history of heavy prenatal exposure to alcohol, a diagnosis of a fetal alcohol spectrum disorder (FASD) should also be considered as a potential contributing factor. If a fetal alcohol spectrum disorder diagnosis is confirmed, this can help guide interventions and management to optimize Edward's future outcomes.

Fetal alcohol spectrum disorders (FASDs) are an umbrella term that describes a variety of conditions characterized by a pattern of atypical facial features, growth restriction, structural physical abnormalities, and brain dysfunction resulting from prenatal alcohol exposure. Because the cognitive and behavioral phenotype of children with fetal alcohol spectrum disorders can be nonspecific [4], and overlap with the phenotype of other neurodevelopmental disorders, and because the majority of individuals with FASDs do not manifest dysmorphic craniofacial features [5], misdiagnosis and underdiagnosis of FASDs are common. [6] To mitigate the long-term morbidities associated with fetal alcohol spectrum disorders, it is important to maintain a heightened index of suspicion for prenatal alcohol exposure and the possibility of an alcohol-related diagnosis in children at risk, as early diagnosis and recognition of the disabilities associated with FASDs can help optimize future outcomes [7].

This chapter will begin with an overview of fetal alcohol spectrum disorders (FASDs) and will provide a rationale for considering a diagnosis of FASD in children with a history of trauma. The chapter will review the pathogenesis and diagnostic criteria of fetal alcohol spectrum disorders, using the recently updated NIAAA Expert Consensus Diagnostic Guidelines [8], and will describe the clinical evaluation of FASDs, including the assessment of the facial features of fetal alcohol syndrome (FAS). The chapter will then highlight the effects of intrauterine alcohol exposure on the developing brain, underscoring the developmental emergence of alcohol-related neurocognitive and behavioral deficits and the phenotypic overlap with other neurodevelopmental disorders. Finally, recognizing that prenatal alcohol exposure and experience of trauma often coexist, the chapter will conclude with suggestions to promote resilience in children with a history of prenatal alcohol exposure.

Overview of Fetal Alcohol Spectrum Disorders and a History of Trauma: Common Comorbidities

Prenatal exposure to alcohol can have numerous adverse effects on a developing fetus, including a spectrum of structural anomalies and neurocognitive and behavioral disabilities that have been termed fetal alcohol spectrum disorders (FASDs). First identified in the United States in 1973 by Kenneth Lyons Jones, M.D. [9, 10], fetal alcohol syndrome (FAS) describes children at the most severe end of this spectrum who display the complete phenotype of characteristic facial anomalies, growth restriction, and developmental abnormalities of the central nervous system. Although FAS is the form of FASD most readily recognized by clinicians, other categories within the continuum of adverse effects due to prenatal alcohol exposure are becoming better defined, including partial fetal alcohol syndrome (p-FAS), alcohol-related neurodevelopmental disorders (ARNDs, also referred to as Other Specified Neurodevelopmental Disorder under *DSM-5*), and alcohol-related birth defects (ARBDs) [11, 12].

FASDs are underdiagnosed in general treatment settings [13–15] and are especially underdiagnosed in at-risk populations, particularly children in foster care [6, 16]. Population-based prevalence studies have estimated that FASDs affect 2.4–4.8% of the general population [5], with prevalence estimates as high as 16.9% for children in the foster care system [16]. Entry into the foster care system is often concomitant with a history of detrimental caregiving experiences, parental substance use, trauma, abuse, neglect, and maltreatment [17–19]. Similarly, these trauma-related risk factors are also associated with a high likelihood of prenatal alcohol exposure [20–23]. Consequently, clinicians should maintain a heightened index of suspicion for the possibility of prenatal alcohol exposure in children with a history of child trauma, maltreatment, or involvement in the child welfare system, and should have a low threshold to pursue an evaluation for a fetal alcohol spectrum disorder, recognizing that an FASD diagnosis can co-occur in children with trauma-related diagnoses. Because FASDs represent a major public health concern, early evaluation of children at risk is important to initiate interventional strategies to optimize outcomes for affected children.

Pathogenesis of Intrauterine Alcohol Exposure on the Developing Fetus

Mechanisms of Alcohol-Related Neurotoxicity

Fetal alcohol spectrum disorders (including FAS, p-FAS, ARBD, or ARND) are disorders of teratogenesis, resulting directly from the effects of maternal alcohol consumption on the developing fetus. The effects of alcohol on the developing fetus are varied and can include a pattern of atypical facial features, growth restriction, structural physical abnormalities, and brain dysfunction, with the pattern of structural and functional aberrations related to the dose, duration, and timing of prenatal alcohol exposure. Alcohol-related central nervous system (CNS) effects can result from heavy alcohol exposure during any period of the pregnancy (Fig. 6.1) [24], while the dysmorphic craniofacial features result from heavy alcohol exposure in the first trimester of pregnancy [25]. The mechanisms by which alcohol disrupts fetal brain development are complex and multifactorial. Alcohol consumed by the mother readily crosses the placenta and enters fetal circulation where it crosses the blood-brain barrier and exerts direct neurotoxic effects on the developing brain [26]. The neurotoxic effects of alcohol are mediated through several mechanisms. Alcohol disrupts neuronal cell-cell adhesion by affecting the gene expression of L1 and other cell adhesion molecules [27]. The neuronal cell adhesion molecule L1 is critical for brain development and plays a role in adult learning and memory and is theorized to play a role in the cerebellar dysfunction associated with fetal alcohol spectrum disorders [28, 29]. In addition, ethanol induces oxidative stress mechanisms resulting in mitochondrial dysfunction and apoptotic cell death in the fetal brain [30, 31]. Decreased activity of fetal antioxidant enzymes is thought to contribute to the heightened susceptibility of the fetal brain to the apoptotic effects of alcohol. [32, 33] Alcohol also interferes with cell division, proliferation, neuronal migration, and proliferation of the cranial neural crest cells [34], which contributes to the midline craniofacial dysmorphology (small palpebral fissure length, lip and philtrum anomalies, described below) seen in children with FAS.

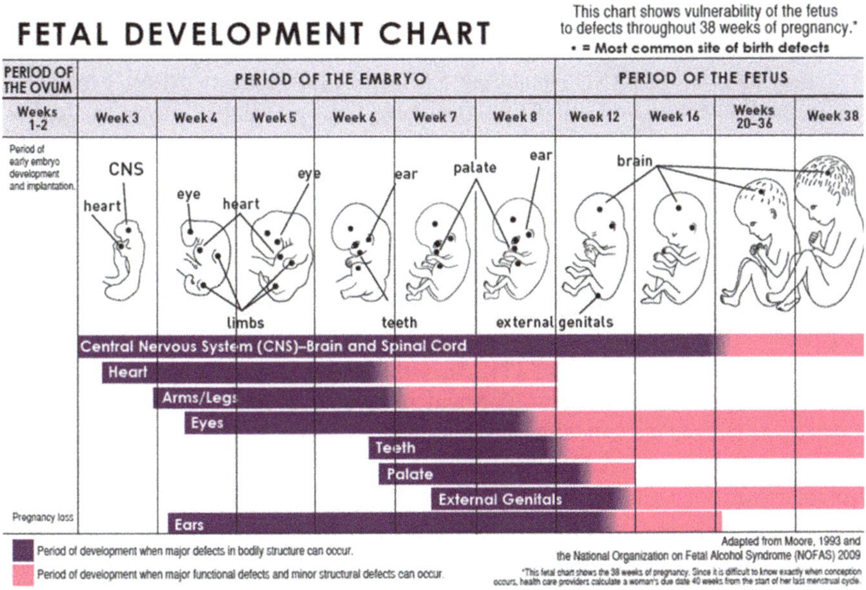

Fig. 6.1 Fetal development chart demonstrating the vulnerability of the fetus to alcohol-related defects throughout pregnancy. Fetal Development Chart downloaded from https://www.cdc.gov/dotw/fasd/images/chart_928px.jpg accessed 10/20/2017

Epigenetics and FASDs

It has long been known that susceptibility to the teratogenic effects of ethanol is dependent on genetic factors in both the mother and fetus. For example, a recent genome-wide single-nucleotide variant (SNV) study in mice identified 900 genes that are downregulated by alcohol exposure in the embryo [35]. Such changes in gene expression are *epigenetic* (gene activation or inactivation initiated by environmental triggers that do not alter the underlying DNA sequence, which in turn affect how cells "read" the genes). Alcohol inhibits gene expression in the developing fetal brain through at least three epigenetic mechanisms: DNA methylation, histone modification, and noncoding RNA (circulating micro-RNA [miRNA])-associated gene silencing [36]. For example, in both animal and human studies, ethanol exposure during pregnancy results in significant elevations in circulating miRNAs in maternal blood. In a recent study of alcohol-exposed pregnancies in Ukraine, 11 miRNAs were significantly elevated in the plasma of heavily alcohol-exposed women who had children with FASDs, compared to both women who drank heavily but had apparently normal children and unexposed women [37]. These data indicate that maternal plasma miRNA profiles predict infant outcomes and may be useful as biomarkers in the diagnosis of FASDs, alleviating the previously discussed difficulty in accuracy of maternal reporting of alcohol intake during pregnancy.

Diagnostic Criteria for Fetal Alcohol Spectrum Disorders

The diagnosis of an FASD (including FAS, p-FAS, ARBD, or ARND) reflects a constellation of symptoms and signs resulting from prenatal exposure to alcohol. Per the recently updated NIAAA Expert Consensus Diagnostic Guidelines [8], the diagnostic evaluation of a child with a potential FASD requires the assessment of four domains: (a) prenatal alcohol exposure, (b) facial structure (assessing the three sentinel facial features of FAS), (c) growth (prenatal and postnatal), and (d) neurodevelopmental impairment (characterized by central nervous system involvement manifested as a small head circumference and evidence of a characteristic pattern of cognitive or neurobehavioral deficits). Although there are several classification systems used for FASD diagnosis [11, 38–40], the Revised IOM Criteria [11] first developed by Hoyme et al. in 2005 and revised in 2016 as the NIAAA Expert Consensus Diagnostic Guidelines [8] have the advantage of having been developed from a medical model and validated through testing in a large multiracial international cohort of children [41–44]. The NIAAA Expert Consensus Diagnostic Guidelines also consider different etiologies for the clinical phenotype including genetic factors, other teratogenic (drug) exposures, and environmental contributions to developmental and behavioral disorders when making an FASD diagnosis [12], and the diagnostic approach is easily taught to physicians and non-physicians with good diagnostic reliability [45, 46].

The NIAAA Expert Consensus Diagnostic Guidelines [8] considers the four criteria noted above to determine whether the child meets diagnostic criteria for one of the four fetal alcohol spectrum disorder diagnoses. A diagnosis of fetal alcohol syndrome (FAS) can be made with or without confirmed alcohol exposure but requires all of the following criteria to be met: (1) the presence of two of the three cardinal facial features associated with prenatal alcohol exposure (short palpebral fissures, smooth philtrum, and flattened upper vermillion border); (2) history of pre- or postnatal growth restriction characterized by height or weight ≤10th centile at any point in time; (3) history of a small head circumference, defined as an occipito-frontal circumference (OFC) ≤10th centile at any point in time, or structural brain abnormalities; and (4) evidence of cognitive or neurobehavioral impairment. A diagnosis of partial-FAS (p-FAS) can also be made with or without confirmed alcohol exposure. If alcohol exposure is confirmed, a diagnosis of p-FAS requires the following two criteria to be met: (1) the presence of two of the three cardinal facial features associated with prenatal alcohol exposure and (2) evidence of cognitive or neurobehavioral impairment. If prenatal alcohol exposure is *not* confirmed, a diagnosis of p-FAS requires the above two criteria and the additional confirmation of growth restriction characterized by *either* (1) history of pre- or postnatal growth restriction or (2) a history of a small head circumference or structural brain abnormalities. A diagnosis of alcohol-related neurodevelopmental disorder (ARND) requires (1) documented prenatal alcohol exposure and (2) evidence of cognitive or neurobehavioral impairment, *with or without* (3) a history of a small head circumference or structural brain abnormalities. ARND is characterized by the presence of the neurobehavioral deficits associated with prenatal alcohol exposure, without the accompanying dysmorphic craniofacial features, and cannot be diagnosed in children <3 years of age [8]. A diagnosis of alcohol-related birth defects (ARBDs) requires documented prenatal alcohol exposure, and the presence of one or more specific major malformations demonstrated in animal models and human studies to be related to prenatal alcohol exposure, including cardiac defects (e.g., atrial septal defects, ventricular septal defects, aberrant great vessels, conotruncal heart defects), skeletal defects (e.g., radioulnar synostosis, vertebral segmentation defects, large joint contractures, scoliosis), renal anomalies (e.g., aplastic/hypoplastic/dysplastic kidneys, "horseshoe" kidneys, ureteral duplications), eye anomalies (e.g., strabismus, ptosis, retinal vascular anomalies, optic nerve hypoplasia), and hearing impairment (e.g., conductive or neurosensory hearing loss) [47, 48] (Table 6.1).

Clinical Evaluation for FASDs

The key elements of clinical evaluation include (a) obtaining an accurate history of prenatal alcohol exposure, (b) providing an accurate assessment of facial features, (c) verifying growth restriction, and (d) identifying central nervous system (CNS) deficits.

History of Prenatal Alcohol Exposure

In order for a child to be diagnosed with an FASD, prenatal alcohol exposure must be confirmed (with the exception of FAS and p-FAS, which can be diagnosed on the basis of the characteristic clinical features with or without confirmation of prenatal alcohol exposure). Accurate determination of prenatal alcohol exposure is often difficult to verify. Due to the stigma associated with drinking during pregnancy [49], mothers may be reluctant to admit to alcohol use during pregnancy, may underreport, or may not recall the amount of alcohol consumed during pregnancy, resulting in maternal self-report data regarding prenatal alcohol use that is often unreliable [50–52]. Because a) prepregnancy alcohol consumption is highly correlated with the presence of alcohol-related diagnoses and neurobehavioral problems [53, 54], and b) mothers may not consider or report alcohol consumption prior to learning of their pregnancies, screening questionnaires such as the T-ACE and its revision, the TACER-3, have been developed to screen for maternal alcohol use in pregnancy. The TACER-3 Risk Drinking Screen [55] demonstrates good sensitivity and specificity and assesses for symptoms of *tolerance* (≥2 drinks to feel high), a*nnoyance* (annoyed if others complained about drinking), *cutting down* (whether the patient felt a need to cut down on drinking), and whether the patient needed a drink as an *eye opener* (first think in the morning).

Table 6.1 Diagnostic criteria of fetal alcohol spectrum disorders

NIAAA Expert Consensus Diagnostic Guidelines						
Alcohol Exposure	**FAS Facial Features [a]**	**Growth Restriction [b]**	**Deficient Brain Growth [c]**	**Neurobehavioral Impairment [d] < 3yo**	**Neurobehavioral Impairment [e] > 3yo**	**Birth Defects [f]**
FAS						
Confirmed OR Unconfirmed Exposure	X	X	X	X	X 1.Global impairment 2. Cognitive Deficit 3. Behavioral Impair.	
P-FAS						
Confirmed Exposure	X			X	X 1.Global impairment 2. Cognitive Deficit 3. Behavioral Impair.	
Unconfirmed Exposure	X	X ⟷ OR	X	X	X 1.Global impairment 2. Cognitive Deficit 3. Behavioral Impair.	
ARND (Alcohol Related Neurodevelopmental Disorder) **						
Confirmed Exposure				N/A	X 1.Global impairment 2. Cognitive Deficit (2) 3. Behavioral Impair. (2)	
ARBD (Alcohol Related Birth Defects)						
Confirmed Exposure						X

[a]Characteristic pattern of facial anomalies characterizes by ≥2 of the following: (1) Short palpebral fissures (≤10th centile), (2) Thin vermillion border (rank of 4 or 5 on racially normed lip/philtrum guide), and (3) Smooth philtrum (rank of 4 or 5 on racially normed lip/philtrum guide)

[b]Prenatal and/or postnatal growth deficiency: Height and/or weight ≤ 10th centile on gender-specific growth curves

[c]Deficient brain growth/morphogenesis/neurophysiology characterized by ≥1 of the following: (1) Head circumference ≤ 10th centile, (2) Structural brain abnormalities, and (3) Recurrent nonfebrile seizures

[d]Evidence of developmental delay ≥1.5 SD below the mean

[e](1) *Global impairment*: general conceptual ability, PIQ, VIQ, or spatial IQ ≥1.5 SD below the mean. (2) *cognitive deficit* in 1 domain ≥1.5 SD below the mean (executive function, specific learning impairment, memory impairment, or visual spatial impairment. (3) *Behavioral impairment without cognitive impairment*: behavioral deficit in 1 domain ≥1.5 SD below the mean in areas of self-regulation (mood or behavioral regulation impairment, attention deficit, or impulse control)

[f]One or more malformations in areas associated with prenatal alcohol exposure: cardiac, skeletal, renal, eyes, ears

[g]For ARND, two domains of impairment are required for either cognitive deficit without behavioral impairment or behavioral impairment without cognitive deficit

Alternatively, because late recognition of pregnancy and drinking in the 3 months *prior* to pregnancy have been associated with the presence of an alcohol-related disorder in the child [5], querying the mother regarding when she learned of her pregnancy may help to further identify a history of prenatal exposures. In maternal interviews, because of potential stigmatization associated with prenatal alcohol use, questions should be asked in a timeline progressing from the broader context of health history to the more sensitive topic of alcohol use [56, 57]. See Appendix for "Sample Interview Questions to Query for Prenatal Alcohol Exposure."

Many times children being assessed for an FASD are in foster care or have been adopted. Depending on the circumstances that led to a child no longer being in the care of the biological mother, medical and familial history may be limited. In these instances, obtaining an accurate history regarding prenatal alcohol exposure can be even more difficult. A child's caregivers may report that the biological mother drank during the pregnancy; however, it is important to determine the source of this information. As information is passed from one source to another, the facts may become distorted, and thus the validity of the information diminishes. Obtaining a child's hospital birth records, medical passport, or court documents regarding termination of parental rights can provide additional information regarding potential prenatal alcohol exposure.

Assessment of Facial Features

Because two of the four categories of FASDs (FAS, p-FAS) require the presence of FAS facial features (see Fig. 6.2), accurate identification of facial dysmorphology is critical to making a diagnosis of an FASD. Accurate identification of FAS facial features is often performed by a physician with specialized training in FAS dysmorphology (e.g., clinical geneticist or developmental pediatrician); however, other health professionals can also be trained to screen for the cardinal dysmorphic facial features associated with FAS [45] and can therefore be instrumental in identifying children who should be referred for further subspecialty evaluation. The guidelines for diagnosis of FAS [8, 11] require two of three characteristic facial features as assessed by a skilled examiner: (a) short palpebral fissure length (≤10th centile compared with published norms), (b) presence of a smooth philtrum, and (c) thin vermilion border of the upper lip when compared to the fullness of the lower lip (characterized by flattening of the Cupid's bow and decreased total area of the upper lip). Lip and philtrum morphology is assessed independently and is scored with a 5-point Likert scale of a racially normed lip-philtrum guide, with scores of 4 or 5 considered compatible with FAS or p-FAS [8, 11, 12] (See Fig. 6.3). Examples of non-FAS and FAS facial features are depicted in Fig. 6.4.

Minor Features

Although not part of the core diagnostic criteria, children with prenatal alcohol exposure have been shown to manifest a pattern of minor structural defects, including midface hypoplasia, epicanthal folds, hypoplastic fingernails, short fifth digits, clinodactyly of fifth fingers, pectus carinatum/excavatum, camptodactyly (inability to completely extend the fingers), "hockey stick" palmar creases, other palmar

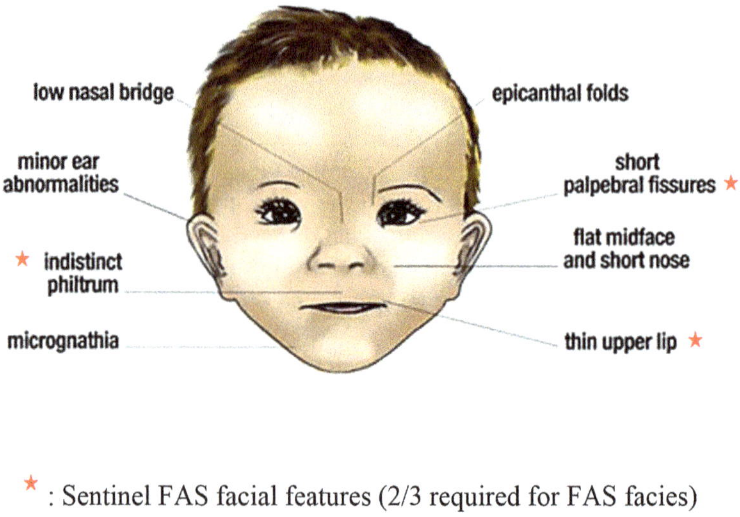

Fig. 6.2 Facial characteristics associated with prenatal alcohol exposure. Alcohol alert number 82: "Fetal alcohol spectrum disorders: understanding the effects of prenatal alcohol exposure," downloaded from http://pubs.niaaa.nih.gov/publications/AA82/AA82.htm accessed 9/25/2015]

crease abnormalities, ptosis, strabismus, heart murmurs, impaired pronation and supination at the elbow, hypertelorism, hypotelorism, elongated philtrum, and "railroad track" ears [11, 58]. The presence of these physical abnormalities can prompt a provider to consider additional evaluation for an alcohol-related diagnosis. Examples of some of these minor anomalies are shown in Fig. 6.5.

Growth Restriction

Growth restriction is characterized by height or weight less than the tenth centile at any point in time (prenatally or postnatally) as plotted on age- and gender-specific growth charts [8, 11, 12].

CNS Abnormalities

CNS dysfunction is characterized by the presence of structural and/or functional abnormalities. Such CNS findings can be reflected in a small head circumference (OFC $\leq$10th centile at any point in time measured on gender-specific head circumference charts), structural anomalies of the brain identified on an MRI scan, or recurrent, nonfebrile seizures.

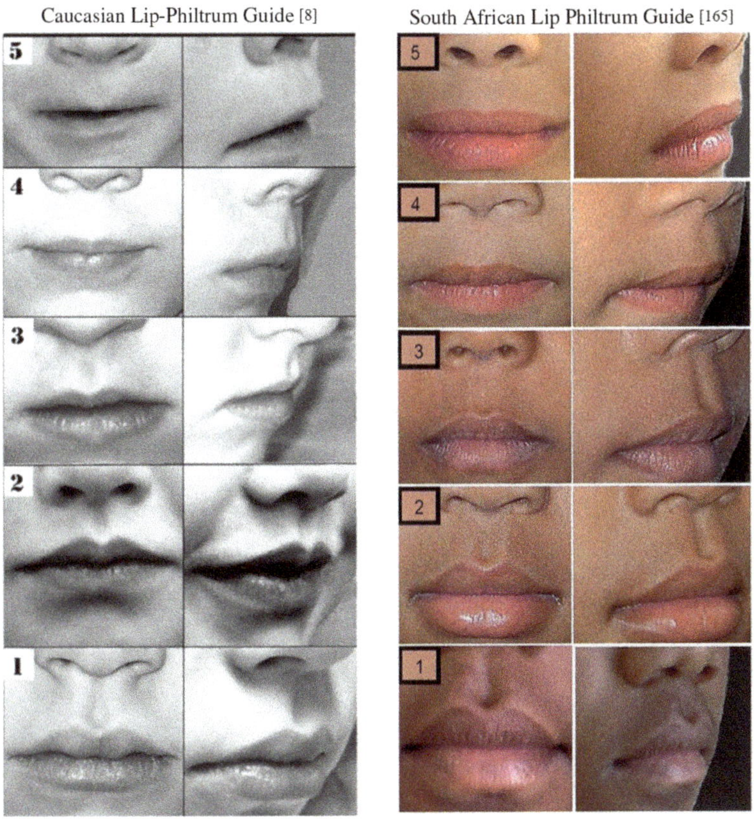

Fig. 6.3 Lip/philtrum morphology

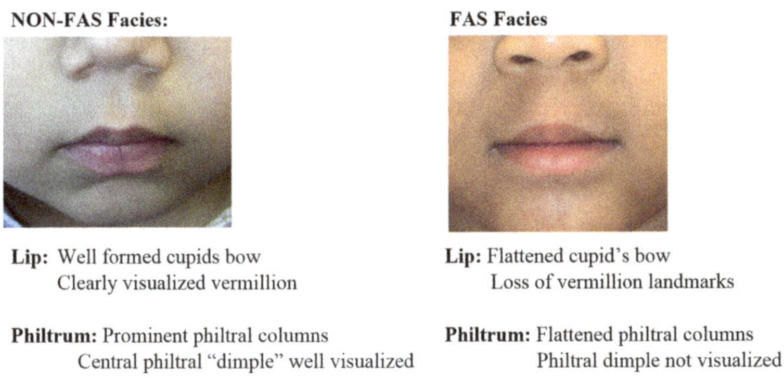

Fig. 6.4 FAS facial features. Photographer, Tedi Milgrom, MPH

Fig. 6.5 Minor features

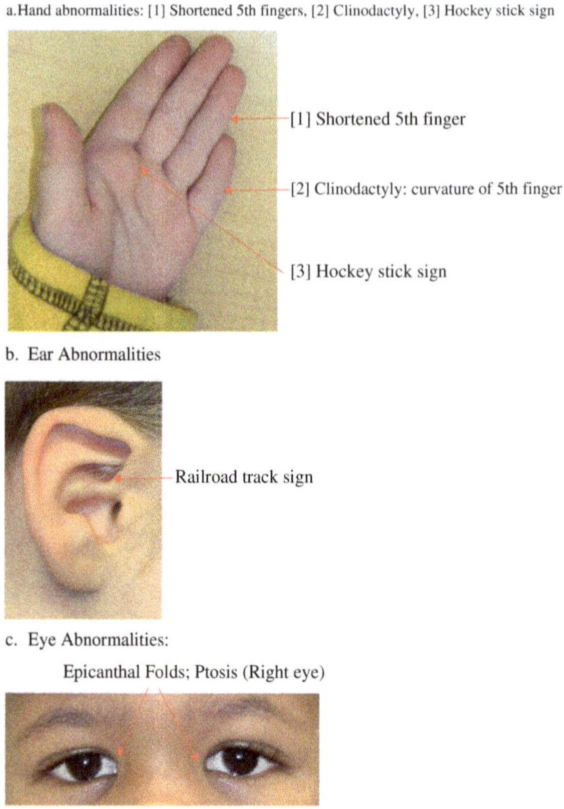

Functional CNS impairments are characterized by evidence of neurobehavioral impairment, defined as either (1) global cognitive impairment defined by general intellectual ability, VIQ or PIQ ≥ 1.5 SD below the mean, or (2) cognitive deficits in at least one neurobehavioral domain including executive functioning, specific learning impairment, memory impairment, or visual impairment or (3) behavioral impairment without cognitive impairment characterized by impairments in self-regulation (mood or behavioral regulation impairment), attention deficit, or impulse control. [8] These areas of CNS impairment overlap with the neurobehavioral features associated with traumatic stress-related disorders [59], which can contribute to the difficulty in making an accurate diagnosis of an FASD, especially in children who do not manifest the craniofacial dysmorphology associated with FAS. Because of the previous ambiguity regarding the neurobehavioral phenotype of heavy prenatal alcohol exposure [60–62], the updated NIAAA Expert Consensus Diagnostic Guidelines sought to clarify the criteria for defining neurobehavioral impairment associated with prenatal alcohol exposure, and have included the requirement of neurobehavioral impairment as part of the diagnostic criteria for diagnoses of FAS, p-FAS and ARND [8] (Table 6.2).

Table 6.2 Neurobehavioral impairments in FASD per the NIAAA expert consensus diagnostic guidelines

Cognitive impairment	
Global impairment	≥3 years old: IQ ≥ 1.5 SD below the mean (FSIQ/VIQ/PIQ) <3 years old: developmental delay ≥1.5 SD below the mean[a]
Cognitive deficits	1 neurobehavioral domain[a] ≥1.5 SD below the mean – Executive function – Specific learning impairment – Memory impairment – Visual spatial impairment
Behavioral impairment without cognitive impairment	
Self-regulation deficits in 1 domain[a] ≥1.5 SD below the mean • Mood • Behavioral regulation • Attention • Impulse control	

[a]ARND requires impairment in two domains and cannot be diagnosed in children <3 year-old

Brain regions Affected by Prenatal Alcohol Exposure

There are select regions of the brain that are especially susceptible to the effects of prenatal alcohol exposure including the frontal lobe, white matter tracts, hippocampus, basal ganglia, cerebellum, and corpus callosum [63–65]. Alcohol-related impairments in these areas are associated with the neurodevelopmental deficits associated with FASDs [66–69], with more severe impairment correlated with the degree of FAS dysmorphology [70]. The effects of alcohol on the frontal lobe include decreased cortical volume [71, 72], and abnormalities in white matter tracts [73], and are thought to contribute to functional deficits in cognition, motor function, response inhibition, attention, and executive function [74–76]. Prenatal alcohol exposure is associated with white matter abnormalities, most notably affecting the corpus callosum, anterior-posterior tracts, cortical spinal tracts, and cerebellum. Abnormalities in these white matter tracts are associated with decreased interhemispheric functional connectivity, contributing to neurocognitive deficits in processing speed, nonverbal abilities, visuomotor skills, verbal learning, and executive function [77, 78]. Prenatal alcohol exposure is also associated with decreased hippocampal volume [72], with associated deficits in working and spatial memory [79, 80], and decreased volume and asymmetry of the basal ganglia [81], contributing to functional deficits in executive function and attention [82], response time [83], inhibitory control [84], spatial memory [85], and higher-order cognitive functioning [86, 87]. The effects of prenatal alcohol exposure on the cerebellum include decreased cerebellar volume [88], potentially contributing to cerebellum-related motor ataxias [89], and deficits in balance, bimanual coordination, attention, and verbal memory [90]. Prenatal alcohol exposure is also associated with structural deficits in the corpus callosum including displacement, hypoplasia, or agenesis of the corpus callosum [87, 91, 92], contributing to deficits in bimanual coordination and impairments in verbal learning and executive function [93]. In summary, prenatal alcohol exposure exerts teratogenic effects on multiple areas of brain structure, contributing to a heterogeneous pattern of impairments in affected children.

Neurobehavioral Profile of Children with FASDs: Developmental Considerations

Although multiple brain structures are susceptible to the effects of prenatal alcohol exposure, the pattern of deficits emerges over time, consistent with brain maturation. As such, the neurocognitive and behavioral deficits of FASDs can manifest differently over the life span, reflecting both heterogeneity and a developmental emergence. Recent efforts to define the range of cognitive and mental health problems occurring in individuals with a history of prenatal alcohol exposure have focused on the three core areas of neurocognition, self-regulation, and adaptive functioning impairments [94–97]. Impairments in the areas of cognition, self-regulation, and adaptive functioning manifest differently according to the child's developmental stage and will vary with the region of the brain that is most affected in that individual child (Table 6.3).

Infancy

The neurobehavioral deficits associated with prenatal alcohol exposure are fairly nonspecific in infancy [4] and are largely characterized by deficits in cognitive and motor development and impairments in emotional and state regulation [98]. Infants with heavy prenatal alcohol exposure have demonstrated dose-dependent lower cognitive development compared to nonexposed infants, on the Bayley Scales of Infant Development [99]. Other infant characteristics associated with heavy prenatal alcohol exposure include delayed motor development and slowed reaction time [100], poorer language and behavioral regulation [101], less complex play [4], poorer feeding, deficits in state regulation, difficulty self-soothing, and increased emotional withdrawal. [102, 103] Because the facial features of FAS may be difficult to identify in infants, and the cognitive and behavioral deficits associated with prenatal alcohol exposure are nonspecific in infancy [4], it is important to maintain a heightened index of suspicion for prenatal alcohol exposure and the possibility of an alcohol-related diagnosis in infants and toddlers at risk.

Table 6.3 Developmental emergence of neurocognitive and behavioral deficits associated with FASDs

Infancy: 0–2 years		
Areas of brain vulnerability with PNAE	Neurocognitive/behavioral deficits associated with developmental stage	
• Cortical synaptogenesis • Development of cortical gray matter	Neurocognitive	• Delayed cognitive development or global developmental delay
• Myelination of sensory pathways	Self-regulation	• Tremulousness, increased jitteriness
• Maturation of the limbic system		• Difficulty with self-soothing and being soothed
		• Emotional withdrawal, decreased infant affective functioning
		• Impaired stress reactivity; deficits in pain regulation
		• Less complex play
• Myelination of motor pathways	Adaptive	• Delayed gross and fine motor milestones
		• Poor feeding: poor sucking. Easily fatigued
Toddler/preschool: 3–5 years		
Areas of brain vulnerability with PNAE	Neurocognitive/behavioral deficits associated with developmental stage	
• Synaptogenesis • Development of cortical gray matter	Neurocognitive	• Delayed cognitive development or global developmental delay
• Development of prefrontal cortex	Self-regulation	• Attention: difficulties with attention regulation; hyperactivity and impulsivity; difficulty shifting attention; impaired visual and auditory attention; difficulty with sustained attention
		• Executive function: difficulty encoding information; difficulty with multi-step directions; difficulty with planning and organization; poor understanding of consequences
• Development of temporal lobes		• Sleep deficits: shortened sleep duration; increased sleep anxiety; parasomnias
		• Sensory processing: difficulty modulating sensory input; sensory seeking

(continued)

Table 6.3 (continued)

• Development of dorsal motor cortex	Adaptive	• Delayed gross motor function: balance, coordination problems; "clumsiness"
		• Poor fine motor skills: difficulty with writing/drawing; poor dexterity; visuospatial deficits; impaired visuomotor coordination
• Development of temporal lobes		• Delayed auditory processing: central auditory delay
		• Speech and language deficits: difficulties with language acquisition; receptive, expressive language delays; deficits in word processing/word recognition; articulation errors; deficits in social pragmatics
		• Memory deficits: difficulty remembering things previously learned
School-age: 6–12 years		
Areas of brain vulnerability with PNAE	Neurocognitive/behavioral deficits associated with developmental stage	
• Decreased intracranial volume: • Decreased volume of parietal and temporal lobes • White matter abnormalities	Neurocognitive	• Lower intellectual quotient • Learning disabilities • Deficits in mathematics (numerical operations/global mathematics skills)
• Prefrontal cortex	Self-regulation	• Executive function deficits: decreased working memory, decreased verbal fluency, poorer planning, sequencing, organization
		• Attention deficits: hyperactivity, impulsivity
• Temporal lobe	Adaptive	• Language: deficits in higher-order language processing.
		• Social pragmatics: deficits in social cognition: inappropriate social initiation/social interaction; inappropriate sexual behaviors
		• Memory: difficulty encoding/consolidating new memory
• Parietal lobe		• Language processing: impaired gestural communication; deficits in social perception
		• Visuospatial: deficits in spatial processing; poor handwriting; impaired visuomotor integration
Adolescence: 13–21 years		
Areas of brain vulnerability with PNAE	Neurocognitive/behavioral deficits associated with developmental stage	

(continued)

Table 6.3 (continued)

• Decreased intracranial volume: • Decreased volume of parietal and temporal lobes • White matter abnormalities	Neurocognitive	• Lower intellectual quotient • Learning disabilities • Deficits in mathematics skills (numerical operations/global mathematics skills)
• Myelination of prefrontal cortex (PFC)	Self-regulation	• Executive function deficits: decreased verbal fluency; poorer planning, sequencing, organization; slow processing; deficits in judgment and metacognition
• Development of connections between PFC and basal ganglia		• Attention deficits: inattention
• Temporal lobe	Adaptive	• Language: deficits in higher-order language processing
		• Social pragmatics: deficits in social cognition: inappropriate social initiation/social interaction; inappropriate sexual behaviors
		• Working memory: difficulty encoding new memories; difficulty with memory recall
• Parietal lobe		• Language processing: deficits in social perception
		• Visuospatial: deficits in spatial processing; poor handwriting; impaired visuomotor integration

Preschool

In the preschool years, children with a history of prenatal alcohol exposure can present with a broad range of cognitive developmental delays involving visuospatial and/or language-based skills as well as deficits in gross and fine motor skills, including problems with gait, balance, and difficulties with handwriting and visuospatial skills [104, 105]. They can also display language delays characterized by speech and language delays [106], articulation problems and language processing dysfunction [107], and delays in auditory processing [108]. The behavioral deficits associated with prenatal alcohol exposure are heterogeneous and can present in the preschool years as difficulties with executive function [109], attention, externalizing behavior problems [110, 111], increased emotional and conduct problems [111], social skills deficits [112], sleep difficulties [113], sensory processing problems, and adaptive behavior deficits [114].

School Age

In the school-age years, brain development is characterized by increased white matter development largely in the parietal and temporal regions of the brain, with increased development of the corpus callosum and hippocampus, and increased functional connectivity to the prefrontal cortex. [115] Prenatal alcohol exposure results in disruption of these normal processes of brain development. In the school-age child, a history of prenatal alcohol exposure has been associated with differences in structural brain development characterized by decreased total intracranial volume, and less robust white matter development, with the greatest areas of impairment observed in the temporal and parietal regions of the brain, including the basal ganglia [70, 116]. These areas of structural brain deficits are associated with various categories of functional impairment including decreased intellectual functioning, the presence of learning disabilities (especially in reading, writing, and math), and impairments in executive functioning including deficits in working memory, processing speed, verbal fluency, planning, sequencing, and organization [116–120]. Operationally, prenatal alcohol exposure can contribute to difficulties encoding and consolidating new information (e.g., children demonstrate difficulty learning and remembering rules and understanding consequences of their behavior), and behaviorally they can present difficulties with attention, impulsivity, and emotion regulation [69, 121, 122]. In addition, prenatal alcohol exposure has also been associated with deficits in higher-order social pragmatic and language skills, including impairments in gestural communication and social perception and emotion recognition, contributing to social-communicative difficulties. Children with prenatal alcohol exposure can also engage in inappropriate social initiations and social interactions, thereby contributing to difficulties with peer relationships [123–125].

Adolescence

These differences in brain morphology and behavior are likely to persist as children with prenatal alcohol exposure transition to adolescence and adulthood. Adolescence is a period of active brain development, characterized by increased myelination of the prefrontal cortex, and increasing functional connectivity between the prefrontal and subcortical (e.g., basal ganglia) regions of the brain [126]. In addition to the language and learning impairments seen in school-age children, the functional and behavioral deficits in adolescence associated with prenatal alcohol exposure are largely related to impairments in functioning of the prefrontal cortex associated with attention and higher-order cognition, including deficits in working memory, attention, executive functioning, information processing, judgment, and metacognition [126], and altered neuro-connectivity in the limbic system, associated with impairments in behavioral regulation [127, 128]. In adolescence, the social, functional, and occupational impairments associated with a fetal alcohol spectrum disorder diagnosis include lower educational attainment and increased school drop-out rates, increased trouble with the law and involvement with the juvenile justice system, and increased risk for and substance and alcohol abuse problems [129].

The Neurobehavioral Similarities between FASDs and Other Neurodevelopmental Disorders

The neurobehavioral deficits associated with fetal alcohol spectrum disorders are broad, and are most notably associated with deficits in attention, executive function, visual and spatial memory, cognitive flexibility, social cognitive deficits [61, 62, 130, 131], and difficulties with emotion regulation, characterized by increased externalizing behavioral problems, aggression, and social problems. [60, 132] The neurobehavioral impairments of FASD are similar to the impairments of other neurodevelopmental disorders, which can contribute to the underdiagnosis or misdiagnosis of FASDs. The attention deficits and externalizing behavioral symptoms seen in children with FASDs can often be misattributed to ADHD, although on measures of sustained attention, inhibitory control, and sluggish cognitive tempo (domains typically impaired in ADHD), children with FASD manifest a different neurocognitive profile compared with children with ADHD [133, 134]. The social skills deficits and sensory processing difficulties seen in children with FASDs are similar to the social-communicative deficits seen in children with autism [135], which may lead to children with an FASD being given a diagnosis of an autism spectrum disorder. Although there are some similarities between FASD and ASD, the social-cognitive deficits of FASD are distinct and distinguishable from ASD. While socially inappropriate behaviors and difficulty with peers are behavioral characteristics seen in both children with FASD and ASD, difficulties in initiating social interaction, sharing affect, and using nonverbal communication are deficits common to children with ASD but are rare in children with FASD [136]. Children who have experienced a history of early pathogenic care and early institutionalization are also more likely to have prenatal alcohol exposure and an FASD diagnosis [137, 138]. However, irrespective of prenatal alcohol exposure, a history of institutionalization also has a well-established association with pathological behaviors described as reactive attachment disorder (RAD) [139–141]. Both sub-types of RAD, the emotionally withdrawn (inhibited type) and indiscriminately social (disinhibited type), are well described in children who have experienced severe psychosocial deprivation and early pathogenic care, with greater severity of symptoms associated with longer duration of institutionalization [142]. The conditions associated with early institutionalization including deprivation, neglect, a lack of individualized caregiving, and failure to form attachments to a caregiver also contribute to the pathogenesis of developmental trauma disorder (DTD). Developmental trauma disorder is characterized by multiple, chronic, or prolonged exposure to developmentally adverse interpersonal trauma in early life [143] and can present with symptoms of severe emotional disturbance, anxiety, oppositionality, and aggression [144]. Because of the phenotypic similarity of FASDs to other psychiatric and neurodevelopmental disorders, an FASD diagnosis may be delayed or missed altogether. Prior to being diagnosed with an FASD, children may be diagnosed with other behavioral or psychiatric disorders [6]. Misattribution of FASD symptoms to another disorder may result in delays in initiating the appropriate treatment and interventions or may result in inappropriate treatment by mental health, educational, and criminal justice systems. [94] With the revision of the DSM-5, a new diagnostic category, Neurobehavioral Disorder Associated with Prenatal Alcohol Exposure (ND-PAE), was created to characterize the neurodevelopmental and mental health symptoms associated with prenatal alcohol exposure [96]. ND-PAE describes three core areas of deficit associated with prenatal alcohol exposure including impairments in neurocognition, self-regulation, and adaptive functioning [145]. Because of the phenotypic similarities in the neurobehavioral impairments of FASDs with other neurodevelopmental disorders, especially DTD, professionals who work with children who have experienced trauma should have a low threshold to pursue further evaluation for an FASD if atypical facial features, growth abnormalities, or cognitive or behavioral concerns are present. Furthermore, if full diagnostic criteria for an FASD are not met (e.g., due to subthreshold facial, cognitive, or behavioral deficits), children should still be provided interventions to address areas of need and should receive ongoing close surveillance and follow-up to monitor for the emergence of neurobehavioral deficits that can appear later in life.

An Update on Edward

On exam, Edward was noted to have microcephaly but manifested no dysmorphic craniofacial features. Given his history of confirmed prenatal alcohol exposure, microcephaly, and deficits in self-regulation and adaptive functioning, Edward met diagnostic criteria for ARND (alcohol-related neurodevelopmental disorder). Prior to receiving an FASD diagnosis, Edward was given multiple psychiatric diagnoses including RAD, ASD, ADHD, conduct disorder, and a learning disability. His history of institutionalization is a well-described risk factor for reactive attachment disorder, and atypical social behaviors (e.g., "quasi-autistic patterns") that bear some phenotypic resemblance to autism [146], but which may not persist across the life span [147]. His history of early, severe, and pervasive traumas contributes to his difficulties with emotion regulation manifest by attention deficits and severe externalizing behavior.

Although he met diagnostic criteria for an FASD, the etiology of his symptoms is likely multifactorial, related to genetic factors, history of significant trauma, abuse, neglect, caregiving inconsistency, as well as prenatal teratogenic (alcohol) exposure. Continued placement in a residential facility was recommended to ensure his safety and consistent treatment for his psychiatric needs. While his psychiatric diagnoses have been instrumental in helping access mental health services, including trauma-focused psychotherapy, an FASD diagnosis is instrumental in helping him access developmental services on an IEP under the qualification of FASD/other health impaired (OHI). In addition, because individuals with an FASD diagnosis have an increased risk of engaging in criminal behavior leading to involvement in the justice system, an FASD diagnosis can provide Edward some protection in the justice system and access to services across systems. [148, 149] In summary, Edward has significant cognitive, social, and functional impairments and will need lifelong supports and services to optimize his health, safety, and well-being.

Fostering Resilience in Children with Prenatal Alcohol Exposure

As previously described, the functional and behavioral deficits associated with a fetal alcohol spectrum disorder diagnosis are heterogeneous and result in lifelong impairments including learning disabilities, impulsivity, hyperactivity, deficits in social skills, judgment, working memory, and metacognition. These deficits can contribute to maladaptive peer relationships and poor judgment and can predispose an individual to an increased risk for victimization and involvement in the criminal justice system. These deficits are compounded when a child has also experienced trauma. There is an extensive literature documenting the effects of early childhood adversity on developing neurobiological systems. These include functional impairments to the hypothalamic-adrenal-pituitary axis, the prefrontal cortex regions involved in executive functioning, and the system involved in threat detection and response, particularly the amygdala, with these deficits exacerbated in children with a history of prenatal alcohol exposure [150]. As such, these areas of brain vulnerability should be the focus of intervention strategies to optimize outcomes.

Early diagnosis and intervention remain the best approaches to optimizing outcomes for children with prenatal alcohol exposure [151], with early diagnosis leading to the receipt of more supports throughout childhood and an enhanced understanding of FASD by family and caregivers [152]. Prevention of FASDs in future pregnancies and the ongoing support of children and families affected with FASDs require multilevel, multisystem intervention strategies to support both the child and caregiver [153–155]. A multidimensional intervention approach should include community education, interventions with caregivers if there is a history of ongoing alcohol abuse, and a focus on parenting [156]. There is evidence to suggest that children with a history of prenatal alcohol exposure benefit from interventions to promote optimal caregiving [4] and that long-term outcomes of children with FASDs are related to the quality and stability of the caregiving environment and level of family functioning [157].

For children with FASDs who remain in the care of their biological parent(s), additional factors should be considered. It is not uncommon for biological mothers with a child exposed to alcohol in utero to report a lack of knowledge about FASDs and to report consumption of alcohol before knowing she was pregnant [158]. Birth mothers also acknowledge feelings of guilt and culpability regarding having "caused" their child's disability, report feeling judged and abandoned by medical and health professionals, and describe feeling alone as they navigate through the educational system to advocate for their child's needs [157, 158]. Interventions with children and their biological caregivers should include a sensitivity to the parent's grief related to the child's diagnosis of an alcohol-related disorder and should consider opportunities to foster the biological parent's sense of competence and efficacy regarding their role in optimizing their child's future outcomes, despite the history of prenatal alcohol exposure.

For all children at risk for FASD, but particularly children with a history of removal from the biological parents (e.g., children in the child welfare system, or children who have been adopted), one should consider the possibility of co-occurring trauma. For individuals who have a history of prenatal alcohol exposure and early childhood adversity, outcomes are optimized with early diagnosis and initiation of targeted developmental, behavioral, and trauma-focused interventions. Interventions should be individualized to the needs of the child and should include interventions to address areas of developmental vulnerability, as well as behavioral- and trauma-focused psychotherapies (to address behavioral symptoms that may be associated with experiences of early pathological care). Through a combination of cognitive, behavioral, and psychosocial strategies, interventions should foster regulatory, relational, emotional, and cognitive functioning while addressing underlying trauma that can contribute to deficits in emotional regulation [159].

Because of the challenges associated with raising a child with a history of prenatal alcohol exposure, attention should be paid to ensure that caregivers have access to social and respite supports. The profile of behavioral, psychological, and cognitive symptoms in this population may make children with FASDs more challenging to parent [160]. As such, caregivers should be educated about the neurological differences of children with FASDs and the deficits that they may manifest in the areas of learning, working memory, executive functioning, processing speed, and behavioral and emotional control, all of which can contribute to maladaptive parent-child interactions and lead to compromised parent-child relationships [161]. Caregivers should also be counseled about the importance of providing responsive, nurturing, and contingent interactions with their children with a history of FASDs and the potential benefits of behaviorally oriented and relationship-focused interventions [160]. In addition, interventions should include a focus on anticipatory guidance, family support, and safety recommendations [162]. Optimal outcomes have been associated with interventions that have included parent education or training; child-directed teaching, with an emphasis on teaching children specific skills they would usually learn by observation or abstraction; and integration into existing systems of treatment [163]. Providers should be attentive to risk factors associated with worse neuropsychiatric outcomes in children with FASD, including a history of trauma, institutionalization, and placement in residential care [164]. In situations where the child is unable to be cared for in the home setting due to severely dysregulated or deviant behaviors, alternative placements should be considered that will optimize the child's safety and facilitate access to comprehensive care and ongoing medical and psychological treatment.

Appendix

Sample Interview Questions to Query for Prenatal Alcohol Exposure

1. How many weeks pregnant were you when you learned of your pregnancy?
2. In the 3 months prior to pregnancy, how many drinks would you typically consume in a week? (*Prompt further, 10–15 drinks? 15–20 drinks?* Etc.)
3. Before you learned of your pregnancy, how many drinks did you drink in one sitting? (*Prompt further, 5–10 drinks? 10–15 drinks?* Etc.)

References

1. Walker SP, Wachs TD, Grantham-McGregor S, et al. Inequality in early childhood: risk and protective factors for early child development. Lancet. 2011;378(9799):1325–38.
2. Wachs TD. Known and potential processes underlying developmental trajectories in childhood and adolescence. Dev Psychol. 1996;32(4):796.
3. Wachs TD. Expanding our view of context: the bio-ecological environment and development. Adv Child Dev. 2003;31:363–409.
4. Molteno CD, Jacobson JL, Carter RC, Jacobson SW. Infant symbolic play as an early indicator of fetal alcohol-related deficit. Infancy. 2010;15(6):586–607.
5. May PA, Baete A, Russo J, et al. Prevalence and characteristics of fetal alcohol spectrum disorders. Pediatrics. 2014;134(5):855–66.
6. Chasnoff IJ, Wells AM, King L. Misdiagnosis and missed diagnoses in foster and Adopted children with prenatal alcohol exposure. Pediatrics. 2015;135(2):264–70.
7. Fast DK, Conry J. Fetal alcohol spectrum disorders and the criminal justice system. Dev Disabil Res Rev. 2009;15(3):250–7.
8. Hoyme HE, Kalberg WO, Elliott AJ, et al. Updated clinical guidelines for diagnosing fetal alcohol spectrum disorders. Pediatrics. 2016;138(2):e20154256.
9. Jones KL. Recognition of the fetal alcohol syndrome in early infancy. Lancet. 1973;302(7836):999.
10. Jones KL, Smith DW. The fetal alcohol syndrome. Teratology. 1975;12(1):1–10.
11. Hoyme HE, May PA, Kalberg WO, et al. A practical clinical approach to diagnosis of fetal alcohol spectrum disorders: clarification of the 1996 institute of medicine criteria. Pediatrics. 2005;115(1):39–47.
12. Manning MA, Eugene Hoyme H. Fetal alcohol spectrum disorders: a practical clinical approach to diagnosis. Neurosci Biobehav Rev. 2007;31(2):230–8.
13. Rojmahamongkol P, Cheema-Hasan A, Weitzman C. Do pediatricians recognize fetal alcohol spectrum disorders in children with developmental and behavioral problems? J Dev Behav Pediatr. 2015;36(3):197–202.
14. Elgen I, Bruaroy S, Laegreid LM. Lack of recognition and complexity of foetal alcohol neuroimpairments. Acta Paediatr. 2007;96(2):237–41.
15. Gahagan S, Sharpe TT, Brimacombe M, et al. Pediatricians' knowledge, training, and experience in the care of children with fetal alcohol syndrome. Pediatrics. 2006;118(3):e657–68.
16. Lange S, Shield K, Rehm J, Popova S. Prevalence of fetal alcohol spectrum disorders in child care settings: a meta-analysis. Pediatrics. 2013;132(4):e980–95.

17. English DJ, Thompson R, White CR. Predicting risk of entry into foster care from early childhood experiences: a survival analysis using LONGSCAN data. Child Abuse Negl. 2015;45(0):57–67.
18. Pelton LH. The continuing role of material factors in child maltreatment and placement. Child Abuse Negl. 2015;41(0):30–9.
19. Chernoff R, Combs-Orme T, Risley-Curtiss C, Heisler A. Assessing the health status of children entering foster care. Pediatrics. 1994;93(4):594–601.
20. Burd L, Cohen C, Shah R, Norris J. A court team model for young children in foster care: the role of prenatal alcohol exposure and fetal alcohol spectrum disorders. J Psychiatry Law. 2011;39(1):179–91.
21. Herrick KHL, Burd L. The elephant in the cradle: fetal alcohol spectrum disorders. Zero Three. 2011;31(3):44–50.
22. Popova S, Lange S, Burd L, Rehm J. Canadian children and youth in care: the cost of fetal alcohol spectrum disorder. Child Youth Care Forum. 2014;43(1):83–96.
23. Kvigne VL, Leonardson GR, Neff-Smith M, Brock E, Borzelleca J, Welty TK. Characteristics of children who have full or incomplete fetal alcohol syndrome. J Pediatr. 2004;145(5):635–40.
24. Centers for Disease Control and Prevention. Fetal development chart. https://www.cdc.gov/dotw/fasd/images/chart_928px.jpg. Accessed 20 Oct 2017.
25. Pruett D, Waterman EH, Caughey AB. Fetal alcohol exposure: consequences, diagnosis, and treatment. Obstet Gynecol Surv. 2013;68(1):62–9.
26. Brien JF, Smith GN. Effects of alcohol (ethanol) on the fetus. J Dev Physiol. 1991;15(1):21–32.
27. Ramanathan R, Wilkemeyer MF, Mittal B, Perides G, Charness ME. Alcohol inhibits cell-cell adhesion mediated by human L1. J Cell Biol. 1996;133(2):381–90.
28. Fitzgerald DM, Charness ME, Leite-Morris KA, Chen S. Effects of ethanol and NAP on cerebellar expression of the neural cell adhesion molecule L1. PLoS One. 2011;6(9):e24364.
29. Dou X, Menkari CE, Shanmugasundararaj S, Miller KW, Charness ME. Two alcohol binding residues interact across a domain interface of the L1 neural cell adhesion molecule and regulate cell adhesion. J Biol Chem. 2011;286(18):16131–9.
30. Ramachandran V, Perez A, Chen J, Senthil D, Schenker S, Henderson GI. In utero ethanol exposure causes mitochondrial dysfunction, which can result in apoptotic cell death in fetal brain: a potential role for 4-hydroxynonenal. Alcohol Clin Exp Res. 2001;25(6):862–71.
31. Ramachandran V, Watts LT, Maffi SK, Chen J, Schenker S, Henderson G. Ethanol-induced oxidative stress precedes mitochondrially mediated apoptotic death of cultured fetal cortical neurons. J Neurosci Res. 2003;74(4):577–88.
32. Cohen-Kerem R, Koren G. Antioxidants and fetal protection against ethanol teratogenicity. I. Review of the experimental data and implications to humans. Neurotoxicol Teratol. 2003;25(1):1–9.
33. Boyadjieva NI, Sarkar DK. Microglia play a role in ethanol-induced oxidative stress and apoptosis in developing hypothalamic neurons. Alcohol Clin Exp Res. 2013;37(2):252–62.
34. Nakatsuji N. Craniofacial malformation in *Xenopus laevis* tadpoles caused by the exposure of early embryos to ethanol. Teratology. 1983;28(2):299–305.
35. Lossie AC, Muir WM, Lo CL, et al. Implications of genomic signatures in the differential vulnerability to fetal alcohol exposure in C57BL/6 and DBA/2 mice. Front Genet. 2014;5:173.
36. Lussier AA, Weinberg J, Kobor MS. Epigenetics studies of fetal alcohol spectrum disorder: where are we now? Epigenomics. 2017;9(3):291–311.
37. Balaraman S, Schafer JJ, Tseng AM, et al. Plasma miRNA profiles in pregnant women predict infant outcomes following prenatal alcohol exposure. PLoS One. 2016;11(11):e0165081.
38. Astley SJSJ. Validation of the fetal alcohol spectrum disorder (FASD) 4-digit diagnostic code. J Popul Ther Clin Pharmacol. 2013;20(3):e416.
39. Chudley AE, Conry J, Cook JL, et al. Fetal alcohol spectrum disorder: Canadian guidelines for diagnosis. CMAJ. 2005;172(5 Suppl):S1–S21.
40. Bertrand JJ. Guidelines for identifying and referring persons with fetal alcohol syndrome. MMWR Recomm Rep. 2005;54(rr-11):1.

41. Moore ES, Ward RE, Wetherill LF, et al. Unique facial features distinguish fetal alcohol syndrome patients and controls in diverse ethnic populations. Alcohol Clin Exp Res. 2007;31(10):1707–13.
42. May PA, Fiorentino D, Coriale G, et al. Prevalence of children with severe fetal alcohol spectrum disorders in communities near Rome, Italy: new estimated rates are higher than previous estimates. Int J Environ Res Public Health. 2011;8(6):2331–51.
43. Autti-Rämö I, Fagerlund Å, Ervalahti N, Loimu L, Korkman M, Hoyme HE. Fetal alcohol spectrum disorders in Finland: clinical delineation of 77 older children and adolescents. Am J Med Genet A. 2006;140((2):137–43.
44. May PA, Blankenship J, Marais AS, et al. Approaching the prevalence of the full spectrum of fetal alcohol Spectrum disorders in a South African population-based study. Alcohol Clin Exp Res. 2013;37(5):818–30.
45. O'Connor MJ, Rotheram-Borus MJ, Tomlinson M, Bill C, LeRoux IM, Stewart IM. Screening for fetal alcohol spectrum disorders by nonmedical community workers. J Popul Ther Clin Pharmacol. 2014;21(3):e442.
46. Jones KL, Robinson LK, Bakhireva LN, et al. Accuracy of the diagnosis of physical features of fetal alcohol syndrome by pediatricians after specialized training. Pediatrics. 2006;118(6):e1734–8.
47. Caputo C, Wood E, Jabbour L. Impact of fetal alcohol exposure on body systems: a systematic review. Birth Defects Res C Embryo Today. 2016;108(2):174–80.
48. Warren KR, Foudin LL. Alcohol-related birth defects—the past, present, and future. Alcohol Res Health. 2001;25(3):153–8.
49. Makelarski JA, Romitti PA, Sun L, et al. Periconceptional maternal alcohol consumption and neural tube defects. Birth Defects Res A Clin Mol Teratol. 2013;97(3):152–60.
50. Jacobson SW, Chiodo LM, Sokol RJ, Jacobson JL. Validity of maternal report of prenatal alcohol, cocaine, and smoking in relation to neurobehavioral outcome. Pediatrics. 2002;109(5):815–25.
51. Czeizel AEA. Smoking and alcohol drinking during pregnancy. The reliability of retrospective maternal self-reported information. Cent Eur J Public Health. 2005;12(4):179.
52. Lange S, Shield K, Koren G, Rehm J, Popova S. A comparison of the prevalence of prenatal alcohol exposure obtained via maternal self-reports versus meconium testing: a systematic literature review and meta-analysis. BMC Pregnancy Childbirth. 2014;14:127.
53. Knudsen AK, Skogen JC, Ystrom E, Sivertsen B, Tell GS, Torgersen L. Maternal pre-pregnancy risk drinking and toddler behavior problems: the Norwegian mother and child cohort study. Eur Child Adolesc Psychiatry. 2014;23(10):901–11.
54. May PA, Blankenship J, Marais A-S, et al. Maternal alcohol consumption producing fetal alcohol spectrum disorders (FASD): quantity, frequency, and timing of drinking. Drug Alcohol Depend. 2013;133(2):502–12.
55. Chiodo LM, Delaney-Black V, Sokol RJ, Janisse J, Pardo Y, Hannigan JH. Increased cut-point of the TACER-3 screen reduces false positives without losing sensitivity in predicting risk alcohol drinking in pregnancy. Alcohol Clin Exp Res. 2014;38(5):1401–8.
56. Sobell LC, Sobell MB, Leo GI, Cancilla A. Reliability of a timeline method: assessing normal drinkers' reports of recent drinking and a comparative evaluation across several populations. Br J Addict. 1988;83(4):393–402.
57. Sobell LC, Agrawal S, Annis H, et al. Cross-cultural evaluation of two drinking assessment instruments: alcohol timeline followback and inventory of drinking situations. Subst Use Misuse. 2001;36(3):313–31.
58. Jones KL, Hoyme HE, Robinson LK, et al. Fetal alcohol spectrum disorders: extending the range of structural defects. Am J Med Genet A. 2010;152A(11):2731–5.
59. Thomason ME, Marusak HA. Toward understanding the impact of trauma on the early developing human brain. Neuroscience. 2017;342:55–67.
60. Mattson SN, Riley EP. The quest for a neurobehavioral profile of heavy prenatal alcohol exposure. Alcohol Res Health. 2011;34(1):51–5.

61. Mattson SN, Roesch SC, Fagerlund Å, et al. Toward a neurobehavioral profile of fetal alcohol spectrum disorders. Alcohol Clin Exp Res. 2010;34(9):1640–50.
62. Mattson SN, Roesch SC, Glass L, et al. Further development of a neurobehavioral profile of fetal alcohol spectrum disorders. Alcohol Clin Exp Res. 2013;37(3):517–28.
63. Riley EP, McGee CL, Sowell ER. Teratogenic effects of alcohol: a decade of brain imaging. Am J Med Genet C Semin Med Genet. 2004;127c(1):35–41.
64. Norman AL, Crocker N, Mattson SN, Riley EP. Neuroimaging and fetal alcohol spectrum disorders. Dev Disabil Res Rev. 2009;15(3):209–17.
65. Fryer SL, Schweinsburg BC, Bjorkquist OA, et al. Characterization of white matter microstructure in fetal alcohol spectrum disorders. Alcohol Clin Exp Res. 2009;33(3):514–21.
66. Guerri C. Neuroanatomical and neurophysiological mechanisms involved in central nervous system dysfunctions induced by prenatal alcohol exposure. Alcohol Clin Exp Res. 1998;22(2):304–12.
67. Roebuck TM, Mattson SN, Riley EP. A review of the neuroanatomical findings in children with fetal alcohol syndrome or prenatal exposure to alcohol. Alcohol Clin Exp Res. 1998;22(2):339–44.
68. Mattson SN, Schoenfeld AM, Riley EP. Teratogenic effects of alcohol on brain and behavior. Alcohol Res Health. 2001;25(3):185–91.
69. Niccols A. Fetal alcohol syndrome and the developing socio-emotional brain. Brain Cogn. 2007;65(1):135–42.
70. Lebel C, Mattson SN, Riley EP, et al. A longitudinal study of the long-term consequences of drinking during pregnancy: heavy in utero alcohol exposure disrupts the normal processes of brain development. J Neurosci. 2012;32(44):15243–51.
71. Rajaprakash M, Chakravarty MM, Lerch JP, Rovet J. Cortical morphology in children with alcohol-related neurodevelopmental disorder. Brain Behav. 2014;4(1):41–50.
72. Donald KA, Fouche JP, Roos A, et al. Alcohol exposure in utero is associated with decreased gray matter volume in neonates. Metab Brain Dis. 2016;31(1):81–91.
73. Sowell ER, Johnson A, Kan E, et al. Mapping white matter integrity and neurobehavioral correlates in children with fetal alcohol spectrum disorders. J Neurosci. 2008;28(6):1313–9.
74. Kodituwakku PW, Kalberg W, May PA. The effects of prenatal alcohol exposure on executive functioning. Alcohol Res Health. 2001;25(3):192–8.
75. Gautam P, Nunez SC, Narr KL, et al. Developmental trajectories for visuo-spatial attention are altered by prenatal alcohol exposure: a longitudinal FMRI study. Cereb Cortex. 2015;25(12):4761–71.
76. Kodali VN, Jacobson JL, Lindinger NM, et al. Differential recruitment of brain regions during response inhibition in children prenatally exposed to alcohol. Alcohol Clin Exp Res. 2017;41(2):334–44.
77. Wozniak JR, Muetzel RL. What does diffusion tensor imaging reveal about the brain and cognition in fetal alcohol spectrum disorders? Neuropsychol Rev. 2011;21(2):133–47.
78. Wozniak JR, Mueller BA, Muetzel RL, et al. Inter-hemispheric functional connectivity disruption in children with prenatal alcohol exposure. Alcohol Clin Exp Res. 2011;35(5):849–61.
79. Coles CD, Goldstein FC, Lynch ME, et al. Memory and brain volume in adults prenatally exposed to alcohol. Brain Cogn. 2011;75(1):67–77.
80. Willoughby KA, Sheard ED, Nash K, Rovet J. Effects of prenatal alcohol exposure on hippocampal volume, verbal learning, and verbal and spatial recall in late childhood. J Int Neuropsychol Soc. 2008;14(6):1022–33.
81. Willford J, Day R, Aizenstein H, Day N. Caudate asymmetry: a neurobiological marker of moderate prenatal alcohol exposure in young adults. Neurotoxicol Teratol. 2010;32(6):589–94.
82. Khoury JE, Milligan K, Girard TA. Executive functioning in children and adolescents prenatally exposed to alcohol: a meta-analytic review. Neuropsychol Rev. 2015;25(2):149–70.
83. Gerhold MM, Jacobson SW, Jacobson JL, Molteno CD, Meintjes EM, Andrew CM. An ERP study of response inhibition in the auditory domain in children with fetal alcohol spectrum disorders. Alcohol Clin Exp Res. 2017;41(1):96–106.

84. Roos LE, Beauchamp KG, Pears KC, Fisher PA, Berkman ET, Capaldi D. Effects of prenatal substance exposure on neurocognitive correlates of inhibitory control success and failure. Appl Neuropsychol Child. 2017;6(4):269–80.
85. du Plooy CP, Malcolm-Smith S, Adnams CM, Stein DJ, Donald KA. The effects of prenatal alcohol exposure on episodic memory functioning: a systematic review. Arch Clin Neuropsychol. 2016;31(7):710–26.
86. Fryer SL, Mattson SN, Jernigan TL, Archibald SL, Jones KL, Riley EP. Caudate volume predicts neurocognitive performance in youth with heavy prenatal alcohol exposure. Alcohol Clin Exp Res. 2012;36(11):1932–41.
87. Donald KA, Eastman E, Howells FM, et al. Neuroimaging effects of prenatal alcohol exposure on the developing human brain: a magnetic resonance imaging review. Acta Neuropsychiatr. 2015;27(5):251–69.
88. Meintjes EM, Narr KL, van der Kouwe AJ, et al. A tensor-based morphometry analysis of regional differences in brain volume in relation to prenatal alcohol exposure. NeuroImage Clin. 2014;5:152–60.
89. Luo J. Effects of ethanol on the cerebellum: advances and prospects. Cerebellum. 2015;14(4):383–5.
90. Valenzuela CF, Lindquist B, Zamudio-Bulcock PA. A review of synaptic plasticity at Purkinje neurons with a focus on ethanol-induced cerebellar dysfunction. Int Rev Neurobiol. 2010;91:339–72.
91. Jacobson SW, Jacobson JL, Molteno CD, et al. Heavy prenatal alcohol exposure is related to smaller corpus callosum in newborn MRI scans. Alcohol Clin Exp Res. 2017;41(5):965–75.
92. Wozniak JR, Muetzel RL, Mueller BA, et al. Microstructural corpus callosum anomalies in children with prenatal alcohol exposure: an extension of previous diffusion tensor imaging findings. Alcohol Clin Exp Res. 2009;33(10):1825–35.
93. Dodge NC, Jacobson JL, Molteno CD, et al. Prenatal alcohol exposure and interhemispheric transfer of tactile information: Detroit and Cape Town findings. Alcohol Clin Exp Res. 2009;33(9):1628–37.
94. Kable JA, O'Connor MJ, Olson HC, et al. Neurobehavioral disorder associated with prenatal alcohol exposure (ND-PAE): proposed DSM-5 diagnosis. Child Psychiatry Hum Dev. 2016;47(2):335–46.
95. Doyle LR, Mattson SN. Neurobehavioral disorder associated with prenatal alcohol exposure (ND-PAE): review of evidence and guidelines for assessment. Curr Dev Disord Rep. 2015;2(3):175–86.
96. Hagan JF, Balachova T, Bertrand J, et al. Neurobehavioral disorder associated with prenatal alcohol exposure. Pediatrics. 2016;138(4):e20151553.
97. Kable JA, Mukherjee RA. Neurodevelopmental disorder associated with prenatal exposure to alcohol (ND-PAE): a proposed diagnostic method of capturing the neurocognitive phenotype of FASD. Eur J Med Genet. 2017;60(1):49–54.
98. Coles CD, Smith IE, Falek A. Prenatal alcohol exposure and infant behavior: immediate effects and implications for later development. Adv Alcohol Subst Abuse. 1987;6(4):87–104.
99. Jacobson JL, Jacobson SW, Sokol RJ, Martier SS, Ager JW, Kaplan-Estrin MG. Teratogenic effects of alcohol on infant development. Alcohol Clin Exp Res. 1993;17(1):174–83.
100. Jacobson SW, Jacobson JL, Sokol RJ. Effects of fetal alcohol exposure on infant reaction time. Alcohol Clin Exp Res. 1994;18(5):1125–32.
101. Coles CD, Kable JA, Drews-Botsch C, Falek A. Early identification of risk for effects of prenatal alcohol exposure. J Stud Alcohol. 2000;61(4):607–16.
102. Molteno CD, Jacobson JL, Carter RC, Dodge NC, Jacobson SW. Infant emotional withdrawal: a precursor of affective and cognitive disturbance in fetal alcohol spectrum disorders. Alcohol Clin Exp Res. 2014;38(2):479–88.
103. Streissguth AP, Sampson PD, Barr HM. Neurobehavioral dose-response effects of prenatal alcohol exposure in humans from infancy to adulthood. Ann N Y Acad Sci. 1989;562(1):145–58.

104. Kalberg WO, Provost B, Tollison SJ, et al. Comparison of motor delays in young children with fetal alcohol syndrome to those with prenatal alcohol exposure and with no prenatal alcohol exposure. Alcohol Clin Exp Res. 2006;30(12):2037–45.
105. Lucas BR, Latimer J, Pinto RZ, et al. Gross motor deficits in children prenatally exposed to alcohol: a meta-analysis. Pediatrics. 2014;134(1):e192–209.
106. McGee CL, Bjorkquist OA, Riley EP, Mattson SN. Impaired language performance in young children with heavy prenatal alcohol exposure. Neurotoxicol Teratol. 2009;31(2):71–5.
107. Cone-Wesson B. Prenatal alcohol and cocaine exposure: influences on cognition, speech, language, and hearing. J Commun Disord. 2005;38(4):279–302.
108. Stephen JM, Kodituwakku PW, Kodituwakku EL, et al. Delays in auditory processing identified in preschool children with FASD. Alcohol Clin Exp Res. 2012;36(10):1720–7.
109. Fuglestad AJ, Whitley ML, Carlson SM, et al. Executive functioning deficits in preschool children with fetal alcohol spectrum disorders. Child Neuropsychol. 2015;21(6):716–31.
110. D'Onofrio BM, Van Hulle CA, Waldman ID, Rodgers JL, Rathouz PJ, Lahey BB. Causal inferences regarding prenatal alcohol exposure and childhood externalizing problems. Arch Gen Psychiatry. 2007;64(11):1296–304.
111. Alvik A, Aalen OO, Lindemann R. Early fetal binge alcohol exposure predicts high behavioral symptom scores in 5.5-year-old children. Alcohol Clin Exp Res. 2013;37(11):1954–62.
112. Rasmussen C, Becker M, McLennan J, Urichuk L, Andrew G. An evaluation of social skills in children with and without prenatal alcohol exposure. Child Care Health Dev. 2011;37(5):711–8.
113. Chen ML, Olson HC, Picciano JF, Starr JR, Owens J. Sleep problems in children with fetal alcohol spectrum disorders. J Clin Sleep Med. 2012;8(4):421–9.
114. Carr JL, Agnihotri S, Keightley M. Sensory processing and adaptive behavior deficits of children across the fetal alcohol spectrum disorder continuum. Alcohol Clin Exp Res. 2010;34(6):1022–32.
115. Lenroot RK, Giedd JN. Brain development in children and adolescents: insights from anatomical magnetic resonance imaging. Neurosci Biobehav Rev. 2006;30(6):718–29.
116. Roussotte FF, Sulik KK, Mattson SN, et al. Regional brain volume reductions relate to facial dysmorphology and neurocognitive function in fetal alcohol spectrum disorders. Hum Brain Mapp. 2012;33(4):920–37.
117. Gautam P, Lebel C, Narr KL, et al. Volume changes and brain-behavior relationships in white matter and subcortical gray matter in children with prenatal alcohol exposure. Hum Brain Mapp. 2015;36(6):2318–29.
118. O'Leary CM, Taylor C, Zubrick SR, Kurinczuk JJ, Bower C. Prenatal alcohol exposure and educational achievement in children aged 8-9 years. Pediatrics. 2013;132(2):e468–75.
119. Carter RC, Jacobson JL, Molteno CD, Dodge NC, Meintjes EM, Jacobson SW. Fetal alcohol growth restriction and cognitive impairment. Pediatrics. 2016;138(2):e20160775.
120. Lewis CE, Thomas KG, Molteno CD, et al. Prospective memory impairment in children with prenatal alcohol exposure. Alcohol Clin Exp Res. 2016;40(5):969–78.
121. Tsang TW, Lucas BR, Carmichael Olson H, Pinto RZ, Elliott EJ. Prenatal alcohol exposure, FASD, and child behavior: a meta-analysis. Pediatrics. 2016;137(3):e20152542.
122. Glass L, Graham DM, Deweese BN, Jones KL, Riley EP, Mattson SN. Correspondence of parent report and laboratory measures of inattention and hyperactivity in children with heavy prenatal alcohol exposure. Neurotoxicol Teratol. 2014;42:43–50.
123. Kully-Martens K, Denys K, Treit S, Tamana S, Rasmussen C. A review of social skills deficits in individuals with fetal alcohol spectrum disorders and prenatal alcohol exposure: profiles, mechanisms, and interventions. Alcohol Clin Exp Res. 2012;36(4):568–76.
124. Keil V, Paley B, Frankel F, O'Connor MJ. Impact of a social skills intervention on the hostile attributions of children with prenatal alcohol exposure. Alcohol Clin Exp Res. 2010;34(2):231–41.
125. Kerns KA, Siklos S, Baker L, Muller U. Emotion recognition in children with fetal alcohol spectrum disorders. Child Neuropsychol. 2016;22(3):255–75.

126. Casey BJ, Getz S, Galvan A. The adolescent brain. Dev Rev. 2008;28(1):62–77.
127. Migliorini R, Moore EM, Glass L, et al. Anterior cingulate cortex surface area relates to behavioral inhibition in adolescents with and without heavy prenatal alcohol exposure. Behav Brain Res. 2015;292:26–35.
128. Day NL, Helsel A, Sonon K, Goldschmidt L. The association between prenatal alcohol exposure and behavior at 22 years of age. Alcohol Clin Exp Res. 2013;37(7):1171–8.
129. Moore EM, Riley EP. What happens when children with Fetal alcohol Spectrum disorders become adults? Curr Dev Disord Rep. 2015;2(3):219–27.
130. Lindinger NM, Malcolm-Smith S, Dodge NC, et al. Theory of mind in children with fetal alcohol spectrum disorders. Alcohol Clin Exp Res. 2016;40(2):367–76.
131. Stevens SA, Clairman H, Nash K, Rovet J. Social perception in children with fetal alcohol spectrum disorder. Child Neuropsychol. 2017;23(8):980–93.
132. Mattson SN, Riley EP. A review of the neurobehavioral deficits in children with fetal alcohol syndrome or prenatal exposure to alcohol. Alcohol Clin Exp Res. 1998;22(2):279.
133. Coles CD. Discriminating the effects of prenatal alcohol exposure from other behavioral and learning disorders. Alcohol Res Health. 2011;34(1):42.
134. Graham DM, Crocker N, Deweese BN, et al. Prenatal alcohol exposure, ADHD, and sluggish cognitive tempo. Alcohol Clin Exp Res. 2013;37(Suppl 1):E338–46.
135. Stevens SA, Nash K, Koren G, Rovet J. Autism characteristics in children with fetal alcohol spectrum disorders. Child Neuropsychol. 2013;19(6):579–87.
136. Bishop S, Gahagan S, Lord C. Re-examining the core features of autism: a comparison of autism spectrum disorder and fetal alcohol spectrum disorder. J Child Psychol Psychiatry. 2007;48(11):1111–21.
137. Miller LC, Chan W, Litvinova A, Rubin A, Tirella L, Cermak S. Medical diagnoses and growth of children residing in Russian orphanages. Acta paediatr. 2007;96(12):1765–9.
138. Miller LC, Chan W, Litvinova A, et al. Fetal alcohol spectrum disorders in children residing in Russian orphanages: a phenotypic survey. Alcohol Clin Exp Res. 2006;30(3):531–8.
139. Chisholm K, Carter MC, Ames EW, Morison SJ. Attachment security and indiscriminately friendly behavior in children adopted from Romanian orphanages. Dev Psychopathol. 2009;7(2):283–94.
140. Rutter M, Colvert E, Kreppner J, et al. Early adolescent outcomes for institutionally-deprived and non-deprived adoptees. I: disinhibited attachment. J Child Psychol Psychiatry. 2007;48(1):17–30.
141. Smyke AT, Zeanah CH, Gleason MM, et al. A randomized controlled trial comparing foster care and institutional care for children with signs of reactive attachment disorder. Am J Psychiatr. 2012;169(5):508–14.
142. Zeanah CH, Smyke AT, Koga SF, Carlson E, The Bucharest Early Intervention Project Core Group. Attachment in institutionalized and community children in Romania. Child Dev. 2005;76(5):1015–28.
143. van der Kolk BA, Roth S, Pelcovitz D, Sunday S, Spinazzola J. Disorders of extreme stress: the empirical foundation of a complex adaptation to trauma. J Trauma Stress. 2005;18(5):389–99.
144. Ackerman PT, Newton JE, McPherson WB, Jones JG, Dykman RA. Prevalence of post traumatic stress disorder and other psychiatric diagnoses in three groups of abused children (sexual, physical, and both). Child Abuse Negl. 1998;22(8):759–74.
145. Kable JA, Coles CD. Evidence supporting the internal validity of the proposed ND-PAE disorder. Child Psychiatry Hum Dev. 2018;49(2):163–75.
146. Rutter M, Andersen-Wood L, Beckett C, et al. Quasi-autistic patterns following severe early global privation. J Child Psychol Psychiatry Allied Discip. 1999;40(4):537.
147. Rutter M, Kreppner J, Croft C, et al. Early adolescent outcomes of institutionally deprived and non-deprived adoptees. III. Quasi-autism. J Child Psychol Psychiatry. 2007;48(12):1200–7.
148. Brown NN, Burd L, Grant T, Edwards W, Adler R, Streissguth A. Prenatal alcohol exposure: an assessment strategy for the legal context. Int J Law Psychiatry. 2015;42-43:144–8.

149. Mutch RC, Jones HM, Bower C, Watkins RE. Fetal alcohol spectrum disorders: using knowledge, attitudes and practice of justice professionals to support their educational needs. J Popul Ther Clin Pharmacol. 2016;23(1):e77–89.
150. Fisher PA, Beauchamp KG, Roos LE, Noll LK, Flannery J, Delker BC. The neurobiology of intervention and prevention in early adversity. Annu Rev Clin Psychol. 2016;12:331–57.
151. Abrams SE. Interventions that protect. Public Health Nurs. 2010;27(3):201–2.
152. Currie BA, Hoy J, Legge L, Temple VK, Tahir M. Adults with fetal alcohol Spectrum disorder: factors associated with positive outcomes and contact with the criminal justice system. J Popul Ther Clin Pharmacol. 2016;23(1):e37–52.
153. Clarke-McMullen DM. Evaluation of a successful fetal alcohol spectrum disorder coalition in Ontario, Canada. Public Health Nurs. 2010;27(3):240–7.
154. Paley B, O'Connor MJ, Frankel F, Marquardt R. Predictors of stress in parents of children with fetal alcohol spectrum disorders. J Dev Behav Pediatr. 2006;27(5):396–404.
155. May PA. A multiple-level, comprehensive approach to the prevention of fetal alcohol syndrome (FAS) and other alcohol-related birth defects (ARBD). Int J Addict. 1995;30(12):1549.
156. Smith IEI. Multilevel intervention for prevention of fetal alcohol syndrome and effects of prenatal alcohol exposure. Recent Dev Alcohol. 1991;9:165.
157. Olson HC, Oti R, Gelo J, Beck S. "Family matters:" Fetal alcohol spectrum disorders and the family. Dev Disabil Res Rev. 2009;15(3):235–49.
158. Salmon JJ. Fetal alcohol spectrum disorder: New Zealand birth mothers' experiences. Can J Clin Pharmacol. 2008;15(2):e191.
159. Zarnegar Z, Hambrick EP, Perry BD, Azen SP, Peterson C. Clinical improvements in adopted children with fetal alcohol spectrum disorders through neurodevelopmentally informed clinical intervention: a pilot study. Clin Child Psychol Psychiatry. 2016;21(4):551–67.
160. Paley B, O'Connor MJ. Intervention for individuals with fetal alcohol spectrum disorders: treatment approaches and case management. Dev Disabil Res Rev. 2009;15(3):258–67.
161. O'Connor MJ, Sigman M, Kasari C. Attachment behavior of infants exposed prenatally to alcohol: mediating effects of infant affect and mother-infant interaction. Dev Psychopathol. 1992;4(02):243–56.
162. Pei J, Baugh L, Andrew G, Rasmussen C. Intervention recommendations and subsequent access to services following clinical assessment for fetal alcohol spectrum disorders. Res Dev Disabil. 2017;60:176–86.
163. Bertrand J. Interventions for children with fetal alcohol spectrum disorders (FASDs): overview of findings for five innovative research projects. Res Dev Disabil. 2009;30(5):986–1006.
164. Fagerlund A, Autti-Ramo I, Hoyme HE, Mattson SN, Korkman M. Risk factors for behavioural problems in foetal alcohol spectrum disorders. Acta Paediatr. 2011;100(11):1481–8.
165. Hoyme HE, Hoyme DB, Elliott AJ, et al. A South African mixed race lip/philtrum guide for diagnosis of fetal alcohol spectrum disorders. Am J Med Genet A. 2015;0(4):752–5.

Chapter 7
Interventions for Trauma- and Stressor-Related Disorders in Preschool-Aged Children

Kelley Munger, Elizabeth C. Loi, and Amelia Roth

> **Vignette #1**
> "Sally" is a vivacious 5-year-old girl who has been placed in a new therapeutic classroom at the Relief Nursery, a program designed for children with significant behavioral challenges. She had been attending Head Start, but her behaviors were determined to be too unmanageable for that environment, prompting the referral. Her teachers and therapists at the Relief Nursery believe she has an autism spectrum disorder (ASD), as she is rigid, impulsive, directive, and aggressive, hoards, often lacks remorse, and has great difficulty engaging successfully with her peers. Drs. Roth and Phelps were consulted to provide diagnostic assessment regarding this question of ASD.
>
> Sally was exposed to methamphetamines and heroin during her first trimester of gestation, until her mother entered a rehabilitation program. She lives with her maternal grandparents, with whom she has lived for most of her life. Sally's mother had been intermittently involved with her and then took Sally from her grandparents' home around the time of her second birthday. During a 3-month span of time, mother and daughter lived together in a hotel with mother's abusive boyfriend, subjecting Sally to drug use and culture, prostitution, neglect, and frequent domestic violence. Child protective services (CPS)

K. Munger
Early Intervention Program, University of Oregon, Eugene, OR, USA
e-mail: kmunger@uoregon.edu

E. C. Loi
Department of Psychology, University of Oregon, Eugene, OR, USA
e-mail: eloi@uoregon.edu

A. Roth (✉)
OHSU Child Development and Rehabilitation Center, Eugene, OR, USA
e-mail: rothame@ohsu.edu

J. M. Fogler, R. A. Phelps (eds.), *Trauma, Autism, and Neurodevelopmental Disorders*, https://doi.org/10.1007/978-3-030-00503-0_7

became involved, and Sally was then placed back with her maternal grandparents, with whom she has lived subsequently. Sally has not seen her mother since CPS placed her back with her grandparents, though she continues to ask about her daily, in a sad and longing manner.

Sally's mother reported to the maternal grandmother that she never really bonded to Sally, while expressing that she did bond readily to her other three children, all sons. A brother, with whom Sally has visitation frequently, often talks about his time with their mother, which is very upsetting for Sally, who openly grieves the loss of her mother. Sally's grandmother has always felt quite sorry for Sally and admits that for years she had failed to set any boundaries for Sally. However, this parenting approach has recently changed at the urging of a therapist. Now, grandmother acknowledges the importance of limit setting and providing behavioral expectations. Grandmother notes that this has worked well and that Sally's behavior has improved significantly (after an initial extinction burst) in only a matter of months. Grandmother freely admits her role in Sally's behavioral difficulties, having initially, inadvertently, reinforced her negative behaviors.

In the classroom, Sally is observed to be talkative and interactive and demonstrates excellent social reciprocity and referencing. She has a reactive affect, appears to have a sense of humor, enjoys imitation, makes frequent eye contact and social referencing, and exhibits joint attention and shared enjoyment. She displays typical prosody of speech and vernacular and engages peers and teachers easily. Drs. Roth and Phelps conclude that Sally's developmental challenges are best conceptualized as a trauma- and stressor-related disorder, as opposed to an ASD, and communicate this impression to Sally's therapist, to which he replies (*somewhat* tongue-in-cheek), "Well, you're wrong!". As Sally graduates from her therapeutic preschool and moves on to a public school kindergarten, her grandmother decides to discontinue necessary mental health treatments, feeling these might set her apart as "different" from other kids. Might her grandmother's attitude toward treatments be different had Sally been diagnosed with an ASD?

Vignette #2

Mark is an energetic 5-year-old boy who presents for a full team evaluation for a possible autism spectrum disorder, strongly suspected by both his school and mother. He is accompanied by his mother and maternal grandparents. The mother is well spoken and able to effectively articulate her many concerns about Mark during a private interview. Her greatest concerns surround his propensity toward violence, sexualized behaviors, hyperactivity and frequent inattention, repetitive behaviors including rocking and flapping, behavioral rigidities, fixation on and unusual level of interest in gems/crystals, and decreased imaginative play. He tends to be irritable and has frequent tantrums, and his aggressive behaviors often appear unprompted. He killed the family hamster recently by throwing it against the wall when angry and has never expressed remorse. He has threatened to kill his dad and makes frequent disturbing comments such as "I want to chop off people's privates and set things on fire." He tends to get into many fights at school and is actually very sneaky about it, covertly hurting/antagonizing others while attempting to avoid punishment. He lies frequently, confabulates elaborate stories, and is prone to running off in an unsafe manner. He has no history of early developmental delays aside from those related to social and emotional functioning. He engages best with peers during physical play and has a strong desire for friends and playmates, though is generally feared by his peers. He lacks personal boundary awareness and is overly friendly with strangers, even being described as a child who might "go home with a complete stranger." He prefers to play with older kids and does seek affection and praise from adults. He tends to be very manipulative with others, as well as inappropriate. He has touched other children's bottoms at school and has a history of "crushing" other children's genitals with his fist, starting in preschool. Mother feels he seems to pick out "weaker" kids to fight with, and he requires constant supervision to keep other children safe.

He was observed in clinic to engage in rough, repetitive play, had infrequent stereotypies, and initially displayed diminished eye contact with examiners. As he warmed up throughout the day, his eye contact improved, and he engaged easily in typical social reciprocity and social referencing throughout the remainder of the day. His repetitive movements diminished as the day progressed, and he displayed a reactive affect during engagement with providers, as well as typical prosody of speech and use of vernacular.

His past medical history is significant for a low initial APGAR score of 3, related to a nuchal cord, with his 5-min score rising to a 7 and without need for NICU. The only toxic in utero exposures revealed were early tobacco use and one cocktail-type drink during the 1st 8 weeks of gestation, prior to mother's knowledge of the pregnancy. He eats well and has grown appropriately. He wakes frequently overnight due to hypervigilance with the need for reassurance from fears. Mother denied Mark having endured any significant past trauma or major social stressors during her interview with the developmental pediatricians.

Mark participated in an assessment using the Autism Diagnostic Observation Schedule, which was found to be clearly inconsistent with an autism spectrum disorder. His structured parent interview (based on DSM-5 criteria) with mother alone was only borderline consistent with an autism spectrum disorder. Many of her answers regarding his behaviors suggestive of autism did not correlate with behaviors directly observed during the clinic day. His full-scale IQ was in the borderline impaired range; though given his extremely oppositional behaviors, this was felt to be a gross underestimate of his true abilities. Fine motor skills and language skills both tested in the average range, and he was noted to have significant sensory seeking and sensory avoidant behaviors. His adaptive skills were found to be in the average range.

The team's medical social worker was able to engage the maternal grandparents in a scheduled interview, during which they revealed that Mark's biological father has been admitted twice to a hospital for drug-induced psychosis and that his father also carries diagnoses of alcoholism and true addictions to both video games and pornography, all of which Mark was exposed to daily during his first 2.5 years of life. It was also disclosed that his mother had a psychotic break while caring for Mark, related to cocaine use. After his biological parents separated when he was 2.5 years old, Mark was then subjected to mother's serial abusive domestic relationships, parental drug use and culture, as well as intermittent periods of homelessness.

It is interesting to note that early on in his full-day evaluation, Mark had presented as a child with a probable ASD, given history reported by his mother and initial observations. However, as the day progressed and he became more relaxed, it became clear that Mark did not in fact meet criteria for an ASD. With the additional information provided by grandparents, he was diagnosed with a trauma- and stressor-related disorder, with prominent anxiety features, ADHD, stereotypic movement disorder, and sensory modulation difficulties.

The mother was very disappointed with the lack of ASD diagnosis and especially with the recommendation to begin intensive mental health therapies for Mark and herself. She called a few months later, still having not engaged with mental health therapies, requesting a repeat ASD evaluation, as she remains certain he meets criteria and that treatments for autism, rather than trauma-based interventions, are what will improve her son's functioning.

Pediatricians are frequently asked by parents, foster parents, and other caregivers for referrals for formal autism evaluations during brief, 10–15-min medical encounters in the primary care setting. Certainly, caregivers' concerns and children's behaviors briefly noted in a sterile, anxiety-provoking medical clinic can be initially concerning for an ASD. Though some progressive clinics are starting to routinely screen for adverse childhood experiences during well and sick child checks, the possibility of childhood trauma is often not considered in determining the first avenue of referral for a child with challenging or unusual behaviors, including social and emotional delays. Long wait lists for medical autism evaluations can further delay access to appropriate therapies, while entrance into mental health therapies tends to include much shorter wait-lists.

The phenomenon of a trauma- and stressor-related disorder masquerading as an autism spectrum disorder seems poorly understood by the majority of primary caregivers, teachers, doctors, and therapists, who are the very persons responsible for identifying kids at risk for ASDs and TSRDs. There is a sense of urgency instilled in pediatricians to provide early detection of children at risk for an autism spectrum disorder, and therefore early diagnosis to ensure rapid acquisition of appropriate therapies, and thus potentially optimized developmental outcomes. However, there does not appear to be an equal sense of urgency assigned to the early identification of TSRDs, despite the growing body of evidence substantiating the biological changes that occur in pathologically stressed children, and the evidence-based therapies available to help steer their developmental trajectories toward that of typicality and health. In this chapter, we will explore the components of effective trauma treatment as well as specific interventions that have demonstrated promising results in preschool populations. Where applicable, we will review the evidence regarding the impacts of early trauma and how these evidence-based treatments were designed to address them.

Trauma Treatment With Preschoolers

In order to counteract the harmful effects of trauma on preschoolers' development, effective treatment is critical. Treatments within this area take on many different forms, with some modalities addressing biological functioning and others addressing behaviors. At this time, intervention research using biological outcome measures are limited, while research describing behavioral outcomes are relatively more common. This section reviews the clinical goals of trauma treatment in general as well as recent studies of treatments within both frameworks designed for use among young children during or around the preschool period.

Clinical Goals of Trauma Treatment

Improved Parent-Child Relationships and Parenting Skills

When trauma is a part of a child's story, the presence of a strong, nurturing, and sensitive caregiver is essential and has the potential to enhance a child's resilience in the face of trauma [1]. Young children in particular look to their caregivers to the "be the answer" in the face of uncertainty and challenge [2], and a secure parent-child relationship can provide a powerful space from which to heal from trauma. Therefore, treatments, *whenever possible,* should not only target the child but also the relational environment of the child, so that both child and parent can benefit from growth in caregivers' capacities. In a dyadic model of therapy, caregivers are supported in how to regulate the environment of the child to create felt safety, while also mentoring a child in how to regulate himself in a developmentally appropriate manner [3].

Addressing Adaptive Concerns

Trauma often impacts the adaptive development of young children, leading to symptoms such as disrupted sleep, feeding, and other problems related to self-care [4]. For instance, some children who have experienced neglect may either hoard or restrict food and may experience dysregulated sleep patterns. Multiple modalities include components that address adaptive concerns, and occupational therapy may also serve a supplemental role in children with particularly disrupted adaptive development or sensory concerns [5].

Addressing Developmental Concerns

Another important goal of treatment should be to help return a child to a healthy developmental trajectory. Trauma can have significant and long-lasting developmental impacts including cognitive, motor, adaptive, and socioemotional delays [1]. As a result, young children who have experienced trauma should receive a comprehensive developmental assessment and be referred to early intervention (EI) or early childhood special education (ECSE) services to address developmental delays. Even when developmental delays are not a pressing concern, treatment modalities should seek to empower caregivers in understanding an individual developmental trajectory and their role in meeting those developmental needs [4]. In addition, any supplemental therapies provided should empower caregivers to support development in the child's natural environments [6]. For example, some children who are evaluated for autism or related concerns may present with developmental delays in one or more area regardless of whether or not an autism-related diagnosis is appropriate. In this case, services addressing developmental delays should be provided according to local eligibility standards and availability of resources. In-home services that address developmental delays in accordance with the recommended practices of early intervention/early childhood special education (EI/ECSE) are inherently focused on a family's strengths, needs, and goals [7] and may provide the opportunity for skill building and respite, especially in areas where intensive family therapy options are severely limited.

Another aspect of returning to a healthy developmental trajectory is play. Play is an essential aspect of developmental flourishing across domains, and often traumatized children display impoverished play patterns. For example, children may withdraw to a corner out of fear, wander about in a "daze," or struggle to play with others due to hypervigilance or struggles with social communication. Because of the primacy of play in a young child's life, therapies that incorporate a return to joyful, playful exploration are critical. Many modalities, such as Child-Parent Psychotherapy (CPP), Trust-based Relational Intervention® (TBRI®), and Theraplay® incorporate playful engagement with young children [8–10]. Whereas toxic stress in humans results from chronic activation of physiological stress responses over time, human play is correlated with activation of the parasympathetic nervous system, which has a calming effect [11].

Restoring Felt Safety

Often children who have experienced trauma do not experience internal safety despite the best efforts of caregivers to provide external safety and emotional support. The paralyzing fear or chronic arousal that a child may have experienced as a result of disorienting or frightening experiences can create enduring internal dysregulation. For a child who has experienced a pervasive lack of safety in the past, any current experiences of safety are experienced alongside memories, both implicit and explicit, of a frightening past [12]. As such, another salient feature of effective trauma treatment involves empowering caregivers to meet a child's need for internal safety that was either not met early on or that has been compromised by the experience of acute trauma (i.e., a house fire or automobile accident). Often, this requires caregivers to provide more nurture, predictability, structure, and care than a preschool-aged child is able to verbally request.

Constructing and Integrating Trauma Narratives

The gradual development of a coherent story about the trauma is at times a powerful component of treating trauma in young children [13]. Constructing a trauma narrative is incorporated into trauma-focused cognitive behavioral therapy (TF-CBT) by guiding children through slowly writing and processing their trauma story while monitoring a child's reaction to this process. The developmentally appropriate creation of a trauma story may serve to slowly desensitize a child to paralyzing or overwhelming feelings associated with traumatic experiences while also allowing a child to integrate frightening experiences into the bigger story of his or her life. Especially important for young children are considerations related to a child's developmental capacity to participate in meta-cognitive processes, such as "zooming out" to see his or her place in a larger story, or the ability to expect better things for the future. Generally speaking, the younger the child, the more difficult it will be to construct a coherent or well-defined story. However, most young children will possess an innate ability to act and "play out" stories that are meaningful to them, while the story is narrated by a parent during a therapy session. The construction of this narrative should take place with the support of a skilled therapist in the context of an appropriate trauma intervention such as TF-CBT or Child-Parent Psychotherapy. For preschool-aged children, whenever possible, a caregiver should be present during this play and can also provide protective elements to the story, such as a lost child being found by his mother [4].

Enhancing Affect Regulation and Coping Skills

Trauma often compromises a child's self-regulatory skills or limits the development of these skills in the first place. As a result, treatment should aim to build and/or restore regulatory capacity in a child. When a child is impacted by early trauma, especially relational trauma, he or she may have missed the opportunity to develop positive relationships in which early regulatory skills are built through nurturing interactions with an attuned caregiver. Additionally, young children with trauma have often been exposed to chaotic and frightening situations which overwhelmed the developing brain's ability to cope, often leaving a child in a more frequent state of trauma-associated dysregulation. This dysregulation over time can become a pattern of affective and behavioral dysregulation that impacts many areas of development and functioning [4, 14]. Finally, young children who have experienced trauma may re-experience early traumatic experiences or have overpowering, intense feelings in response to trauma reminders [15]. Effective trauma treatments must address both the physiological and emotional dysregulation common in trauma-exposed children by simultaneously enlisting parents as "co-regulators" while also training children in self-regulatory skills when developmentally appropriate. Effective therapeutic approaches seek to understand a child's history and context in order to determine the amount of regulatory support required by a child. Some older preschoolers may lack the developmental experience of being almost entirely regulated by another (as is typically the case for infants in the entire first year of life). These children will require more intensive supports in order to effectively build regulatory capital in order to deal with trauma-related dysregulation.

Trauma Treatment Models with Preschoolers

When complex trauma has been identified in a preschool-aged child, the developmental, bodily, behavioral, and relational impacts of trauma should be addressed through a treatment plan designed to meet the needs of the affected child within that child's particular context and unique set of needs. Identifying appropriate treatment options that can be accessed with ease is essential to initiating a successful healing process. Often families need to access intensive mental health supports as well as accommodations within their current daily environments (i.e., home, preschool). In this section will examine evidence-based intensive therapeutic models as well as second-tier supports intended to enhance the relational environment of traumatized children in their homes and schools.

Intensive Treatment Models

Trauma-Focused Cognitive Behavioral Treatment (TF-CBT)

Trauma-focused cognitive behavioral treatment (TF-CBT) is a manualized treatment designed to reduce trauma-related symptoms in children through a treatment model that includes both parent and child. Developed by Anthony Mannarino, Judith Cohen, and Esther Deblinger, TF-CBT targets ages 3–21 and generally requires 12–25 sessions in an outpatient setting with a mental health practitioner trained in TF-CBT (free training available at http://www.musc.edu/tfcbtconsult). TF-CBT takes into account the significance of the caregiving relationship in providing safety and co-regulation for children with trauma histories as well as the developing nature of emotional regulation in young children [16]. TF-CBT provides parents and children with a structured environment in which children can process trauma with the support of their non-offending caregivers while also developing skills for behavioral, thought, and emotional regulation in the aftermath of trauma. TF-CBT also seeks to enhance trust, safety, and communication within parent-child relationships. TF-CBT has been widely used and adapted for various cultural settings and provides a flexible framework for a variety of contexts including preschool-aged settings [16].

TF-CBT has developed a substantial evidence base since the manualized version of TF-CBT was first published in 2006. Although no systematic review of TF-CBT with preschoolers specifically has been conducted to date, Ramirez de Arellano et al. examined ten high-quality randomized controlled trials examining the effectiveness of TF-CBT and found a high level of evidence of TF-CBT's effectiveness in producing positive outcomes for a variety of trauma-related symptoms in children of all ages. Scheeringa et al. found a significant decrease in PTSD symptoms in 3- to 6-year-olds compared to a waitlist control group [17]. In the same study, the authors found that PTSD effect sizes increased at 6-month follow-up, indicating that TF-CBT may provide long-lasting effects for trauma symptoms in young children.

Strengths: manualized, free training, large evidence base

Training information: https://tfcbt.musc.edu/

Child-Parent Psychotherapy (CPP)

Alicia Lieberman and Patricia van Horn developed Child-Parent Psychotherapy (CPP) as relationship-based treatment designed specifically to address trauma in children prenatally up to 5 years old [4]. CPP is rooted in attachment theory but also incorporates psychodynamic, developmental, social learning, and cognitive behavioral principles [18]. The focus of treatment is to help caregivers to provide appropriate safety and protection against both internal and external dangers to children while repairing the attachment relationship that may have been disturbed by interpersonal trauma. Generally speaking, CPP is conducted with parent-child conjoint play sessions. Based on previous RCTs, treatment lasts an average of 1 year with an average of approximately 32.82 sessions across all participants [19]. The CPP-trained therapist acts as an emotional and developmental "translator" between caregiver and child and employs simple strategies to promote understanding, trust, shared joy, and competent parenting practices in addition to helping the parent and child construct coherent trauma stories and cope with trauma reminders. Therapists also provide emotional support, concrete assistance, and crisis intervention when necessary.

Three randomized controlled trials and several additional studies have demonstrated the effectiveness of CPP for impacting a variety of outcomes including trauma-related symptomatology and security of attachment [18]. Lieberman et al. conducted a randomized controlled trial with children who had been exposed to domestic violence [20]. At posttreatment follow-up, children receiving CPP demonstrated a greater reduction in behavior problems and trauma-related symptoms, and mothers demonstrated greater reduction in avoidant symptomatology. Further analysis revealed that children and mothers with four or more traumatic or stressful life events also demonstrated decreased depression, PTSD symptoms, and behavior problems as well as lower rates of PTSD and co-occurring diagnoses, indicating that CPP may be appropriate for families experiencing multiple traumas and stressors [21]. In a study of young children with histories of maltreatment, Cicchetti et al. found that CPP participants were significantly more likely to experience changes in attachment security when compared to standard treatment [22]. CPP is one of the few trauma-specific treatments designed with young children in mind that has been extensively validated in populations of young children who have experienced complex trauma.

Strengths: Has been validated across cultures and actively honors cultural variations, designed specifically for very young children, strong parent component

Training information: http://childtrauma.ucsf.edu/child-parent-psychotherapy-training

Parent-Child Interaction Therapy (PCIT)

Parent-child interaction therapy (PCIT) is an evidence-based treatment for children ages 2–7 with emotional and behavioral disorders, including trauma-related behavior disorders [23]. Goals of PCIT include strengthening the caregiver-child relationship while decreasing behavior problems and increasing prosocial behavior in children. Goals for caregivers include increased positive parenting and reduced parental stress. PCIT can be conducted in an average of 12–20 sessions. In standard PCIT, coaches provide "live" coaching from behind a one-way mirror to parents interacting with their children via a transmitter and receiver device. In the first phase, treatment is focused on enhancing relationship-building skills in parents. Once relationship-based criteria are met, the second phase of treatment focuses on helping caregivers to provide positive discipline to their children. One goal of PCIT is to reduce negative caregiver-child interactions and reduce potential for future maltreatment, making it an appropriate training model for families with histories of or at-risk for interpersonal trauma by way of maltreatment [24].

PCIT has been evaluated extensively. In a meta-analysis examining 13 studies, Thomas and Zimmer-Gembeck found medium to large effect sizes for improving problem behavior with PCIT treatment [25]. Chaffin et al. randomly assigned parents with histories of abuse to PCIT, PCIT plus enhanced services, and standard community care control group [26]. This study found a significant reduction in re-report for abuse in the group receiving PCIT. Researchers found that a reduction in negative caregiver-child interactions mediated the reduction in re-reports, indicating that PCIT may reduce the likelihood of future maltreatment and trauma by inducing positive changes in the caregiver-child relationship.

Strengths: may reduce future maltreatment experiences, large evidence base

Training information: http://www.pcit.org/

Supplemental Supports

Often young children experiencing the aftermath of trauma require intensive environmental supports at home and school to support the healing process initiated by more intensive treatments such as those mentioned previously. Multicomponent and parent training programs that seek to enhance regulatory capacities in and between both parent and child are an essential part of a well-coordinated response to trauma, particularly for families who have been impacted by chronic and/or complex trauma and stress. In this section, we will review programs that provide supplemental or ongoing support to families with histories of complex trauma. The following sidebar and list of interventions are not intended to be exhaustive but rather intended to provide a sampling of beneficial approaches to enhancing development and functioning in young children with trauma histories.

Circle of Security

The Circle of Security intervention is a parent group designed to enhance attachment relationships between caregivers and young children ages birth to 5 who are at risk for a variety of problems. Circle of Security takes place over 8 sessions and provides parents with psychoeducation about early social and emotional development as well as opportunities to reflect on the roots of insecurity in their attachment relationships. The intervention seeks to increase sensitivity and responsivity through reflections about videotaped interactions between caregivers and their child [27, 28]. Circle of Security has developed a strong evidence base, with several evaluations demonstrating positive effects on security of attachment [29].

Strengths: Relationship-focused, short-term

Training Information: https://www.circleofsecurityinternational.com/trainings

Trust-Based Relational Intervention

Trust-Based Relational Intervention® (TBRI®) was developed by Karyn Purvis and David Cross to treat complex trauma, particularly in children who have experienced relational trauma such as institutionalization, foster care, and subsequent adoption [9]. TBRI® targets caregivers (including teachers) of children ages 0–17 and employs a holistic, multidisciplinary approach designed to meet the needs of children "from hard places." TBRI® consists of three sets of complementary principles intended to help caregivers build deeper connections (connecting principles), empower their child's body by meeting needs (empowering principles), and promote prosocial behavior (correcting principles). This approach is delivered through an intensive caregiver training in which participants receive psychoeducation about the complex needs of trauma-exposed children as well as practical strategies for providing an environment of "felt safety" in order to promote optimal development [9].

In a randomized study of TBRI® caregiver training, Purvis et al. found significant decreases in trauma symptoms as well as behavioral problems post-intervention in the group receiving intervention compared with no changes in the control group [30]. Other studies of TBRI® employing a pre-post research design have found decreases in salivary cortisol, depression symptoms, aggressive behavior, and negative attachment behaviors [31, 32]. Although TBRI® has been used extensively with preschool-aged children, no extensive evaluation to date has been conducted using only preschool-aged children.

Strengths: Involves all caregivers including extended family and teachers and addresses body-based symptoms

Training Information: https://child.tcu.edu/professionals/tbri-training/#sthash.H0INHQ2H.dpbs

Theraplay®

Theraplay® is a short-term family therapy model focused on building trust and attachment between parent and child through healthy and playful parent-child interactions [33]. During sessions, therapists guide dyads through a sequence of playful games and nurturing activities designed to enhance four dimensions of healthy attachment relationships: structure, nurture, engagement, and challenge. Throughout sessions, the therapist guides the parent in regulating child behavior while also communicating delight and safety to the child. Theraplay® also offers formats for school-based groups and may be an appropriate choice for increasing regulation and safety within preschool settings serving children with trauma histories.

Siu conducted a randomized controlled trial evaluating Theraplay® with children in grades 2–4 [34]. Findings indicated a decrease in internalizing behaviors in children receiving Theraplay® treatment compared to a waitlist control group. Although more empirical research is needed in preschool-aged children, the nonverbal and dyadic nature of this treatment modality is highly appropriate for both preschool-aged and trauma-affected children.

Strengths: Focused on nonverbal development, caregiver fully incorporated, short-term

Training: https://www.Theraplay.org/index.php/training

Therapeutic Preschools and Childcare

Children with complex trauma and/or many layers of risk (i.e., poverty, future maltreatment risk) may benefit from a "wraparound" environment of care that is trauma-informed. Multicomponent programs such as Childhaven Childhood Trauma Treatment (CCT) and Children's Relief Nursery (CRN) provide therapeutic childcare/preschool options that include optional specialized services and treatments in addition to a day-to-day environment designed to the meet the safety and regulatory needs of children with trauma histories. Service options may also include treatments such as parent-child therapy, respite care, support groups, home visits, and assistance accessing basic resources.

Body-Based Treatments

Children with trauma histories may have experienced unhealthy or painful touch or may have been deprived of touch early in life. Children may have also experienced chronic dysregulation related to the sensory world. Thus, therapeutic modalities that provide healthy experiences of touch and other sensory experiences may be appropriate for children with trauma histories. Therapeutic options include occupational therapy, sensory-motor affect regulation therapy (SMART), massage therapy, and animal-assisted therapy.

Trauma Treatment with Preschoolers Targeting Biological Outcomes

Extensive research has documented the disruptive effect of early life trauma on the developing body's systems, such as the brain and the hypothalamic-pituitary-adrenal (HPA) axis, in preschoolers. As these systems support critical functions, such as cognition and stress reactivity and regulation, early insults compromise the body's capacity for optimal growth and well-being. The need for the establishment of interventions that address these critical facets of children's development is clear. In addition, more research is needed regarding previously mentioned interventions and the biological impacts of these evidence-based practices. It may be that various features, such as "restoring felt safety," strongly correlate with, for example, a return to optimal HPA axis functioning; however, more research is needed to establish the biological effects of already established evidence-based trauma treatments. Intervention research that measures the biological impacts on young children are at this time scarce. More research in the future on this topic would provide additional insight on effective strategies to improve the overall course of development and further understand "active ingredients" of treatment for children at risk due to trauma.

Research by Fisher et al. [35] demonstrates how effective treatment can support adaptive HPA regulation. Fisher et al. examined the impact of Multidimensional Treatment Foster Care for Preschoolers versus regular foster care on diurnal cortisol levels. A third group of children without a history of maltreatment and not in foster care constituted another comparison cohort. Multidimensional Treatment Foster Care for Preschoolers targets socioemotional skills and development more generally through education with foster parents in anticipation of and following placement and through therapy with children. The findings of the study showed that families who had undergone Multidimensional Treatment Foster Care for Preschoolers had children who displayed cortisol trajectories similar to those of children without a history of maltreatment, whereas families who had undergone regular foster care had children who displayed dampened cortisol trajectories. These results provide support for the ability of an intervention focused on enhancing the relational quality of foster care to shape HPA regulation in young children. Additional research in this area would provide new insight into how treatments can shape the biological effects of trauma in other systems, as the effects can be multifaceted and varied.

The Biological Embedding of Early Life Trauma

The associations observed between early trauma and later adverse developmental outcomes have been shown to be influenced in part by dysregulated biological mechanisms. Biological systems are *interwoven* with the child's experience of his or her environment: mounting evidence from research suggests that multiple biological systems are sensitive to the effects of trauma and, in response, display changes in various markers of functioning. Here, we review recent research findings on the effects of trauma on the physiology of preschool-aged children (see Table 7.1).

The Brain

The brain undergoes astounding developmental changes during childhood, setting the stage for effective cognitive functioning in adulthood. Experience plays a key role in modulating brain development, with safe, supportive, and stimulating environments supporting the healthy development of the brain. In contrast, threatening, dismissive, and neglectful environments disrupt the healthy development of the brain. While the brain is largely regarded as plastic, that is, open to change and adaptation, research data suggest that early trauma may have an enduring impact on the brain development trajectory of children. Understanding the specific impacts

Table 7.1 Summary of biological findings in children who have experienced developmental trauma

Study	Intervention study?	ROI	Sample characteristics	Key findings	Implications
Tottenham et al. [36]	No	Amygdala volume	34 children with history of institutionalization 28 children without history of institutionalization Ages: 5–11 years	Children adopted at older age had greater amygdala volumes	Inconclusive: Does larger volume correspond to over- or underactivity?
Hodel et al. [37]	No	Amygdala volume Hippocampus volume Prefrontal cortex volume	110 children with history of institutionalization 62 children without history of institutionalization Ages: 12–14 years	No significant differences in amygdala volume; hippocampal and prefrontal cortex volumes diminished in institutionalized children and children adopted at older age	Early adversity is associated with altered brain structure that persists into early adolescence
Demir-Lira et al. [38]	No	Left lateral frontal cortex (fMRI)	28 children from a community sample Ages: 4–7 years	Decrements on a reversal learning paradigm associated with greater regional homogeneity, alterations in the right temporal/parahippocampal areas	Early life stress could be linked to later cognitive control
Curtis & Cicchetti [39]	No	Parietal lobe (EEG)	44 maltreated children 43 children with no history of maltreatment Ages: 6–12 years	EEG results indicated that children without a history of maltreatment displayed more activity in the left hemisphere, whereas children with a history of maltreatment displayed more activity in the right hemisphere	As elevated activation in the right hemisphere is implicated in post-traumatic stress disorder (PTSD), the authors suggested that the findings in the study may well indicate that children in the maltreated group may have had a relatively higher incidence of PTSD
Bruce et al. [40]	No	Hypothalamic-pituitary-adrenal (HPA) axis	177 children in foster care 60 children not in foster care and without a history of maltreatment Ages: 3–6 years	Children in the foster care group demonstrated morning cortisol levels that were lower; this group also displayed different patterns in cortisol levels according to the form of maltreatment–extreme physical neglect related to low levels, extreme emotional maltreatment related to elevated levels	cortisol secretion may be blunted among children with a history of maltreatment relative to controls, but within children who have contended with maltreatment, the form of the maltreatment appears to shape HPA regulation

(continued)

Table 7.1 (continued)

Study	Intervention study?	ROI	Sample characteristics	Key findings	Implications
Cutuli et al. [41]	No	Hypothalamic-pituitary-adrenal (HPA) axis	66 children growing up within a homeless shelter Ages: 4–7 years	elevated morning and pre-task cortisol levels and a different task-related cortisol trajectory were associated with the index of negative lifetime events	type and quantity of trauma may be important for how the early stress response system adapts to the environmental circumstances
Cicchetti et al. [42]	No	Hypothalamic-pituitary-adrenal (HPA) axis	265 children who had been maltreated 288 children who had been maltreated Ages: 7–13 years	children with early past physical or sexual abuse in addition to elevated levels of depressive or internalizing scores demonstrated a reduced lowering of cortisol between the morning and afternoon	A history of physical or sexual abuse disrupted the HPA axis such that cortisol levels remained elevated, indicating that children who had experienced this form of abuse may remain hypervigilant to potential threats
Davies et al. [43]	No	Hypothalamic-pituitary-adrenal (HPA) axis	208 children in the first grade from a community sample Age: 6.6 years (mean age)	Participants' distress responses accounted for unique variance in heightened cortisol levels over the course of a staged conflict paradigm, the Simulated Phone Argument Task, in the laboratory between their mother and father	Other elements of a child's psychological constitution may play an important role in how biological systems interact with traumatic circumstances
Gunnar et al. [44]	No	Hypothalamic-pituitary-adrenal (HPA) axis	44 children who had been adopted early 42 children who been adopted later 38 children had never been given up for adoption Ages: 10–12 years	participants who had experienced moderate early life stress (i.e., children who had been adopted early on) displayed a lowered cortisol response	Absolute cortisol level may be less important than relative levels when evaluating HPA reactivity among groups of individuals. It may be important to also examine the association between cortisol levels and other measures of adaptation, such as behavior profiles and mental health criteria

Fisher et al. [35]	Yes	Hypothalamic-pituitary-adrenal (HPA) axis	57 children placed in Multidimensional Treatment Foster Care 60 children placed in regular foster care 60 children without a history of maltreatment and not in foster care	Families who had undergone Multidimensional Treatment Foster Care for Preschoolers had children who displayed cortisol trajectories similar to those of children without a history of maltreatment, whereas families who had undergone regular foster care had children who displayed cortisol trajectories dampened cortisol trajectories	Provides support for the ability of an intervention focused on enhancing the relational quality of foster care to shape HPA regulation in young children
Asok et al. [45]	No	Telomeres	51 high risk children 38 low risk children Ages: 3–6 years	Compared to children who were at low risk for abuse, children at heightened risk demonstrated shorter telomeres; within the high-risk group, elevated levels of parental responsiveness were related to longer telomeres	Parents can wield a buffering influence in the face of early stress
Troller-Renfree et al. [46]	Yes	Error-related negativity	49 children placed in the Care As Usual Group 54 children placed in the Foster Care Group 47 children in the Never Institutionalized Group Age: 8 years	Children in foster care who exhibited small error-related negativity, a measure of self-control, displayed worse academic and psychopathology outcomes compared to children in foster care who exhibited greater error-related negativity. This differential effect was not detected among children who received care as usual	Foster care could influence the development of cognitive control and its relation to adaptation
Tyrka et al. [47]	No	Immune system	18 children with a history of maltreatment 22 children without a history of maltreatment Ages: 3–5 years	Along with other indices of early adversity, including recent contextual stressors, traumatic life events were related to elevated levels of IL-1B, a proinflammatory cytokine	Even at this young age (3–5 years), trauma can be reflected in alterations to children's immune system

ROI Region of Interest

that trauma has on the body's developing systems is a critical initial step for justifying intervention efforts and identifying potential targets of intervention. The brain undisputedly plays a central role in optimal functioning, and research data show that early life stress exerts an influence on the course of its development.

Several structures of the brain have been examined with the goal of detecting possible changes as a function of early trauma. These structures have included the amygdala, the prefrontal cortex, and the hippocampus. The amygdala serves as the emotion processing center of the brain. The prefrontal cortex, a brain structure that continues to grow through adolescence and into early adulthood, underlies critical cognitive processes, such as executive function. The hippocampus primarily subserves memory.

Several neuroimaging studies on children who have experienced trauma in the form of institutionalization have been conducted. Research has observed changes in the amygdala following a history of this type of early trauma, suggesting that children's ability to regulate emotions may be impacted. Tottenham et al. [36] investigated the effect of previous institutionalization on the brain development of children between the ages of 5 and 11 years. The results of this magnetic resonance imaging (MRI) study, in which they were able to collect imaging data from 34 children who had a history of institutionalization and 28 children who did not, revealed that children who were adopted at a relatively older age exhibited greater amygdala volumes. The implications of the relatively larger size of the amygdala volumes are difficult to discern without further research. Data on the functional significance of greater amygdala size paints an inconsistent picture, with some work suggesting that it is associated with elevated reactivity and other work suggesting that it is associated with dampened activity. Future neuroscience research linking the relation between neural structures and behavioral phenotypes will enhance our appreciation of what these observed differences in amygdala volumes mean for children who have undergone the trauma associated with institutionalization.

Another study following the Tottenham et al. efforts also examined the impact of early institutionalization on several brain structures, including the amygdala. This later study from Hodel et al. had a larger sample of children—110 children, who had been institutionalized (the mean age was 13.01 years), and 62 children, who had not been institutionalized [37]. In contrast to the finding of the previous study, the children in this particular study who had been institutionalized did not exhibit greater amygdala volumes. These results suggest that additional research must be done in order to fully understand how early trauma shapes this particular region of the brain. Is the amygdala affected by early trauma? If so, what can be done to enhance the functioning of children who display greater volumes? Would the amygdala volume sizes change in response to targeted treatment? With respect to other areas of the brain, this study did find that the volumes of the prefrontal cortex and the hippocampus were diminished among children who had been institutionalized and children who were relatively older at the time of adoption, respectively. These observed differences also invoke the question of whether these differences represent clinically relevant consequences for cognition or behavior. This study deepens our understanding of the enduring impact of early trauma on the developing brain, and additional research to aid in elucidating the associations with other domains of development would support intervention efforts to facilitate optimal brain development.

Emerging research suggests that early-life stress may negatively impact the development of the prefrontal cortex. Demir-Lira et al. [38] investigated the relation between early life stress and left lateral frontal cortex regional homogeneity within a sample of children who were between 4 and 7 years old. The children completed resting-state functional magnetic resonance imaging (fMRI) and a reversal-learning paradigm. The results indicated that greater regional homogeneity, along with alterations in the right temporal/parahippocampal areas, was linked to decrements on the behavioral paradigm. Such findings underscore the potent adverse effect that early-life stress can have on the developing brain.

The parietal lobe, an area of the brain important for visuomotor function, has also been shown to be affected by early trauma. Curtis and Cicchetti [39] explored resilience and emotion regulation among a sample of children between the ages of 6 and 12 years using electroencephalogram (EEG) technology. In this study, one group of children ($n = 44$) had experienced maltreatment, while the other group of children ($n = 43$) had not experienced maltreatment. The EEG results indicated that children without a history of maltreatment displayed more activity in the left hemisphere, while children with a history of maltreatment displayed more activity in the right hemisphere. As elevated activation in the right hemisphere is implicated in posttraumatic stress disorder (PTSD), the authors suggested that the findings in the study may well indicate that children in the maltreated group may have had a relatively higher incidence of PTSD. It is notable that the children in this study were young (between 6 and 12 years of age), and yet, indications of the detrimental impact of trauma on their mental health could be identified during this early period prior to adolescence. This lends support to early intervention efforts that could help stymie the trajectory of adverse outcomes of young children who have had to endure elevated levels of stress over the course of the first several years of their lives.

The caregiving environment might be one potential target of intervention. EEG data from the Bucharest Early Intervention Project show that in comparing 8-year-old children who had been institutionalized and then went on to either receive foster care or care as usual, foster care could influence the development of cognitive control and its relation to adaptation [46]. In particular, the results from the study showed that children in foster care who exhibited small error-related negativity, a measure of self-control, displayed worse academic and psychopathology outcomes compared to children in foster care who exhibited greater error-related negativity. This differential effect was not detected among children who received care as usual. If children can be identified, whether with neuroscience methods or otherwise, as being at risk for compromised mental health, the process of providing support can begin early and hopefully prevent unfavorable outcomes in these children's futures.

The results of numerous types of neuroscience studies present evidence suggesting that the developing brain may be particularly sensitive to the detrimental effects of trauma. It is critical to take on a holistic view of how a young child's mental and physical health could be impacted by early adverse conditions. Brain development during the early years shapes the course of how a child may function in the years ahead. Therefore, brain development within the context of early trauma is a major public health concern that calls for scrutiny and support. Prompt and effective treatment could mitigate the emergence of poor health in adulthood.

The Hypothalamic-Pituitary-Adrenal Axis

The hypothalamic-pituitary-adrenal (HPA) axis is one of the body's stress regulation systems. When individuals confront stress, the HPA axis is activated, and a series of reactions results in the secretion of the hormone, cortisol. Cortisol marshals the body's resources to contend with stress. In particular, the release of cortisol triggers an infusion of glucose into the body's bloodstream, leading to a higher level of energy that the body can draw upon in the face of stress. While a robust stress response is indicative of a healthy stress regulation system, chronically elevated levels of cortisol, such as the type observed in the context of trauma, have been shown to be related to a host of adverse health outcomes, such as obesity, disrupted immune function, and later psychopathology. On the other hand, chronically blunted levels of cortisol have also been observed in individuals with a history of trauma. While the specific mechanism for this pattern remains to be fully understood, it has been conjectured that perhaps the body has habituated to chronic activation of the HPA axis and has effectively "turned off" and resorted to a downregulated response. Taken together, these patterns in HPA axis functioning suggest trauma may be related to over- and under-activation of the HPA axis. Optimal functioning may be represented by levels that are between the extremes of high and low cortisol levels. The extant literature on HPA axis regulation among children with a history of early trauma suggests that children who have experienced early adverse experiences show atypical HPA functioning, even at ages as young as 3 years. This demonstrates that individual differences in cortisol secretion may become evident quite early, prompting the question of what may happen if trauma persists over the long term.

Two types of cortisol have been investigated in relation to early trauma: diurnal cortisol and cortisol following a stressor. Diurnal cortisol provides an index of HPA functioning over the course of a day. This class of cortisol is typically measured in the morning shortly after awakening and/or in the afternoon. The typical course of cortisol throughout the day is such that cortisol levels peak in the morning after awakening and taper off over the course of the ensuing hours, with the lowest levels typically observed at night before individuals go to bed. In the face of acute stress, however, the typical rhythm of cortisol may be disrupted, and an elevation in cortisol levels may be observed. Conversely, activation of the stress response system over a protracted period of time may result in an overall blunting of cortisol response.

Diurnal cortisol levels in children have been shown to exhibit marked changes in relation to early trauma. Bruce et al. [40] examined the morning cortisol levels of children who were between the ages of 3 and 6 years and were either (1) in foster care or (2) not in foster care and without a history of maltreatment. The results of this study showed that children in the foster care group demonstrated morning cortisol levels that were lower relative to children who were not in foster care. Furthermore, among children in the foster care group, different patterns in cortisol levels were found according to the form of maltreatment. In particular, extreme physical neglect was related to low levels, while extreme emotional maltreatment was related to elevated levels. Levels at these two ends of the spectrum may both be maladaptive and predispose children to later challenges. These findings suggest that overall, cortisol secretion may be blunted among children with a history of maltreatment relative to controls, but within children who have contended with maltreatment, the form of the maltreatment appears to shape HPA regulation. These data indicate that the relation between early trauma and stress reactivity may not constitute a straightforward story. Rather, multiple factors, such as the type of trauma, must be taken into consideration to form a nuanced picture of how the body is responding to an environment of stress.

Trauma may indeed take on different forms, and it is imperative that empirical studies consider trauma across diverse contexts in order to fully construct a cogent appreciation of how it may affect development. Cutuli et al. [41] also investigated the morning cortisol levels of children growing up within a stressful environment, a homeless shelter. In this sample of 4- to 7-year-old children, morning cortisol and cortisol reactivity were assessed in relation to two risk categories: socioeconomic risk and negative life events. Researchers sampled saliva in the morning (mean sample time was 46 min following wake up) and throughout several cognitive tasks. This study found that elevated morning and pre-task cortisol levels and a different task-related cortisol trajectory were associated with the index of negative lifetime events. The authors reported that further research would be necessary to explicate the observed result with respect to the differential cortisol task response. These findings indicate that the type and quantity of trauma may be important for how the early stress response system adapts to the environmental circumstances. In regard to the HPA axis, the type of risk that a child is experiencing appears to be integral to how a child reacts to the associated stress, with some types of risk exerting a more detrimental effect than others.

Research consistently demonstrates the harmful effects of early trauma to children's stress response systems. Cicchetti et al. [42] explored the diurnal patterns of cortisol among children with and without early (i.e., before 5 years) physical or sexual abuse. Saliva samples from participants were collected twice daily over the course of 5 days, within the context of a summer camp. The results revealed that children with early past physical or sexual abuse in addition to elevated levels of depressive or internalizing scores demonstrated a reduced lowering of cortisol between the morning and afternoon. This study found that a history of physical or sexual abuse disrupted the HPA axis such that the typical reduction in cortisol levels did not occur. Rather, the cortisol levels remained elevated, indicating that children who had experienced this form of abuse may remain hypervigilant to potential threats.

As young children spend much of their time within the context of the family, it is important to understand how trauma specific to that environment can shape biological systems. Children's stress responses to conflict between caregivers have also been investigated. Davies et al. [43] investigated predictors of first graders' cortisol responses to interparental conflict. The results revealed that over and above demographic variables, participants' distress responses accounted for unique variance in heightened cortisol levels over the course of a staged conflict paradigm, the simulated phone argument task, in the laboratory between their mother and father. These findings indicate that other elements of a child's psychological constitution, such as personality, may play an important role in how biological systems interact with traumatic circumstances. Individual differences may be observed among children who may have experienced the same type of potentially traumatic event, so it is critical to identify what may underlie these differences, as it may inform how treatment unfolds.

A critical reason for addressing trauma symptoms early on is the potential for the consequences of trauma to persist in the many years ahead. Gunnar et al. [44] examined the impact of different levels of early life stress (i.e., low, moderate, and severe) on the cortisol reactivity in groups of preadolescents who had either been adopted early or later or who had never been given up for adoption. The participants completed the Trier Social Stress Test for Children (TSST-C) in the laboratory and cortisol was assessed before, during, and after the task. The results revealed that participants who had experienced moderate early-life stress (i.e., children who had been adopted early on) displayed a lowered cortisol response. This evidence suggests that the absolute cortisol level may be less important than relative levels when evaluating HPA reactivity among groups of individuals. It may be important to also examine the association between cortisol levels and other measures of adaptation, such as behavior profiles and mental health criteria. This study provides empirical support for the enduring quality of trauma and the necessity of intervention for children to achieve optimal development.

Genes

Early trauma has also been found to adversely impact genes. Telomeres, chromosome sections that prevent damage to DNA when it undergoes replication, have been the target of recent research that has sought to find new biomarkers of early life stress. Asok et al. investigated telomere length among young children, ages 3–6 years, who were at heightened risk for abuse [45]. Compared to children who were at low risk for abuse, children at heightened risk demonstrated shorter telomeres. However, within the high-risk children, elevated levels of parental responsiveness were related to longer telomeres, demonstrating the buffering influence parents can wield in the face of early stress. This type of research opens up a promising new avenue of inquiry on the role of early trauma on young children's physiology.

The Immune System

Recent research has highlighted the role of early trauma on the immune function of preschoolers. Chronic inflammation in primarily studies of adults has been implicated in the development of cardiovascular disease [48, 49]. It has been proposed that increased markers of inflammation in early childhood places children at risk for later adverse health outcomes. Emerging evidence from the psychoneuroimmunology literature suggests that early trauma exerts a negative influence on preschoolers' developing immune system. Tyrka et al. [47] investigated the association between trauma and Interleukin-1B (IL-1B), a pro-inflammatory cytokine. In this study of 3- to 5-year-olds with and without a history of maltreatment ($N = 40$), IL-1B was assayed from saliva samples. The authors showed that along with other indices of early adversity, including recent contextual stressors, traumatic life events were related to elevated levels of IL-1B. These data indicate that even at this young age, trauma can be reflected in alterations to children's immune system.

Future Directions for Understanding the Biological Correlates of Trauma

As this overview has indicated, the body's various systems appear to be acutely sensitive to the distressing impact of early trauma. Key systems and organs that are integral for children to thrive may buckle under the strain of early adversity. In particular, the brain, HPA axis, genes, and immune system have been shown to be structurally or functionally different in children with a history of significant early stress. Research into other domains of biological functioning will serve to enhance our understanding of how the developing body contends with trauma. Additional avenues for empirical work include the epigenetics of trauma and the impact of trauma that occurs while the child is developing in utero.

The early years of a child's life are characterized by rapid growth and development and great plasticity. Trauma represents a disruptive force that poses serious threats to the burgeoning biological systems that are preparing the child to function in the immediate environment. Atypical shifts in development and dysregulation of the various systems place a child at risk for a host of adverse outcomes. More work is needed to fully uncover the full range of ways in which the body's systems may react to challenging experiences. This work is critical as limited knowledge constricts our capacity to inform and design effective interventions to counter the harmful effects of trauma. Research on the biological underpinnings of early trauma symptoms indicate that the consequences of trauma are multifold and complex. Differences observed between young children with a history of trauma and children without such a history may be unique to various characteristics associated with the type of trauma, rendering it difficult to arrive at generalizations about the consequences of trauma. It is therefore imperative that multiple factors are considered to fully elaborate on how the effects may be produced. Concurrent intervention efforts to stem the development of trauma's adverse consequences on preschoolers' biology represent a critical area of related research.

Conclusion

The importance of early diagnosis and treatment of autism spectrum disorders has been paralleled to that of the early diagnosis and treatment of childhood cancers by some leaders in the field, such as Amy Wetherby, PhD, given that in both cases intensive treatment is known to significantly impact outcomes. However, in the case of childhood trauma- and stressor-related disorders, not only are caregivers generally not clamoring for this type of diagnosis (and may even be withholding background key social information which might suggest this); pediatricians have tended to be undereducated in both the symptoms of such and the devastating impact of delayed diagnosis and treatment. As in the cases of Sally and Mark, outlined in the beginning of this chapter, children's acquisition of valuable, intensive mental health therapies can frequently be delayed or even thwarted when TSRDs are interpreted to be ASDs by parents, therapists, and providers. A better understanding of the etiology, prevalence, and natural course of untreated TSRD's among parents and professionals is imperative, if appropriate allocation of treatments for both children with ASDs and TSRDs is to be achieved, thus optimizing their individual potential for health and a high quality of life.

References

1. Yoches M, Summers SJ, Beeber LS, Harden BJ, Malik NM. Exposure to direct and indirect trauma. In: Summer SJ, Chazan-Cohen R, editors. Understanding early childhood mental health: a practical guide for professionals. Baltimore, MD: Brookes; 2012. p. 79–98.
2. MacNamara D. Rest play grow. Vancouver: Aona; 2016.
3. Cross DR, Purvis, KB. Lectures on TBRI® and attachment. Fort Worth, TX; 2014.
4. Lieberman AF, van Horn P. Psychotherapy with infants and young children: repairing the effects of stress and trauma on early attachment. New York: Guilford; 2008.
5. Ogden P, Goldstein B, Fisher J. Brain-to-brain, body-to-body: a sensorimotor psychotherapy perspective on the treatment of children and adolescents. In: Longo RE, Prescott DS, Bergman J, Creeden K, editors. Current perspectives and applications in neurobiology: working with young persons who are victims and perpetrators of sexual abuse. Holyoke: NEARI Press; 2012.
6. Odom SL, Wolery M. A unified theory of practice in early intervention/early childhood special education: evidence-based practices. J Spec Educ. 2013;37(3):164–73.
7. Division of Early Childhood (DEC) Recommended Practices Commission. DEC recommended practices. 2014. https://divisionearlychildhood.egnyte.com/dl/tgv6GUXhVo.
8. Diaz MA, Lieberman AF. Use of play in child-parent psychotherapy with preschoolers traumatized by domestic violence. In: Schaefer CE, editor. Play therapy for preschool children. Washington, DC: APA; 2010. p. 131–56.

9. Purvis KB, Cross DR, Dansereau DF, Parris SR. Trust-based relational intervention (TBRI): a systematic approach to complex developmental trauma. Child Youth Serv. 2013;34(4):360–86.
10. The Theraplay Institute. How theraplay differs from other child therapies. https://www.Theraplay.org/index.php/how-Theraplay-differs. Accessed 16 Nov 2017.
11. Cozolino L. The neuroscience of human relationships. New York: WW Norton; 2006.
12. van der Kolk B. The body keeps the score: brain, mind, and body in the healing of trauma. New York: Penguin; 2014.
13. Cohen JA, Mannarino AP, Deblinger E. Treating trauma and traumatic grief in children and adolescents. New York: Guilford; 2006.
14. van der Kolk BA, Roth S, Pelcovitz D, Sunday S, Spinazzola J. Disorders of extreme stress: the empirical foundation of a complex adaptation to trauma. J Trauma Stress. 2015;18(5):389–99.
15. van der Kolk BA. The neurobiology of childhood trauma and abuse. Child Adolesc Psychiatr Clin N Am. 2003;12:293–317.
16. Ramirez de Arellano MA, Lyman DR, Jobe-Shields L, George P, Dougherty RH, Daniels AS, Ghose SS, Huang L, Delphin-Rittmon ME. Trauma-focused cognitive-behavioral therapy for children and adolescents: assessing the evidence. Psychiatr Serv. 2014;65(3):1–12.
17. Scheeringa MS, Weems CF, Cohen JA, Amaya-Jackson L, Guthrie D. Trauma-focused cognitive-behavioral therapy for posttraumatic stress disorder in three-through six year-old children: a randomized clinical trial. J Child Psychol Psychiatry Allied Discip. 2017;52(8):853–60.
18. National Child Traumatic Stress Network. Trauma-informed interventions: CPP. 2012. http://nctsn.org/sites/default/files/assets/pdfs/cpp_general.pdf. Accessed 1 Nov 2017.
19. University of California San Francisco. Child trauma research program. https://childtrauma.ucsf.edu/. Accessed 16 Nov 2017.
20. Lieberman AF, van Horn P, Ippen CG. Toward evidence-based treatment: child-parent psychotherapy with preschoolers exposed to marital violence. J Am Acad Child Adolesc Psychiatry. 2005;44(12):1241–8.
21. Ippen CG, Harris WW, van Horn P, Lieberman AF. Traumatic and stressful events in early childhood: can treatment help those at highest risk? Child Abuse Negl. 2011;35:504–13.
22. Cicchetti D, Rogosch FA, Toth SL. Fostering secure attachment in infant in maltreating families through preventive interventions. Dev Psychopathol. 2006;18:623–50.
23. PCIT International. Parent-child interaction therapy. 2015. http://www.pcit.org/. Accessed 16 Nov 2017.
24. National Child Traumatic Stress Network. Trauma-informed interventions: PCIT. 2008. http://www.nctsn.org/sites/default/files/assets/pdfs/pcit_general.pdf. Accessed 16 Nov 2017.
25. Thomas R, Zimmer-Gembeck MJ. Behavioral outcomes of parent-child interaction therapy and triple P-positive parenting program: a review and meta-analysis. J Abnorm Child Psychol. 2007;35(3):475–95.
26. Chaffin M, Silovsky JF, Funderburk B, Valle LA, Brestan EV, Balachova T, Jackson S, Lensgraf J, Bonner BL. Parent-child interaction therapy with physically abusive parents: efficacy for reducing future abuse reports. J Consult Clin Psychol. 2014;72(3):500–10.
27. Circle of Security International. https://www.circleofsecurityinternational.com/. Accessed 16 Nov 2017.
28. Powell B, Cooper G, Hoffman K, Marvin B. The circle of security intervention: enhancing attachment in early parent-child relationships. New York: Guilford; 2014.
29. Berlin LJ, Zeanah CH, Lieberman AF. Prevention and intervention programs to support early attachment security. In: Cassidy J, Shaver PR, editors. Handbook of attachment: theory, research, and clinical applications. New York: Guilford; 2016. p. 739–58.
30. Purvis KB, Razuri EB, Howard AR, Call C, DeLuna J, Hall JS, Cross DR. Decrease in behavioral problems and trauma symptoms among at-risk adopted children following trauma-informed parent training intervention. J Child Adolesc Trauma. 2015;8(3):201–10.
31. Purvis KB, Cross DR. Improvements in salivary cortisol, depression, and representations of family relationships in at-risk adopted children utilizing a short-term therapeutic intervention. Adopt Q. 2006;10(1):25–43.

32. Purvis KB, Cross DR, Federici R, Johnson D, McKenzie LB. The hope connection: a therapeutic summer day camp for adopted and at-risk children with special socio-emotional needs. Adopt Foster. 2007;31(4):38–48.
33. The Theraplay Institute. Building better relationships. 2017. https://www.Theraplay.org/. Accessed 16 Nov 2017.
34. Siu AFY. Theraplay in the Chinese world: an intervention program for Hong Kong children with internalizing problems. Int J Play Therapy. 2009;18(1):1–12.
35. Fisher PA, Stoolmiller M, Gunnar MR, Burraston BO. Effects of a therapeutic intervention for foster preschoolers on diurnal cortisol activity. Psychoneuroendocrinology. 2007;32(8–10):892–905.
36. Tottenham N, Hare TA, Quinn BT, et al. Prolonged institutional rearing is associated with atypically large amygdala volume and difficulties in emotion regulation. Dev Sci. 2010;13(1):46–61.
37. Hodel AS, Hunt RH, Cowell RA, van den Heuvel SE, Gunnar MR, Thomas KM. Duration of early adversity and structural brain development in post-institutionalized adolescents. NeuroImage. 2015;105:112–9.
38. Demir-Lira ÖE, Voss JL, O'Neil JT, Briggs-Gowan MJ, Wakschlag LS, Booth JR. Early-life stress exposure associated with altered prefrontal resting-state fMRI connectivity in young children. Dev Cogn Neurosci. 2016;19:107–14.
39. Curtis WJ, Cicchetti D. Emotion and resilience: a multilevel investigation of hemispheric electroencephalogram asymmetry and emotion regulation in maltreated and nonmaltreated children. Dev Psychopathol. 2007;19(3):811–40.
40. Bruce J, Fisher PA, Pears KC, Levine S. Morning cortisol Levels in preschool-aged foster children: differential effects of maltreatment type. Dev Psychobiol. 2009;51(1):14–23.
41. Cutuli JJ, Wiik KL, Herbers JE, Gunnar MR, Masten AS. Cortisol function among early school-aged homeless children. Psychoneuroendocrinology. 2010;35(6):833–45.
42. Cicchetti D, Rogosch FA, Gunnar MR, Toth SL. The differential impacts of early physical and sexual abuse and internalizing problems on daytime cortisol rhythm in school-aged children. Child Dev. 2010;81(1):252–69.
43. Davies PT, Sturge-Apple ML, Cicchetti D, Cummings EM. Adrenocortical underpinnings of children's psychological reactivity to interparental conflict. Child Dev. 2008;79(6):1693–706.
44. Gunnar MR, Frenn K, Wewerka SS, van Ryzin MJ. Moderate versus severe early life stress: associations with stress reactivity and regulation in 10–12-year-old children. Psychoneuroendocrinology. 2009;34(1):62–75.
45. Asok A, Bernard K, Roth TL, Rosen JB, Dozier M. Parental responsiveness moderates the association between early-life stress and reduced telomere length. Dev Psychopathol. 2013;25(3):577–85.
46. Troller-Renfree S, Zeanah CH, Nelson CA, Fox NA. Neural and cognitive factors influencing the emergence of psychopathology: insights from the Bucharest Early Intervention Project. Child Dev Perspect. 2017;12:28–33.
47. Tyrka AR, Parade SH, Valentine TR, Eslinger NM, Seifer R. Adversity in preschool-aged children: effects on salivary interleukin-1β. Dev Psychopathol. 2015;27(2):567–76.
48. Cain BS, Meldrum DR, Dinarello CA, et al. Tumor necrosis factor-alpha and interleukin-1beta synergistically depress human myocardial function. Crit Care Med. 1999;27(7):1309–18.
49. Fearon WF, Fearon DT. Inflammation and cardiovascular disease: role of the interleukin-1 receptor antagonist. Circulation. 2008;117(20):2577–9.

Chapter 8
Reactive Attachment Disorder and Autism Spectrum Disorder: Diagnosis and Care in a Cultural Context

Jorge Benavides-Rawson and Roy Richard Grinker

Vignette: Spain

In an illustrative case from Spain, in the community of Cantabria, a team of clinical psychologists found themselves limited in the options for treatment for a young patient with what they diagnosed as reactive attachment disorder of infancy. In this report, Portugal-Fernández and Balsa-Vidal [1] describe the case of a 2-year and 4-month-old child that was sent to the Spanish equivalent of Child Protective Services by his pediatrician. The child presented "delays in almost all areas of development" without a possible medical cause. Additionally, the treating physician had reported a "strange relationship between the mother and child." After several visits to the child's home and school that included interviews with the mother and teachers, the team of psychologists reported delays in language, motor skills, eating habits, and sleeping patterns. The attachment patterns of the child, while different from the team's age-normed expectations, did not show a refusal of attachment, rather a "low attachment selectivity." The child would jump to embrace almost any adult that approached him.

Since the diagnosis of RAD requires identification of an etiologic factor, the Spanish psychologists spent time with the mother-child duo and found that the mother indeed refused to care for the child, show affection, or spend time with him. The mother of the child expressed that she did not like small children and that the expected behaviors of a mother *no le salían* (they don't come out of her naturally). The treating psychologists report not being able to find a possible treatment protocol in the literature besides the recommendation

J. Benavides-Rawson (✉) · R. R. Grinker
Department of Anthropology, The George Washington University, Washington, DC, USA
e-mail: jbenavides@gwmail.gwu.edu; rgrink@gwu.edu

J. M. Fogler, R. A. Phelps (eds.), *Trauma, Autism, and Neurodevelopmental Disorders*, https://doi.org/10.1007/978-3-030-00503-0_8

to separate the mother from the child. Eventually they created a "social learning-based intervention" [1] that helped the mother learn through modeling and imitation how to interact with her child. The authors report that the child did show improvements after the intervention.

Korea

In Korea, many Korean mothers not only accept the diagnosis of an attachment disorder, and seek psychiatric treatment for their own "inability" to relate properly to their children, but may be culturally predisposed to accept and seek it more than a diagnosis of autism spectrum disorder (ASD). They may be culturally predisposed to accept the diagnosis of RAD for at least three reasons. First, whereas scientists have demonstrated that ASD has a significant genetic basis—either through heredity or de novo mutations—RAD is associated instead with the behavior of the parents only. As a diagnosis, RAD thus removes from the other family members, especially their other children, the fear of passing on the condition to their own children. Under a heredity model, ASD threatens to impugn the family lineage. Indeed, many of the parents the second author interviewed who contemplated autism as a label for their children ultimately rejected it if they could not find a history of it in the extended family. Second, if it is the mother and not the child who is truly "ill," then there is an assumption of a greater chance for recovery. In this model, the mother may take the blame for a child's impairments in order to save the rest of the family from stigma. (Of course, either diagnosis does damage to the mother). Third, the diagnosis of RAD makes sense for Koreans who have witnessed rapid social and economic change since the Korean War and often wonder if modernity—including working mothers—threatens to destroy good parenting and social connectedness more generally [2]. Over the last 10–15 years, in large part as the result of a group of Korean clinicians who have popularized the concept of RAD in Korea, programs began to appear in the Seoul area to help mothers learn how to attach to their children. Mental health experts sometimes encourage mothers of children with RAD to quit their jobs. If the child gets better, the diagnosis and the treatment are validated. If the mother refuses to quit and the child improves nonetheless, the diagnosis is validated on the argument that the therapeutic relationship helped the child.

Confusion over the diagnosis and causes of autism and other neuropsychiatric conditions leads parents to question the accuracy of clinical assessments. For example, in Korea, some children have numerous different diagnoses from an array that included ASD, reactive attachment disorder, ADHD, "nonverbal language disorder," anxiety disorder, obsessive-compulsive disorder, and conduct disorder, among others. Mothers organize support groups in Korea in part to discuss their children but largely to discuss their doctors. One group in Seoul, studied by the second author, eagerly discussed which diagnoses are associated with which doctors. (One doctor is known to favor "nonverbal language disorder," another RAD, and so on). In addition, they complained that the lack of authority of medical discourse in psychology and psychiatry exacerbates their suspicions of the psychiatric community and validates conspiracy theories, such as the discredited belief that vaccines can cause autism, they derived from US websites [3].

The topic of misdiagnosis is one that confronts psychiatry perhaps more than any other field of medicine, in large part because of the lack of biomarkers and because, with the exception of a few conditions (grief disorder, post-traumatic stress disorder, reactive attachment disorder), nearly all psychiatric conditions are, technically, idiopathic, at least as characterized by the DSM. The idiopathic nature of disorder introduces a more pronounced element of subjectivity, and by extension, cultural influence, to what is usually conceptualized as a scientific, data-driven conversation about disease and disability. Perceived stigma and cultural beliefs about the cause and remedy of different disorders have a powerful influence over whether a family will seek help for a child's difficulties, what form that help will take (e.g., medical treatment vs. home- vs. school-based remedies), and who will administer it (e.g., physician vs. tutor vs. nonmedical healer). Studying these phenomena in a culture other than our own can offer helpful insights into our own, official and unofficial, diagnostic processes, in part because we are able to distance ourselves from such biases as self-justification.

Through the lens of two quite different cultures (Korea and Spain), this chapter considers reactive attachment disorder (RAD), an unusual psychiatric condition in its presumption of an etiology of pathological caretaking (the evidence for which is often hidden from the clinician), and its curious historical linkage to autism spectrum disorder (ASD), a condition that many now consider to be rooted in neurobiology but which historically (and psychodynamically) was initially linked to the same etiology. We explore the cultural, systemic, and (soft) scientific factors contributing to diagnostic variability generally and between these arguably emotionally charged diagnostic categories particularly. We conclude with an argument and recommendations for culturally sensitive assessment of trauma- and stressor-related disorder, with or without co-occurring neurodevelopmental disorder.

Reactive Attachment Disorder: Diagnostic Criteria and Historical Linkage to Autism Spectrum Disorder

DSM-V guidelines for the diagnosis of RAD include the following:

The child has experienced a pattern of extremes of insufficient care as evidenced by at least one of the following:

1. Social neglect or deprivation in the form of persistent lack of having basic emotional needs for comfort, stimulation, and affection met by caring adults
2. Repeated changes of primary caregivers that limit opportunities to form stable attachments (e.g., frequent changes in foster care)

3. Rearing in unusual settings that severely limit opportunities to form selective attachments (e.g., institutions with high child to caregiver ratios)

Because of the diagnostic requirement for some form of evidence that the child in question has experienced "extremes of insufficient care," the diagnosis remains uncommon in most countries. Nonetheless, clinicians do make diagnoses of RAD even in the absence of empirical evidence. How is this possible?

RAD first appeared in the DSM-III in 1980 but had traction in clinical circles much earlier, even in the era of the DSM-I (first published in 1952), due to the dominance of the psychoanalytic paradigm that considered mental illnesses to be an unhealthy reaction to one's environment. Schizophrenia, for example, was a "schizophrenic reaction," explainable in terms of an individual's pathological response to a range of stressors. Consistent with psychoanalytic thinking, RAD was an outgrowth of the belief that psychopathology was often caused by deprivation, whether parental or otherwise. Following the two world wars, and increased and detailed documentation of abusive institutions, such as prisoner-of-war camps and large orphanages, psychologists posited that certain environmental conditions could explain the lack of social responsiveness and failure to thrive among some children, conditions observable even in infancy [4]. The diagnosis of RAD was more likely to be given to children with a history of sexual, physical, or emotional abuse [5], but this association warrants a closer look. Diagnosis of RAD in cases of presumed abuse could have been a diagnostic artifact: children with a history of abuse have higher rates of RAD because neglect and abuse are parts of the diagnostic criteria. More problematic, the psychodynamic conceptualization of RAD was arguably overextended to include developmental delays and the characteristic social communication deficits of autism spectrum disorder (ASD). Bruno Bettelheim, for example, popularized the idea that young children with developmental delays and autistic symptoms in particular benefited from being removed from what he termed the mother's "black milk" (by which he meant a lack of love). Such children were treated by being separated from their mothers and enrolled in residential schools.

For Bettelheim, children with autistic syndromes suffered distress due to the conflicting emotional cues they received from their mother and from the external environment. This conflict of perceived emotions would trigger a state of overwhelming anxiety in the child leading him or her to shut down communication with the outside world [6]. Therefore, maternal psychopathology was the cause of autism, and as a result a generation of mothers came to believe they were to blame for their children's suffering [7].

As the second author has written elsewhere, RAD is often glossed in Korea as "lack of love" (aejeong kyolpib), a term strikingly similar to Bettelheim's concept of the "refrigerator mother." Despite the received view within psychology and psychiatry (and of course, within the DSM itself) that RAD should be diagnosed only when there is evidence of pathological caretaking, interviews with Korean mental health professionals, especially those without training in the United States, showed a strong bias toward diagnosing an attachment disorder in children exhibiting the triad of impairments associated with autism especially when the clinician believes the mother was not engaged with her child or who was separated from the child for financial or healthcare reasons. Some professionals in Korea have gone so far as to write that RAD mimics autism and that, therefore, RAD is misdiagnosed as ASD [2, 8, 9]. Indeed, Shin et al. [9] report on 25 children (ages 2–4) who presented with attachment difficulties, social and linguistic delays, beginning at between 9 and 12 months of age, and appeared to qualify for a diagnosis of a pervasive developmental disorder. Focusing on the maternal characteristics, the authors write that nine of the mothers met the criteria for depression on the Beck Depression Inventory and others exhibited subclinical symptoms of a range of other mental illnesses. Twenty Korean mothers in this study had "high scores" on the Korean version of the Minnesota Multiphasic Personality Inventory (MMPI), on items relating to depression, paranoia, psychopathic deviance, obsession, and social deviance. Other conclusions were drawn based on interpretation rather than systematic scoring. For example, 18 mothers were noted to be "suspicious in their statements." When mothers sought additional opinions from experts, this was interpreted as "avoiding consistent relationships with evaluators." Echoing Richters and Volkmar [4], the diagnosis of RAD was made because the clinicians observed improvement of ten of these children over the course of approximately 1 year's treatment. That is, successful treatment to help build relationships with both therapists and mothers, in what the authors call "infant-mother psychotherapy," justified the diagnosis of RAD. The diagnoses were made despite the fact that the most common interventions for children with autism, and no evidence of ASD, are quite similar: the vast majority of recommended interventions for ASD and RAD, throughout the world, focus on building social relationships and developing social communication skills for individuals diagnosed with ASD and on building attachment to caregivers for individuals diagnosed with RAD.

There are clearly several problems with this Korean study claiming successful diagnosis and treatment of RAD. The most obvious is the practice of diagnosing RAD in the absence of compelling evidence of pathological caretaking. The observations are made in the clinic, not in naturalized settings like the home. The evidence of maternal pathology appeared within the artificial clinical setting, and maternal behaviors in that setting were interpreted in pathological terms. Also problematic is the underlying assumption that RAD involves lack of attachment or social relatedness. As Powell and Bettes [10] note, RAD, as operationalized in this Korean study, need not involve a specific attachment disorder but rather the development of strategies of attachment in order to cope with the deprivation or inconsistencies in their caretaking environment. In addition, it is unclear if any other children from these same mothers suffered from attachment issues. Fathers were neither observed nor interviewed in the study because, the authors point out, Korean fathers are seldom involved in child care. Any naturalistic observation in a Korean home will, however, show that fathers and other relatives are essential players in the drama of household life. Furthermore, without evidence, the authors infer that mothers used videotapes in the home as a way "to avoid direct interaction with their children."

In a fascinating twist, the researchers resuscitate the Freudian concept of the "ghosts in the nursery" to argue for a culturally constituted, historically contingent, pattern of mothering deriving from the Korean War. To make the case, they first note, described as well-known culture-bound Korean disorder among women, *hwa-byung*. This is a somatic syndrome marked by a host of symptoms ranging from dysphoria, fatigue, and headaches to insomnia, a burning sensation in the body, and gastrointestinal complaints. Among Korean clinicians, hwa-byung is often attributed to the withholding of emotion, especially anger. If the inhibition of expression of emotion is related to hwa-byung, could there be another culture-bound disorder, perhaps one that resembles autism but is distinctively Korean? They conclude that Korean women have long inhibited expressions of anger—about the colonization of their country by Japan between 1910 and 1945, the national division of Korea, and the Korean war. Perhaps the mothers of the Korean mothers in the study themselves responded to the trauma of the past by being emotionally unavailable to their children. And now, their grandchildren, the children in this study, suffer from that legacy by being raised by mothers who continue this culturally bound type of emotional repression (and, as a result, emotional unavailability).

Autism Spectrum Disorder: The Quest for an Explanation

One could argue that the "appeal" of a psychodynamic conceptualization of autism, even one that so badly pathologizes innocent mothers, is that it provides a definitive explanation for a child's baffling, and sometimes frightening, socially disconnected behavior. It is important to understand that not only is autism an ever-changing construct, but cross-cultural variations in diagnostic practices for autism have been found, even among communities whose scientific traditions are often assumed to be similar, such as the United States and western European countries. While the American Psychiatric Association removed autism from the category of "psychosis" in 1980, the French child psychiatric establishment, in their own indigenous manual of mental disorders, the *Classification Française des Troubles Mentaux de l'Enfant et de l'Adolescent* (CFTMEA), classified autism as a psychosis until November 2004. French health professionals have been much more likely than those in North America and other European nations to conceptualize autism in more traditionally psychoanalytic terms, as a problem that lies within family social relationships and with the mother-child relationship in particular. Disturbingly, numerous therapies for autism in France blur the line between reactive attachment disorder and autism by relying on therapies that share many of the assumptions in Bettelheim's original project. Wet-packing in France, for example, involves wrapping the child (often naked) in towels that have been soaked in cold water and then warming the child up. The goal is to help break down the child's defenses that he or she has built up against very primitive anxieties and to realize a sense of self. The practice is difficult to watch, as it appears traumatic for the children, and while practiced in France and other French-speaking countries, wet-packing remains controversial [11].

Underdiagnosis of autism and referral bias among children from ethnic minorities is a known reality in developed nations. Begeer et al. [12] reported that children of Turkish and Moroccan origin in the Netherlands had a lower diagnosis rate (2.2%) compared to ethnically Dutch children (4.4%). Additionally, the authors found that pediatricians in the Netherlands were more likely to refer nonminority children to a psychiatrist after evaluating clinical vignettes. Within the United States, race, ethnicity, and socioeconomic status all play a role in which children are identified as having autism. Mandell et al. [13] found that African-American children subsequently diagnosed with autism are at least 2.5 times less likely to receive a diagnosis at their first specialty visit than a white child with autism. Work by Jarquin et al. [14] found that non-Hispanic Black children receive only the most severe diagnosis of ASD, in contrast to non-Hispanic White children who receive the diagnosis at all levels of severity. Using data collected from states on the number of children eligible for special education services under the category of autism, Morrier and Hess [15] found significant underrepresentation for Hispanic children in 95% of US states. Travers et al. [16] were able to document this particular finding has persisted between 1998 and 2006, while the likelihood of eligibility based on ASD varied across time for other minority groups.

We note that educational eligibility is not equivalent to diagnosis, although these findings are consistent with the recommendation by Mandell and Novak [13] to conduct research on "the complex relationship between culture and treatment, focusing on cultural differences in the behavioral phenotype of ASD, recognition of symptoms, interpretation of symptoms, families' decisions regarding medical and educational interventions, and interactions between families and the healthcare system" [13]. This intricate network of factors is illustrated by the research conducted by Colbert and colleagues [17] on the influence of knowledge of autism among Hispanic families in Texas. The authors found a positive correlation between the level of acculturation and knowledge about ASD, mainly in relation to the adoption of English over Spanish. Socioeconomic status (SES) was also correlated to knowledge levels. While this correlation might be present in minority and majority groups, it becomes a notable factor when we consider that rates of low SES are higher among Hispanic and other minorities in the United States. Certain culturally specific traits of Hispanic families had conflicting effect in this study. On the one hand, the presence of social support, a well-known trait of Hispanic culture, increased the level of knowledge of ASD. On the other hand, religiosity, also of high cultural value, correlated negatively with ASD knowledge. This last finding is consistent with other observations that Latin American parents—particularly mothers—might see their child's autism as either a gift from God to prove themselves or as a punishment from God for a previous transgression. These religious explanatory models of mental health can prevent parents from seeking behavioral healthcare services for their children [18–20].

It would not be surprising, then, to find that diagnostic confusion is linked to cultural context. It is axiomatic that societies conceptualize the symptoms of autism in ways that are meaningful to them—for example, Navajo mothers in the American Southwest viewing autism as "perpetual childhood"—because this idea fits within the expectations of a matrilineal society to preserve the bonds between the child and his or her mother's family. But cultural context also includes the culture of science, as the DSM is no less a cultural construct than any other form of disease classification.

Healthcare Discrepancies in Cultural Context: The Politics and Cultural Ecology of Psychodiagnostic Assessment

Diagnosis and treatment are also influenced by the position of an individual along various axes, such as ethnicity, class, and gender. Individuals from ethnic and racial minorities are less likely to receive the same number and kind of diagnostic tests as their nonminority counterparts and undergo fewer major procedures. African-Americans with peripheral vascular diseases are more likely to undergo amputations and less likely to undergo revascularization procedures. Hispanic patients receive less pain medication than their non-Hispanic counterparts for the same orthopedic injuries, and Hispanic children are less likely to have health insurance in the United States, which translates to reduced access to diagnostic services and treatment [21]. These differences also hold for people already within the healthcare system [22]. Immigrants in the United States receive only about half of the available healthcare services when compared with their native-born counterparts, regardless of their insurance coverage [23].

Psychiatry as a field has been especially fraught with diagnostic variability, and also misdiagnosis, often due to cognitive and implicit biases, as well as the limitations of its existing technology (i.e., rating scales rather than biomarkers). Perhaps the best known example of such variability is the diagnosis of psychotic disorders instead of affective disorders among African-American men [24, 25]. African-American men at first admission to state psychiatric hospitals are five times more likely to be diagnosed with schizophrenia than their white counterparts, even when they do not fulfill the diagnostic criteria, and this pattern exists independent of the race of the clinician [26]. The misdiagnosis often results from an interpretation of depressive symptoms as the negative symptoms of schizophrenia (apathy, blunting of affect, low motivation, etc.) and psychosis related to mood disorders interpreted as positive symptoms of schizophrenia. Other examples include the preference for diagnoses of emotional disturbance and conduct disorder for children with organic brain syndromes or autism, as is the case with the vignette about autism in Korea at the beginning of this chapter [3, 27]. Often, behaviors that are considered normative in one society (e.g., hearing the voice of a deceased loved one within several days of the person's death among some American Indian groups) are mistaken for psychopathology [28].

Misdiagnosis in psychiatry can also be seen as part of a larger issue with disparities in mental health on a global scale. Neuropsychiatric disorders represent 37% of healthy life years lost due to morbidity and disproportionally impact low- and middle-income countries [29]. Differences in access to healthcare professionals, reduced number of specialists, and different cultural understandings of mental health are some of the factors leading to this unequal burden of mental health in developing nations. In Ethiopia, for example, Tekola et al. [30] found that there are only 60 psychiatrists serving a population of 96 million; of those only 2 are pediatric psychiatrists. Additionally, there is a very limited popular understanding of autism in Ethiopia, which, together with fear of stigma and parental blame, prevents parents from seeking a clinical diagnosis for their children. While studied locally, these inequities have a global effect. Many of these individuals migrate to the United States and other developed nations where they face an already biased healthcare system that continues to limit their access to care. Seemingly objective differences in resources between developed and undeveloped countries become irrelevant, even invisible, to the individual who cannot access or use them.

Any clinician knows how often medical diagnoses are based not on empirical clinical tests but on the basis of symptoms, patterns of symptoms, and patient history or even in order to justify a treatment or intervention. A clinician may diagnose malaria in someone who lives in or recently visited a tropical rainforest and who has a fever, chills, and enlarged spleen, even without identifying the actual parasite under a microscope. The context and the symptom profile are sufficient evidence to support a diagnosis and a treatment plan; even where the differential diagnosis is broad, if a treatment for a possible condition works, one may often assume the diagnosis was correct. Not surprisingly, then, medical misdiagnosis is common. Cardiac episodes are often confused with anxiety or panic attacks, Lyme disease is confused with any number of other conditions, and thyroid cancers are now famously overdiagnosed in a number of countries [31]. Some misdiagnoses are motivated by often unconscious ethnic, gender, or racial biases. Misdiagnoses may be partially the result of different kinds of treatment plans for different kinds of individuals, since the desired treatment often drives the diagnosis. In the cases of children who have RAD but not ASD, as illustrated by the Spanish case at the beginning of our chapter, families can "fall through the cracks" in the healthcare system due to a reduced pool of effective treatments.

Giving a child a diagnosis of RAD over ASD or vice versa can prevent a child from receiving appropriate psychological and education services, yet differentiation between the two is often established less through systematic or evidence-based assessments than through highly subjective, culturally constituted factors, such as clinicians' perceptions or feelings. The Coventry Grid is a case in point. Coventry Child and Adolescent Mental Health Services (CAMHS) in the United Kingdom developed the Coventry Grid, a tool designed to identify behavioral differences to distinguish between ASD and attachment problems in children. In her description of this tool, Moran [32] explains that while the main features of autism are also present in attachment disorders, a closer look at the behavior patterns of the child can shine light on the difference between the two diagnoses. One of the key differences, according to the author, lies in the relationship with the therapy provider. According to the clinicians working at CAMHS, relationships with children with development problems had a more "emotional feel," while children in autism spectrum developed relationships with their therapy providers that had a more "matter-of-fact feel." In these interactions, they found that children with attachment problems would develop "relationships" more quickly and were able to maintain them, while children with ASD required more time and work to develop relationships with the clinicians. On the other hand, emotional boundaries were less of an issue with children with ASD since they "were not usually setting out to test those boundaries."

The Coventry Grid is an attempt to separate the more cognitive-led behaviors of children with ASD from the more emotional-led ones found in attachment disorders. Nevertheless, it fails to take into account possible cultural framings of such behaviors. For example, the tool lists a set of differences with the relation between children and possessions (usually toys). One such difference is that children with attachment problems "may seek social approval/envy from others for possessions," while a child with ASD makes collections of objects but does not seek such approval. This item in the grid has the embedded assumption that having a possession is inherently a positive trait that can elicit approval, but this is not true in all cultures. For children from large families in Latin America, toys and clothes are perceived as collective property among all the siblings and even with larger groups of kin-related children; therefore, displays of possession might elicit the opposite emotional response from peers and adults. Language cues used in the Coventry Grid can also be misleading since children in different societies learn specific aspects of their language at different times [27]. The concept of a relationship is also highly variable. What defines a common sociality or social engagement? Can an encounter in a clinical setting be compared to one in a more naturalistic setting? Even though this tool was developed within the United Kingdom, present-day western societies include families from a variety of origins who might continue to enculturate their children within their own cultural norms, and new definitions of sociality now comprise technological and interspecies communications.

Conclusion

Clinicians, psychologists, educators, and policy makers must take into account the cultural background of children presenting with symptoms of autism and/or attachment disturbance and their families. Understanding cultural differences must be central for all professionals who work with children and adults with psychiatric and neurodevelopmental conditions, not just because it promotes a respectful and sensitive interaction but because it can be vital for the adequate and successful management and care of these individuals. We used the example of ASD vs. RAD for this particular chapter, but a "one-size-fits-all" approach to the care of people with any condition can hinder the interventions designed to improve their and their families' lives; furthermore, it can inhibit families from seeking professional assistance in the first place if they feel their beliefs and cultural norms are not being understood. As it pertains to this chapter, the diagnosis of autism versus reactive attachment disorder can be influenced by cultural nuances that might not be known or apparent to the diagnostician. These differences include not only culturally constructed forms of social interaction but also a diagnostic preference from the parents who might lean toward one diagnosis or the other based on expectations of care, services available, or culture-specific biases.

References

1. Portugal-Fernández R, Balsa-Vidal H. Un caso de trastorno reactivo de la vinculación en la infancia. Rev Psiquiatr Psicol Niño Adolesc. 2004;4:1–10.
2. Hong K. Impacts of rapid social and family changes on the mental health of children in Korea. Psychiatry Invest. 2006;3:6–25.
3. Grinker RR, Cho K. Border children: interpreting autism spectrum disorder in South Korea. Ethos. 2013;41:46–74.
4. Richters MM, Volkmar FR. Reactive attachment disorder of infancy or early childhood. J Am Acad Child Adolesc Psychiatry. 1994;33:328–32.
5. Hanson RF, Spratt EG. Reactive attachment disorder: what we know about the disorder and implications for treatment. Child Maltreat. 2000;5:137–46.
6. Coto-Choto M. Autismo infantil: el estado de la cuestión. Revi Cienc Soc. 2007;116:169–80.
7. Bettelheim B. The empty fortress: infantile autism and the birth of the self. New York: The Free Press; 1967.
8. Grinker RR. Unstrange minds: remapping the world of autism. New York: Basic Books; 2007.
9. Shin Y, Lee K, Min S, Emde RN. A Korean syndrome of attachment disturbance mimicking symptoms of pervasive developmental disorder. Infant Ment Health J. 1999;20:60–76.
10. Powell GF, Bettes BA. Infantile depression, nonorganic failure to thrive, and DSM-III-R: a different perspective. Child Psychiatry Hum Dev. 1992;22:185–98.
11. Spinney L. Therapy for autistic children causes outcry in France. Lancet. 2007;370:645–6.
12. Begeer S, Bouk SE, Boussaid W, Terwogt MM, Koot HM. Underdiagnosis and referral bias of autism in ethnic minorities. J Autism Dev Disord. 2009;39:142–8.
13. Mandell DS, Listerud J, Levy SE, Pinto-Martin JA. Race differences in the age at diagnosis among Medicaid-eligible children with autism. J Am Acad Child Adolesc Psychiatry. 2002;41:1447–53.
14. Jarquin VG, Wiggins LD, Schieve LA, Van Naarden-Braun K. Racial disparities in community identification of autism spectrum disorders over time; Metropolitan Atlanta, Georgia, 2000–2006. J Dev Behav Pediatr. 2011;32:179–87.
15. Morrier MJ, Hess KL. Ethnic differences in autism eligibility in the United States public schools. J Spec Educ. 2012;46:49–63.
16. Travers JC, Higgins K, Pierce T, Boone R, Miller S, Tandy R. Emergent literacy skills of preschool students with autism: a comparison of teacher-led and computer-assisted instruction. Educ Train Autism Dev Disord. 2011;46:326–38.
17. Colbert AM, Webber J, Graham R. Factors that influence autism knowledge in hispanic cultures: a pilot study. J Racial Ethn Health Disparities. 2016;4(2):156–64.
18. Dyches TT, Wilder LK, Sudweeks RR. Multicultural issues in autism. J Autism Dev Disord. 2004;34:211–22.
19. Pizarro HC. Esquema corporal: una conducta básica para el aprendizaje del niño con autismo. Rev Educ. 2005;29:207–15.
20. Salkas K, Magaña S, Marques I, Mirza M. Spirituality in Latino families of children with autism spectrum disorder. J Fam Soc Work. 2016;19:38–55.
21. Alegria M, Vallas M, Pumariega AJ. Racial and ethnic disparities in pediatric mental health. Child Adolesc Psychiatr Clin N Am. 2010;19:759–74.
22. Geiger HJ. Unequal treatment: confronting racial and ethnic disparities in health care. Washington DC: The National Academies; 2003. p. 415–54.
23. Edberg M, Cleary S, Vyas A. A trajectory model for understanding and assessing health disparities in immigrant/refugee communities. J Immigr Minor Health. 2011;13:576–84.
24. Bell CC, Jackson WM, Bell BH. Misdiagnosis of African-Americans with psychiatric issues–part I. J Natl Med Assoc. 2015;107:25–34.
25. Schwartz RC, Blankenship DM. Racial disparities in psychotic disorder diagnosis: a review of empirical literature. World J Psychiatry. 2014;4:133–40.

26. Barnes A. Race, schizophrenia, and admission to state psychiatric hospitals. Admin Pol Ment Health. 2004;31:241–52.
27. Grinker RR, Yeargin-Allsopp M, Boyle C. Culture and autism spectrum disorders: the impact on prevalence and recognition. In: Amaral DG, Geschwind G, Daniel H, editors. Autism spectrum disorders. Oxford: Oxford University Press; 2011.
28. Adeponle AB, Thombs BD, Groleau D, Jarvis E, Kirmayer LJ. Using the cultural formulation to resolve uncertainty in diagnoses of psychosis among ethnoculturally diverse patients. Psychiatr Serv. 2012;63:147–53.
29. Wang PS, Aguilar-Gaxiola S, Alonso J. Use of mental health services for anxiety, mood, and substance disorders in 17 countries in the WHO world mental health surveys. Lancet. 2007;370:841–50.
30. Tekola B, Baheretibeb Y, Roth I, Tilahun D, Fekadu A, Hanlon C, Hoekstra RA. Challenges and opportunities to improve autism services in low-income countries: lessons from a situational analysis in Ethiopia. Global Ment Health. 2016;3:1–11.
31. Ahn HS, Kim HJ, Welch HG. Korea's thyroid-cancer epidemic--screening and overdiagnosis. N Engl J Med. 2014;371:1765.
32. Moran H. Clinical observations of the differences between children on the autism spectrum and those with attachment problems: the Coventry grid. Good Autism Pract. 2010;11:46–59.

Chapter 9
Special Population Consideration in ASD Identification and Treatment

Alison Chavez, Lark Huang-Storms, and Katharine Zuckerman

Introduction

Vignette

Maria is a 15-year-old Latina girl, accompanied by her father for a developmental-behavioral pediatrics assessment in a large suburban area of the USA. Maria's father, Mr. J., relates that he and Maria's mother have been concerned about Maria since she was 3 or 4 years of age but, due to various insurance issues, had not pursued an assessment earlier. Mr. J. notes that Maria seemed to achieve all of her early developmental milestones on time. However, around age 4, he began to notice that Maria seemed very withdrawn, choosing to play by herself even when other children were around. Maria even tended to avoid playing with siblings and cousins and seemed to prefer to be alone. Mr. J. recalled that a teacher once remarked that other children laughed at Maria on the playground and perhaps this is why she was withdrawn; Mr. J. remembers dismissing the concern as harmless teasing. Furthermore, Mr. J. notes that the play Maria would do by herself was odd—that she would sort or line up her toys, sometimes to examine them minutely, but not necessarily to play with them as other children her age would do.

A. Chavez (✉)
Department of Psychology, University of Massachusetts Boston, Boston, MA, USA
e-mail: alison.chavez001@umb.edu

L. Huang-Storms
Department of Pediatrics, Oregon Health and Science University, Portland, OR, USA
e-mail: huangsto@ohsu.edu

K. Zuckerman
Division of General Pediatrics, Oregon Health and Science University, Portland, OR, USA
e-mail: zuckerma@ohsu.edu

J. M. Fogler, R. A. Phelps (eds.), *Trauma, Autism, and Neurodevelopmental Disorders*, https://doi.org/10.1007/978-3-030-00503-0_9

At times, Maria would sit by herself and not play with her toys at all, but would instead wiggle her fingers and talk to herself. While relating the history, Mr. J. became tearful, reporting that he has always been too busy with work, always working two to three jobs at a time throughout Maria's childhood, which is a big part of the reason that Maria was not brought in for an assessment a decade earlier. Mr. J. expresses concern that Maria is the way she is because he, as a father, did not have the time to play with her. He also expresses guilt over not addressing the teacher's bullying concerns because the victimization could have caused Maria to become withdrawn.

Currently, Maria is doing very well in many respects. She attends high school; she is in the ninth grade. Academically, she does quite well in school, earning As and Bs. Her teachers describe her as more hardworking than her peers. Her teachers also note that she does seem capable of understanding the content of the work, but perhaps struggles to keep up with the pace. She is taking a full workload of mainstream coursework. She particularly enjoys math and science. She does not have an Individualized Educational Program (IEP), although she is in a study skills class with a special education teacher. Mr. J. is unsure why Maria does not have an IEP. He notes that the school has requested a formal evaluation for autism spectrum disorder, but this has not yet been accomplished. It is mentioned that Maria enjoys drawing horses and reading graphic novels. When asked what she likes to do with her free time, Maria says she likes to watch YouTube videos on her phone, yet has a difficult time describing exactly what she likes to watch. She is very organized. Her room is very clean. She is very careful with her appearance, but has always preferred clothing that is comfortable and soft in texture. Maria is helpful around the house and is good about completing her chores.

On the other hand, there are a number of persistent concerns. Socially, Maria is somewhat of a loner and does not have any close friends. Maria reports that she usually hangs out by herself during school lunch, or goes to the library, and asserts she is happy that way. She describes that when she did find herself becoming friends with other girls, she thinks that they mocked her mannerisms and teased her about her hobbies. Maria vaguely described boys being physically mean and says that these experiences taught her to keep to herself to avoid being taunted. Maria often struggles to follow along with conversations. She does not understand the content of conversations often and has difficulty engaging in conversations. She remarks that she struggles with eye contact and feels like she mumbles. She has difficulty understanding jokes and sometimes thinks teachers are upset with her when they are only teasing. Mr. J. reports that Maria shows little facial expression. When Maria is frustrated, she often hits her head with her hands. Even when not frustrated, when perfectly calm, she does have some other repetitive behaviors, which include repetitive shaking of her hands and combing through her hair with her fingers. Mr. J. adds that he cannot remember if Maria's repetitive behaviors started before she was teased in school; he wonders if the behaviors are the result of students bullying his daughter.

Past medical history, review of systems, family history, and social history were all non-contributory, except as described that Mr. J. expresses great guilt over his heavy workload and wonders how that might have impacted his daughter's development since he was not available when she may have needed him and that intermittent insurance coverage contributed to deferral of this assessment for some years. During the interview, Maria maintained flat affect with minimal variability in facial expression and variable, often avoidant, eye contact. She used few gestures, but when she did, they seemed somewhat exaggerated. She responded to questions appropriately but often seemed confused by questions and would often go off on non-sequiturs. She made no spontaneous overtures and rarely responded to social bids. However, she was generally pleasant and fully cooperative with exam and interview. Structured observations, using the Autism Diagnostic Observation Schedule (ADOS), suggest impairments of social interaction skills and social communication skills, as well as restricted imagination, and observation of some repetitive movements and behaviors. Adaptive assessment indicates borderline-impaired skills overall, with relatively strong skills in subdomains of functional academics and self-care and relatively low skills in social and communication skills. At the end of the assessment, Maria and her father are presented with a diagnosis: autism spectrum disorder (ASD).

According to current estimates, approximately 1 in 68 children in the USA has an ASD [1–4]. This prevalence rate suggests recent stabilization after a large prevalence increase over the past two decades. The large and recent change in ASD prevalence is likely multifactorial in nature, relating to changes in ASD diagnostic criteria over the past 20 years (including a broader range of phenotype and severity), diagnostic shifts from intellectual disability to ASD, and improved case capture due to overall broader ASD service access [5]. Additionally, enhanced awareness of the condition [6, 7], and greater exposure to environmental risk factors [8, 9], may play a role in increasing prevalence.

Closer analysis of ASD prevalence rate by demographic characteristics such as sex, race, and ethnicity reveals significant variation in ASD diagnosis rates in the USA. More specifically, estimates from the Centers for Disease Control and Prevention (CDC) indicate that the ASD prevalence in 8-year-old males (1 in 42) is higher than that in same-aged females (1 in 189) [4]. Compared to non-Latino White boys, people of color in the USA (i.e., individuals who identify as racial and ethnic minorities) also experience delays and lower rates of ASD diagnosis. In addition to delays in diagnosis, both girls and children of color also are diagnosed at lower rates than White children overall, even when they meet diagnostic criteria for ASD; furthermore, those that are diagnosed are more likely to have comorbid intellectual disability [10–12]. As a result, children like Maria, who experience difficulties in mainstream educational systems but are functioning well enough to "make do," never receive the educational supports that might allow them to achieve their developmental potential.

Individuals with autism spectrum disorder (ASD) also commonly experience comorbid mental disorders such as anxiety, attention-deficit/hyperactivity disorder (ADHD), and trauma- and stressor-related disorders (TSRD) [13, 14]. Deficits in social awareness associated with ASD may increase the risk of interpersonal victimization across the lifespan, with resulting elevated risk for TSRDs such as posttraumatic stress disorder (PTSD) subsequent to traumatic experiences [15–17]. Alexithymia, characterized by a reduced ability to identify and describe one's own emotional states, is strongly associated with ASD, with between 40% and 65% of adults with ASD meeting criteria [18]. These challenges may impede recognition of self-protective discomfort or fear states in response to others' inappropriate social behaviors, thus placing individuals with ASD at higher risk for interpersonal abuse [19]. In addition, research has indicated that individuals with ASD may experience poorer emotional regulation in the face of adverse events [20], as well as stronger biological responses to stressors as compared to individuals without ASD [21]. Increased stress reactivity and emotional dysregulation have been found to be potential risk factors for PTSD [22], which places individuals with ASD at risk for comorbid anxiety or TSRD symptoms.

This chapter discusses perspectives on ASD among females and racial and ethnic minority people: two populations where there continue to be troubling disparities in the diagnosis of ASD. The first portion of the chapter examines prevalence differences between males and females with ASD and explores the biological and sociological reasons for these differences. The second part of the chapter more specifically examines racial and ethnic differences in ASD prevalence and hypothesized family-, community-, provider-, and system-level reasons for these disparities. The final section of this chapter discusses implications for practice and policy concerning autism care, advocacy, future research, and ethical issues. We conclude the chapter with a note from the editors that further illuminates why issues related to females and racial and ethnic minorities are important to include in the conversation on ASD and TSRD.

Part 1: Sex Discrepancies in ASD Prevalence and Diagnosis

ASD Prevalence in Males and Females

The underlying sex ratio bias in ASD is a long-standing phenomenon, which consistently demonstrates that more males are impacted than females. The *Diagnostic and Statistical Manual of Mental Disorders, Fifth Edition* (*DSM-5*), states that "autism spectrum disorder is diagnosed four times more often in males than in females" [23] and this 4:1 ratio is widely cited as the mean male-to-female ratio in population prevalence studies of ASD [24–26]. Indeed, from the first published descriptions of autism in the 1940s, it has been described as a male-typical disorder [27, 28], and this clinical observation has held constant over the past decades. Autism studies have reported wide variability in the male-to-female ratio, ranging from 1.65:1 in a high-risk sibling cohort [29] to greater than 8:1 in higher-functioning samples [30]. However, male skew in ASD rates is consistently found. In spite of historical changes in nosological details of the diagnostic criteria, empirical research also indicates similar male-to-female ratio in ASD over time [1] and across the DSM-IV and DSM-5 criteria [31, 32].

It should be noted that averages of sex ratios do not capture the substantial variability found across ASD prevalence research, even among epidemiological studies implementing similar inclusion criteria and recruitment methods. This heterogeneity raises questions about sex-determined biological differences and possible differences in clinical correlates, such as cognitive function, across the sexes. Intellectual functioning, in particular, appears to affect the ASD sex ratio [33]. An early review of epidemiological surveys of autism published over three decades indicated a median sex ratio of 6:1 among individuals with average intellectual functioning and 1.7:1 among individuals with moderate to severe intellectual disability [34]. This trend has continued to hold, with males consistently and substantially overrepresented among high-functioning samples and more equally balanced male-to-female ratios among samples with significant cognitive impairment [35–37].

Impact of Racial and Ethnic Variables on the ASD Sex Ratio

International prevalence research in ASD indicates that birth-identified sex has a strong influence on rates of ASD across various national, ethnic, and racial backgrounds [38]. These associations persist across epidemiological studies [39], regardless of immigrant status, nationality, or racial/ethnic composition. International studies also tend to replicate the finding that the boy-to-girl ratio is correlated with severity of intellectual disability (e.g., findings using the national disability registry of Taiwan) [40]. However, disparities do exist for certain demographic groups in terms of timely access to ASD diagnosis and treatment, as clearly outlined elsewhere in this chapter [41]. It may well be that in certain racial or ethnic populations, females have increased risk for diagnostic and treatment delays or clinical oversight as compared to males. This seems especially likely in demographic groups that do not emphasize educational access for girls and women, as it is often the school setting where developmental concerns around intellectual ability and social communication are noted and evaluation referrals are initiated [42].

Recent research also suggests it may be possible that overall male prevalence rates in ASD could be lessened in demographic groups supportive of older fathering. Research by Anello and colleagues [43] involving a large series of multiplex families indicated that the ASD male-to-female ratio may significantly attenuate with increasing paternal age, after adjusting for maternal age. Results mirrored descriptive observations of the reduction in the male-to-female ratio with increasing paternal age found in other population-based studies [44, 45]. Current literature has only begun to explore cultural factors like educational access and paternal age that may impact ASD prevalence ratios. It also remains unclear to what degree the male-skewed ratio in ASD may reflect unbalanced sampling of demographic and clinical factors across populations. For example, females of lower socioeconomic strata and non-dominant cultural groups are likely differentially underrepresented across grouping in the autism research literature, but the interplay of these variables with sex has yet to be delineated.

Sex-Differential Biological Factors of ASD Risk

Several biological factors have been postulated that could help explain higher male prevalence rates in ASD. One popular theory, referred to as the "female protective effect," is a variation of a multiple threshold liability model for ASD risk [46]. According to this model, males and females have different genetic liability thresholds, or minimum variant loads, at which they present an ASD phenotype [47, 48]. Thus, affected females would be expected to carry a greater risk variant load, on average, than affected males. This would also increase the likelihood of global cognitive deficits in females with ASD, which has been a consistent finding [49].

Sibling recurrence risk estimates from multiplex families and infant sibling studies are consistent with the effects of a biological mechanism that protects females from manifesting an ASD phenotype. Zhao and colleagues [50] and Ozonoff and colleagues [51] have found ASD recurrence in nearly half of later-born brothers in families; however, these studies report far lower risk (approximately 20%) to later-born sisters from multiplex families. This model is further supported by a 2013 study by Robinson et al. [52] using a general population dizygotic twin cohort, which indicated that sex of the autistic proband influenced the level of autistic traits in the twin sibling. Specifically, higher autistic traits were measured in a sibling when the proband was female, suggesting a greater etiological load in females with ASD and their relatives.

Sex chromosomal genes have been proposed as potential players in molecular mechanisms driving the female protective effect, as conferred by specific risk loci and/or by genome-wide mutational load. An early theory proposed that ASD might be an X-linked disorder, by which females would be protected from X chromosomal mutation effects through compensatory transcription from an intact, second X chromosome. However, ASD transmission in most families does not follow an X-linked pattern [53]. Furthermore, while several ASD risk genes have been identified on the X chromosome (e.g., MECP2, PTCHD1, TMLHE, NLGN3, and NLGN4X [54, 55]), all cause significant cognitive impairment, indicating a more general role for X chromosome gene dosage in neural development. Increasingly, there is evidence for heritable loci with sex-differential penetrance, linkage peaks, and microdeletions [56]. High heritability with distinct genetic influences has also been identified for various ASD diagnostic subdomains (i.e., social impairments, communication impairments, restricted repetitive behaviors, and interests), which may be differentially represented across sexes or manifest as sex- and domain-specific protective factors [57].

Neurodevelopmental hormonal mechanisms have also been proposed to explain the male bias of ASD, including testosterone-related effects on brain development in prenatal life [58]. Baron-Cohen contributed the "Extreme Male Brain" theory of autism, which suggests testosterone modulates effects of genetic variation on the presentation of an autism phenotype. This model proposes that ASD arises from hyper-masculinization of the brain, defined psychometrically as skills for systemizing (i.e., drive to interact with and understand rule-based systems) that are significantly more developed than skills for empathizing. Given that testosterone secreted by fetal testes during gestation drives human sexual differentiation, it has been proposed that fetal testosterone levels may predispose the differentiating brain toward an ASD phenotype. While the mechanisms of these hormonal and genetic findings are not thoroughly elaborated and cannot fully explain the male bias in ASD, research increasingly elucidates possible biological variants that may confer sex-differential risk.

Emergence of a Female ASD Phenotype

As described above, comorbid intellectual disability increases females' likelihood of acquiring an ASD diagnosis. Conversely, cognitively higher-functioning females may go undiagnosed. Research by Dworzynski et al. [59] suggests that, in the absence of additional intellectual or behavioral problems, girls are less likely than boys to meet diagnostic criteria for ASD at equivalently high levels of autistic traits. Posserud et al. [42] observed in a general population sample the tendency for parents of girls to report more ASD symptom concerns than their teachers, but this pattern was not found for boys. Some females with ASD, especially those with strong language and cognitive skills, may be more adept than their male counterparts at compensating for their difficulties in certain contexts such as school [60]. There is emerging evidence that females are more likely to mask their ASD-related difficulties by a process of studying and mimicking social behaviors (a process described as "camouflaging") which may make timely and accurate diagnosis more challenging [61]. Thus, for girls, intellectual disability may be the key salient issue prompting educational evaluation and eventual diagnosis.

In contrast with the higher proportion of diagnosed autistic females than males with intellectual disability, studies find no sex differences in global composite scores of core ASD symptoms as measured by standard autism assessment tools [60]. A range of associated ASD features (including sleep difficulties, eating problems, sensory sensitivities, gross motor impairment, and dyspraxia) also seem to be experienced to a similar degree in both sexes [62]. However, differences emerge when each core symptom domain of ASD is considered separately, with behavioral presentation patterns tending to reflect sex differences that are observed in the broader population literature [63]. Specifically, females tend to demonstrate more significant internalizing emotional difficulties, and males tend to have greater externalizing and interpersonal problems.

Looking at a toddler sample, Hartley and Sikora [64] found that girls showed greater internalizing difficulties than boys on a broad behavioral parent rating scale in the areas of anxiety, social withdrawal, social problems, and thought problems, as well as more attention problems. Older girls with ASD also tend to show greater internalizing symptoms than boys, including anxiety, depression, and other emotional symptoms as reported by parents [65]. Frazier et al. [66] additionally found poorer adaptive functioning in females with ASD ages 4–18 years as compared to their male counterparts. Using an ASD screening questionnaire, Kopp and Gillberg [60] found that parents more frequently endorsed task avoidance for school-aged girls, perhaps reflecting girls' tendency for passive misbehavior. Conversely, males with ASD have been found to show more externalizing behavior problems, such as aggression, hyperactivity, and asocial behavior, as well as increased repetitive/restricted behaviors and interests.

Dworzynski et al. [59] further assessed the potential female diagnosis gap by characterizing children in the UK with high ASD traits who met or fell short of the threshold for ASD diagnosis. A significantly smaller proportion of high-scoring girls met full ASD diagnostic criteria than boys (38% versus 56%), whereas ASD-diagnosed girls had a higher mean total problem score (a composite of hyperactivity, anxiety, conduct, peer, and prosocial problems). Girls who fell below the ASD threshold showed increased communication difficulties, but reduced social impairments as compared to non-diagnosed boys. This suggests that relatively higher levels of social ability in females may preclude full diagnosis of ASD, particularly for those girls who have intact cognition and fewer behavior problems. Because male-typical externalizing behaviors are generally more disruptive in the home or school setting than female-typical internalizing behaviors, males may be more frequently referred for evaluation and diagnosis, especially as compared to females with no intellectual impairment.

A number of studies have indicated that the type and intensity of repetitive behaviors and interests demonstrated by girls tend to be less overt than those of boys with ASD and thus may appear less socially discrepant from their peers [64]. For example, preoccupying interests for girls may appear to be more gender normative and age-typical in terms of topic (e.g., animals, animé), in spite of their circumscribed nature and intensity [65]. In an early large study of sex differences in ASD, Lord et al. [24] found that females with autism had lower levels of unusual visual interests. Contemporary studies have confirmed lower levels of repetitive sensory motor behavior in older girls with ASD, for whom repetitive behaviors are often more obvious and impairing in a peer setting [64]. It is not yet clear whether this reduction is more broadly present across all diagnostic subdomains, such as repetitive sensory motor behaviors, need for sameness, and restricted interests. However, work by Mandy and colleagues [30] found that sex differences were most pronounced for repetitive symptoms more characteristic of higher-functioning individuals, such as cataloguing facts and information about intense areas of interest. As females with ASD tend to have less atypical preoccupying interests that are more aligned with those of their peers, this further increases the risk that higher-functioning females may "fly under the radar" of ASD diagnosis.

Ascertainment and Diagnostic Bias

It is increasingly understood that the high sex ratio in ASD reflects at least some level of bias in the diagnostic criteria currently used, as well as the way these criteria are interpreted differentially for males and females. Original autism descriptions, subsequent diagnostic criteria, and the vast majority of phenotypic data are derived from male samples with ASD. This has made it challenging to assess whether sex ratios reflect true differences in symptom expression or a measurement artifact given that diagnostic criteria were primarily based on male-centric descriptions. However, the contrast between active and passive case ascertainment studies may hint broadly at underdiagnosis of females. In their meta-analysis, Loomes et al. [25] found that in studies that actively sought cases of ASD (i.e., regardless of whether individuals had been previously identified), there were significantly more females as compared to passive studies that included only previously diagnosed cases. The authors assert that a portion of females exist in the general population who would likely meet criteria for ASD if evaluated, but who have not been consistently referred for clinical diagnosis.

Regardless of etiology, clinical awareness of the male-skewed sex ratio in ASD frames expectations around a prototypical male norm. Not only in research but also in publicly recognized film and other media, individuals with ASD are usually male. Being male is, indeed, the strongest risk factor for ASD. This fact influences the clinical expectation that males represent the at-risk group, while lowering the index of suspicion for females and potentially contributing to female under-identification [65]. Clinicians and researchers may find it harder to recognize some manifestations of ASD in girls compared to boys, especially if impairments are more subtle or are better compensated for in certain settings (e.g., structured testing environments with adult clinicians). Less circumscribed, atypical preoccupying interests may also be a protective factor or may represent a less obviously identifiable phenotype during clinical evaluation [67, 68]. At present, diagnostic instruments are anchored on historically male symptom features and do not include behavioral features that may be more characteristic of a female ASD phenotype.

Comorbidity of ASD and Trauma in Females

It is well supported that bullying and teasing victimization is common for individuals with ASD, and these experiences have been found to mediate the relationship between autistic traits and anxiety symptoms [69]. It has also been hypothesized that behavioral rigidities exhibited by children with ASD may be perceived by parents as oppositional, potentially increasing risk for overly punitive parental reactions to behavioral problems [70]. Individuals with ASD may be at increased risk of interpersonal victimization due to weaknesses in emotional and social cognition, which make it more challenging to perceive departures from social norms around intimacy and romantic relationships, including potentially abusive behaviors [71, 72]. Victimization and TSRDs may be more common among females with ASD compared to males with ASD. A retrospective study of childhood abuse, trauma victimization, and PTSD symptoms by autistic traits among adult women in a large US population-based longitudinal cohort found that women with the highest level of autistic traits had 1.5 times the prevalence of sexual abuse, almost twice the prevalence of physical/emotional abuse, and higher PTSD symptoms, as compared to women with the lowest level of autistic traits [73]. Furthermore, higher exposure to childhood abuse accounted for nearly one-third of the higher risk of PTSD symptoms in the upper quintile of women with the highest autistic traits. The authors suggest that higher exposure to chronic stressors from lifelong challenges in social interactions may increase risk for PTSD symptoms in women, which aligns with other research suggesting that chronic exposure to stressors may be a risk factor for PTSD.

Summary

Although most developmental disorders are more common in males [74], the consistency of the male preponderance in ASD across time and populations implicates the involvement of sex-specific biological factors in ASD etiology. Research supports the influence of sex-differential genetic and hormonal factors and etiologic protective factors in females, including higher genetic liability for expression of ASD in females. Factors unique to different ASD symptom domains have also been identified by behavioral genetic studies, further supporting the potential for domain-specific protective factors that may differ across sex. In recent years, increased priority has been placed on the inclusion of females in ASD research. However, the majority of studies of sex differences on the ASD phenotype have included only modest female sample sizes, have focused exclusively on adults, or have assessed a limited number of domains (e.g., cognition or neuropsychological function).

While researchers have made considerable progress identifying novel genetic risk variants for ASD, it has been increasingly recognized that the male predominance in ASD likely also reflects some level of ascertainment bias and male-centric diagnostic nosology. Increasingly, a specific female ASD phenotype is emerging that cannot entirely be accounted for by differential symptom measurement or correlations with intellectual functioning. Research suggests that females may be under-identified and may show different behavioral, cognitive, and developmental patterns of ASD symptom expression. In particular, high-functioning females without restricted interests but with social communication difficulties and need for sameness may not meet full criteria under current diagnostic criteria using standard

ASD instruments. It remains to be seen if this subset of girls and women may be better described by the newer diagnostic addition to the DSM-5 of Social Communication Disorder or if nosological adjustments or sex-specific algorithms will be further developed to inform more encompassing diagnostic criteria for ASD.

Part 2: Racial and Ethnic Disparities in the Prevalence, Diagnosis, and Treatment of ASD

Prior to launching into a discussion of racial/ethnic differences in ASD, it is necessary to define the terms used to describe racial and ethnic minorities. Race describes social categories that have been historically used to categorize humans based on biological markers, although there is scant scientific evidence for such biological markers [75]. Ethnicity designates groups that share a common ancestry, culture, or language. The US Census separates race and ethnicity (e.g., Latino/Hispanic is an ethnicity and not a race, while Asian is a race and not an ethnicity), and consequently many research studies on US populations also adopt this distinction. Racial and ethnic minorities in the USA are defined as those who are non-White; White people are currently being defined as those originating from Europe, the Middle East, or North Africa [76]. We will use the term "people of color" to broadly refer to individuals who identify as racial and ethnic minorities. The terms race and ethnicity or race/ethnicity can be used to describe these groups of people. The term "White" will describe non-Latino White populations.

Multiple studies show variability in ASD prevalence when the population is examined by child race and ethnicity. In the USA, most studies show higher rates of ASD in White compared to non-Hispanic Black/African-American children ("Black"), Hispanic/Latino children ("Latino"), and Asian/Pacific Islander ("Asian/PI") children [77]. Research on ASD prevalence by race/ethnicity in other countries is more mixed. In particular, studies in settings where access to educational and healthcare services is more equitable have shown less difference between racial/ethnic groups or even a slight increase in prevalence among immigrant and/or racial/ethnic minority populations [78–80]. Research on racial/ethnic differences in ASD prevalence is also limited by the fact that race/ethnicity is often confounded by other measures of socioeconomic status (e.g., parental income, parental education), which also show strong prevalence trends, especially in US samples [81, 82] (see further discussion below). Nonetheless, more recent analyses have suggested that, at least in the USA, minority race/ethnicity contributes to lower prevalence even once parental socioeconomic status is taken into account [78, 83].

Unlike identified hormonal and genetic etiological associations between sex and ASD, there is little research to support an association between race-/ethnicity-linked biological variables and occurrence of ASD. In fact, recent genetic research suggests that race is not a meaningful biological construct in general and specifically in mental health research [84, 85]. Furthermore, no plausible biological mechanism has been put forth as to how race/ethnicity might alter risk for ASD. As a result, the low incidence of ASD among non-White groups in national prevalence rates in the USA is thought to be primarily an *under-identification* or *ascertainment bias* in racial and ethnic minority populations [86, 87]. However, it should be recognized that racial/ethnic differences could also be explained by *over-identification* of White children. This may be particularly the case because families have better overall access to educational and health services generally [88, 89] and thus may have greater access to ASD diagnostic resources. To our knowledge, no research has addressed whether over-identification of White children in the USA can explain prevalence differences. However, similar research with ADHD has suggested that under-identification of racial/ethnic minorities is a stronger prevalence driver [90].

The hypothesis of ascertainment bias in children of color is supported by research suggesting that racial and ethnic minorities also are less likely to receive an early ASD diagnosis. With signs and symptoms usually being notable by age 2 [91, 92], a reliable ASD diagnosis can often be made early in childhood. Studies conducted in the USA suggest that the mean age of diagnosis for ASD generally ranges from 3.1 years to 7.4 years [93], with substantial variation attributed to region of the USA sampled, diagnoses examined (e.g., inclusion of Asperger's disorder and pervasive developmental disorder—not otherwise specified [PDD-NOS][1]), and years of records examined [93].

However, studies suggest that children of color tend to be diagnosed at later ages than their White peers [41]. For instance, in a study of Medicaid-eligible children with ASD in the Philadelphia area, Mandell and colleagues [41] found that White children received their first ASD diagnosis at 6.3 years of age, compared with 7.9 years for Black children and 8.8 years for Latino children. While these exact numbers tend to fluctuate from study to study, recent investigations on this topic have identified similar patterns in cohorts of children across different US regions [94] and in national multi-site studies [95, 96].

In addition to experiencing delays in diagnosis, it appears that children of color with ASD also tend to be diagnosed at the point of more severe symptoms than their White peers [97]. This holds true, even when samples are controlled for socioeconomic status [98, 99]. Also, children of color are more likely to have comorbid intellectual disability than White peers [4, 100]. Children of color with ASD who receive delayed diagnoses often do not receive any other diagnosis. However, there is some evidence that Black children tend to receive misdiagnoses of conduct disorder or adjustment disorder prior to being diagnosed with ASD [101, 102].

Racial/ethnic differences are also found in rates of use of ASD treatment [103, 104], which is often one way that ASD prevalence is measured in epidemiologic studies [105]. Access to treatment is also important because studies suggest that early intensive treatment targeting ASD's core features and associated symptoms

[1] Prior to the release of the fifth edition of the *Diagnostic and Statistical Manual of Mental Disorders* (DSM-5) in 2013, autism spectrum disorders included autistic disorder, PDD-NOS, Asperger's disorder, Rett disorder, and childhood disintegrative disorder. The general label "autism spectrum disorder" in the DSM-5 supplanted these labels, and they are no longer current. We will use these labels when referring to studies published before 2013 that differentiated these diagnoses.

(e.g., applied behavioral analysis [ABA]) as well as more general use of therapies such as speech-language and occupational therapy may be associated with superior long-term developmental outcomes [106–108]. As a result, early intensive treatment is recommended by many organizations [109–111].

For instance, a large recent study by Leigh showed that public spending on services for ASD in California differed sharply by race/ethnicity, with Latino or Black children receiving fewer public funds for services than White children ($11,480 versus $9571 and $9482, respectively) [111]. Another study by Liptak reported on national parent survey data demonstrating that Black and Latino families were less likely to report having access to ASD services [10]. Palmer's 2010 Texas study also showed that when a school district has more Latino children, that school district has a lower treated prevalence of ASD [78]. Together, these results suggest that even when developmental treatment services are publicly funded and of no direct cost to families, as in the case of Early Intevention [112] and special education services [113], racial and ethnic minority families tend to be disproportionately underrepresented in utilization rates.

As noted above, however, not all US studies have identified racial and ethnic differences in the diagnosis of ASD [94, 96], and among those that have detected such differences, there is an important secondary discussion of other measures of disparity to be jointly considered. For instance, in one study that found no racial or ethnic disparities in age at first ASD diagnosis, Wiggins et al. [94] examined diagnostic patterns among a large sample of children with ASD in the metropolitan Atlanta area. The study's sample was categorized as White, Black, not stated, and Other—which included racial groups such as Asian/PI and American Indian. Though the study did uncover that White children were more likely to be diagnosed with Asperger's disorder than Black children and that Black children were more likely to be diagnosed with autistic disorder than White children, the researchers ultimately did not identify statistically significant differences in the mean age of diagnosis based on racial and ethnic characteristics. The study sample was drawn heavily from a middle-class Black population, which may have accounted for the lack of differences based on race in the findings. In another large-scale study based on an online national registry of families of children diagnosed with an ASD between 1994 and 2010, researchers identified disparities in age of ASD diagnosis by race but not by Latino ethnicity [114]. However, the registry was a self-selecting group that only included families who spoke English, therefore Spanish-speaking Latino families or Latino families who are less acculturated may not have been represented in the sample. English proficiency among Latinos may be an important predictor of ASD-related healthcare outcomes [115], and thus their exclusion may have underestimated population-level differences. Finally, in a survey of caregivers of individuals with ASD in Pennsylvania, Mandell et al. [93] revealed that in lieu of race and ethnicity, factors such as ASD subtype (i.e., Asperger's disorder, PDD-NOS, and autistic disorder), household income, and urbanicity seemed associated with later age of diagnosis. This study related that members of racial and ethnic minority populations did not receive an ASD diagnosis at an older age than White individuals.

Other Correlates to Consider in Measuring Disparity

A common thread in the aforementioned studies that did not identify differences in ASD diagnosis by race and ethnicity is the potential for race and ethnicity to be confounded with other sociodemographic characteristics. Socioeconomic status (SES) may be one alternative measure of disparity to consider when identifying the causes for the difference in rates of ASD diagnosis and treatment among racial and ethnic groups. SES has been inconsistently defined across health disparity studies [116], capturing elements such as household income, educational attainment, and employment status; some even approach SES by creating a composite variable of the aforementioned factors. Higher levels of household income and parental education have been associated with higher diagnostic rates [117], earlier diagnosis [118], greater satisfaction with the diagnostic process [118, 119], and increased utilization of autism services [120]. Analogously, in studies comparing family impact among children with special healthcare needs (CSHCN), families of children with ASD seem to fare worse in terms of employment status and earnings than families of children with other special healthcare needs [121–123]. Like race and ethnicity, SES may consequently play a role in a family's ability to access diagnostic and treatment services for ASD, particularly since these services are of limited supply. Since racial and ethnic minority families are more likely than White families in the USA to live in poverty, have lower household income, have higher unemployment rates, make fewer earnings, and have lower educational attainment, the concepts of race, ethnicity, and SES are closely intertwined [79, 80].

Parental nativity and immigrant status are other measures of disparity that have been considered alongside race and ethnicity in accounting for disparities in ASD diagnosis and treatment. Though it may be appealing to categorize families into broad groups such as Black and Asian/PI, accounting for parents' place(s) of birth has revealed nuances within these larger racial and ethnic groups. For instance, an analysis of ASD prevalence in Latino children with two foreign-born parents, versus Latinos with two US-born parents, suggested that children with foreign-born parents are diagnosed at lower rates [124]. Similar differences have been identified among other ethnic groups. In a nationally representative sample of parents of children with ASD and other developmental disabilities [125], children with ASD from immigrant households were more likely to lack access to healthcare insurance, lack a usual source of care, not have enough clinician time, and need extra help with healthcare coordination. Immigrant households in Lin and colleagues' study were defined as those with at least one foreign-born parent; nearly 70% of the immigrant households in the study were of Latino origin [125].

In one study that focused on maternal nativity while reviewing assessment records of children with autistic disorder in Los Angeles County, California, Becerra et al. [126] observed that risk of being diagnosed with autistic disorder and exhibiting certain autism phenotypes varied by maternal race, ethnicity, and nativity. More specifically, the study revealed that children of mothers who immigrated from Central America, South America, and Vietnam were most likely to experience greater delays in diagnosis (i.e., these children were diagnosed at later ages).

Results also indicated that compared to US-born White, Black, and Latina mothers, children of foreign-born Black, Filipino, and Vietnamese mothers had the highest risks of experiencing severe autism phenotypes. Due to less information about autism's incidence in lower- and middle-income countries abroad [127–130], it is difficult to resolve whether these results are due to etiological factors (e.g., greater exposure to risks during early childhood development prior to migration to the USA) or due to differences in accessing and receiving care. Besides unveiling crucial differences in ASD risk factors by nativity, Becerra and colleague's study [126] additionally highlights the idea that beyond measuring a family's race and ethnicity in general strokes, it is imperative to examine intra-group variations within larger ethnic groups. A closer examination of subsets of Asian/PIs or Latinos, for instance, may reveal that cultural minorities exist within ethnic groups.

English proficiency may also be an essential measure to account for when evaluating racial and ethnic disparities in the USA. Save for a few regions of the country with heavy concentrations of residents with limited English proficiency [131], being proficient in English strongly facilitates access to healthcare and educational resources for ASD. In focus groups conducted in English and Spanish of parents of Latino children with ASD, Zuckerman et al. [132] found that a common theme in parents' barriers to an ASD diagnosis was limited English proficiency. Limited English proficiency was described as "making every step of the diagnostic process more difficult" by both English- and Spanish-speaking Latino parents. This language barrier to ASD care was additionally corroborated in a later study by the same research group [132] among Latino parents of typically developing children. In the same way that limited English proficiency was revealed to be a barrier to ASD care in the Latino community, one study has also identified English proficiency to be an obstacle among the Chinese-American community as well. While investigating heritage-language use among Mandarin-speaking Chinese parents of children with ASD living in the USA, Yu [133] identified that a major theme in parents' reflections on their home language practices was the importance of English for accessing ASD interventions. Parents cited the lack of interventions and resources available in their native Chinese dialect as a motivating force to learning English in order to help their children. Some parents did acknowledge that lack of fluency in English prevented them from fully supporting their children's development and learning. Since English proficiency, like immigrant status or parental nativity, can be a proxy measure for acculturation [134], more studies are needed on the effects of limited English proficiency in accessing ASD resources to confirm that this is a barrier experienced in multiple communities nationwide [135].

Summary

All in all, it appears that there are several factors to consider when interpreting racial and ethnic differences in the ASD literature. In addition to the factors of SES, nativity, and English proficiency mentioned, there are several others not listed (e.g., comorbid conditions, Medicaid eligibility, urbanicity of region of residence, state regulations around ASD care) that could contribute to differences in how individuals access care for ASD. Understanding these various disparity is only the first step to identifying the causes for differences in diagnosis and care of ASD among racial and ethnic groups in the USA.

Part 3: Public Health Relevance of ASD Disparities

ASD has become a prevalent childhood condition and, as current children become adults, will become a prevalent chronic condition of adulthood. Similarly, the USA is becoming increasingly diverse in race, ethnicity, and language [136], and women are taking on greater roles in the US economy [137]. As a result, disparities in ASD diagnosis and treatment will have growing economic and public health impacts.

Healthcare and Larger Systems Perspective: Access to Care Issues

Factors pertaining to the US educational and healthcare systems of care for children with ASD may contribute to ASD diagnostic and treatment disparities. In particular, access to ASD care is complicated, and process complexity may exacerbate racial, ethnic, and sex differences in care access [138]. In most states in the USA, children and families need to seek ASD diagnostic and therapy services through both the educational system (i.e., via the Individuals with Disabilities Educational Act of 1990, Parts B and C) and through the medical system (i.e., via medical insurance). Both the educational and medical process for ASD service eligibility generally entail specialist evaluation; thus, families must pursue two parallel sets of specialty evaluations in order to receive comprehensive services for their child, which can be particularly challenging for families with less job flexibility or healthcare systems understanding [138]. Furthermore, the eligibility processes for ASD services in these two systems differ. In the medical system, a diagnosis based on DSM criteria is generally required in order to access services. However, educational system requirements for ASD service eligibility are generally more broad [139], and currently only two states (Maine and West Virginia) specifically require DSM criteria for educational eligibility assessment [140]. As a result, it is possible for a child to become eligible for ASD services through one system but not the other, which can be confusing to families. Since an educational eligibility determination is generally more rapid than a medical diagnosis, some families may only pursue services in the educational system even though additional benefits may be obtained by receiving a medical diagnosis. Successfully accessing treatment services for ASD thus often involves significant health and educational system knowledge, communication, and parental advocacy, all of which may be more challenging for low-income or racial and ethnic minority families [134].

Other health system factors may also modulate people of color's access to ASD care; for instance, geographic disparities have been noted in the location of mental health services, which may make ASD care relatively inaccessible to families living outside of major urban centers [141, 142]. Even when ASD evaluation centers are located close to where families live, lack of transportation options or bureaucratic hurdles may make these services relatively inaccessible [143].Additionally, for families with limited English proficiency, there may be shortages of bilingual diagnostic or therapy providers who can provide appropriate treatment services.

More generally, factors such as lack of access to health insurance, insurance inadequacy, and gaps in coverage may particularly affect racial/ethnic minority families [144, 145], making care for ASD via the medical system inaccessible or unaffordable. Finally, immigrant families may face particular challenges due to their documentation status: in most states, undocumented children have few care options through the healthcare system. Even among children who have legal US residence, families may avoid seeking services due to concerns about the documentation status of parents or other family members.

Provider Perspective: Behavioral Factors

Healthcare providers also play an important role in the early identification and subsequent treatment of ASD. Beginning in early childhood, an estimated 91.4% of US children are reported to have a regular source of care when they are sick and 90.3% report having a personal doctor or nurse [146]. Since a majority of children see a pediatric primary care provider (PCP), these providers may be the only developmental professional that a child and his/her family interact with on a regular basis prior to school enrollment, and this may be particularly true for children of color and children whose parents have low educational attainment [147]. As access to ASD diagnosis and specialty services often necessitates referrals from PCPs across an individual's lifespan, healthcare providers are gatekeepers when it comes to right of entry to many ASD resources.

Provider Influence at the Pre-diagnosis Stage

In early childhood, when parents suspect that their child might be on the autism spectrum, conversations with their child's PCP may mediate access to further medical services for ASD. Investigations of parents' medical experiences prior to attaining a diagnosis for their child ("pre-diagnostic experiences") suggest that parents commonly receive reassurance from the child's providers when they bring up developmental concerns and parents oftentimes see multiple providers before their concerns are earnestly addressed [118]. Parents of children of color and those who have low income, are uninsured, and are older, however, are less likely to have their developmental concerns elicited by a healthcare provider [148]. Similar factors may also be present for families of girls [35]. Provider factors are important to note as they may contribute to delays in the diagnosis of ASD [134], and delays have been established to be connected with long-term developmental and family outcomes [149].

In a study using nationally representative data of US children with ASD, intellectual disability (ID) and developmental delay (DD), Zuckerman et al. [134] observed that parents of children with ASD reported to have initial concerns and discussions of their concerns with providers earlier than parents of children with ID and DD. When Zuckerman et al. [134] categorized and analyzed provider responses to parental concerns as "proactive" (i.e., taking initiative toward diagnostic screening/evaluation) or "reassuring/passive" (i.e., falsely reassuring or non-response to parental concerns), they uncovered that parents of children with ASD were overall less likely to receive proactive responses to their concerns and more likely to receive reassuring/passive responses from providers than parents of children with ID and DD. Among parents of children with ASD, those who received more proactive responses to their concerns were also more likely to experience shorter delays in ASD diagnosis versus parents who received reassuring/passive provider responses. The study's results indicate that the manner in which providers respond to parental concerns may influence delays in ASD diagnosis. The study's results additionally suggest that compared to parents of children with other developmental conditions, parents of children with ASD may be at risk for lesser-quality provider responses to their developmental concerns.

Receiving false reassurance from providers has been noted to occur more when a child has a less severe form of ASD [150], and it seems to be dependent on how a parent presents his/her concerns [151]. A qualitative study of pre-diagnostic experiences of parents of children on the autism spectrum in the UK [151] identified three types of parental experiences: those with no concerns pre-diagnosis, those with passive concerns pre-diagnosis (i.e., parents with general worries but unable to articulate concerns using specific examples), and those with active concerns (i.e., parents with specific worries about their child). Analyses of parental experiences suggested that parents who presented active concerns to their child's PCP were most likely to be referred for an assessment in a shorter period. Though Ryan and Salisbury's study [151] did not examine the role of parents' sociodemographic characteristics, other studies have noted that Latino, Black, and Asian parents may have limited knowledge of child development compared to White parents [152–155] and may present with more general and less specific ASD-related concerns [156]. Educational attainment, age, and immigrant status may also predict parent knowledge of child development [152, 157]. If parents do not have much knowledge on child development, it is possible that they may use less detailed and more general descriptions when sharing their developmental concerns in the primary care setting. In addressing parental concerns, healthcare providers therefore need to not only be aware of how they respond to concerns but they also must be tuned in to how parents present their concerns—whether such concerns are presented in great detail or as general apprehensions may be reflective of a parent's knowledge of child development and his/her sociodemographic background.

Identifying parental concerns are only the first step to receiving an ASD diagnosis and treatment. There are behavioral factors that may contribute to disparities in the screening stage of ASD identification. The most current guidelines from the American Academy of Pediatrics (AAP) recommends the PCPs conduct developmental screenings at three time points in early childhood (9-, 18-, and 24- or 30-month visits) and autism-specific screenings at two similar time points (18- and 24- or 30-month visits) [158]. Of note, the US Preventive Services Task Force, as well as several other international bodies, do not currently recommend specific ASD screening. Many providers do not offer specific screening for ASD, and providers may have difficulty recognizing signs of ASD among different racial and ethnic groups [159]. A random sampling of pediatricians in California [160] revealed that while most (80.5%) pediatricians perform some kind of developmental screening at any routine visit, a small percentage (15.2%) of them offer both recommended screenings per the AAP guidelines. An even smaller percentage (10.3%) of pediatricians reported offering both screenings in Spanish. When asked how difficult it was to recognize the signs and symptoms of ASD among various racial and ethnic groups, most pediatricians reported having more trouble identifying signs of ASD in Latinos who primarily speak Spanish and Black children than in White children.

Provider Influence at Time of Diagnosis and in Service Utilization

During the evaluation process for ASD, diagnosing providers may additionally contribute to disparities in ASD diagnosis by inadvertently mistaking signs of ASD for other conditions among females or children of color. For instance, a study of Medicaid-eligible children with autism in the Philadelphia area revealed that an approximately 56.2% of children do not receive an autism diagnosis on their first visit to a diagnosing provider [41]. Black children, in particular, were almost three times more likely than White children to not receive an autism diagnosis at an initial visit (i.e., to be given another diagnosis first). Among the children receiving a diagnosis other than autism, results suggested that Black children were more likely than White children to receive a diagnosis of conduct or adjustment disorder [41], the latter of which has now been re-categorized as a TSRD in DSM-V. Though not statistically significant at the $p < 0.05$ level, the study results also indicated that children in the other race/ethnicity group (including American Indians, Asians, and Latinos) were more likely than White children to receive a diagnosis of adjustment disorder. The results of the study [41] may be interpreted in several ways. First, the results may suggest that differences in diagnostic labels may be a product of clinicians' incorrect beliefs about the occurrence of ASD among different racial and ethnic groups. These results may be accounted for by clinicians' misinterpretation of parental concerns—perhaps there exists difficulties in cross-cultural communications. Another interpretation of the results may look to parents: perhaps there exist racial and ethnic differences in how families interpret signs of ASD and in how they relate these signs to healthcare providers. Finally, the results could be interpreted in the context of TSRD: children of color and low-income children may be at increased risk to experiencing stress and adversity over their lifetimes, which can contribute to the development of TSRDs. However, clinicians may be prematurely making a diagnosis of TSRD by not also considering how ASD may contribute to a child's symptomology.

Though there have been inconsistencies in the literature, some studies suggest that like girls, racial and ethnic minority individuals with ASD may also have distinct clinical presentations of the condition than White individuals, which may additionally account for receiving a false initial diagnosis. Tek and Landa's study [100] of White, Black, Asian, and Latino children with ASD, for instance, observed that children of color tend to have more delayed scores on communications and gross motor sections of standardized measures of ASD. Comparisons of externalizing behaviors reported on autism screening tools [161] have similarly identified differences in scores of Black children with autism compared to White children on the spectrum such that Black children tend to have greater externalizing behaviors such as aggression. Black children have also been noted to present fewer restricted interests and repetitive behaviors than White children [162] when symptoms were compared using DSM-IV criteria. However, several studies have suggested no differences exist between racial and ethnic groups in social communication [162, 163] or externalizing behaviors [162] related to ASD.

Beyond considering differences in clinical presentation of ASD and how providers may misdiagnose people of color, considering how providers interact with families after the diagnosis may give insight into ASD disparities. A survey of the experiences of caregivers in Virginia with ASD diagnosing professionals (e.g., developmental pediatricians, neurologists, psychiatrists) suggested that among 40% of respondents, the diagnosing professional provided some additional information and resources about ASD at the time of diagnosis [164]. However, 18% of families reported that the professional provided no additional information beyond the diagnosis. Analyses of the factors involved in the provision of information at the time of diagnosis suggested that while there were no significant effects of family demographic variables, the type of provider to make the diagnosis was a significant factor [164]. In particular, developmental pediatricians were more likely than other healthcare professionals to present families with additional information on ASD at the time of the evaluation. The differences in the provision of information on ASD by healthcare providers may be reflective of specialized training developmental pediatricians on developmental disabilities compared to other healthcare professionals. Even among physicians who actively provide medical care to adults on the autism spectrum, lack of training and education on working with individuals with ASD seems to be a challenge [165].

Interactions with healthcare providers at the time of diagnosis and in healthcare visits afterward are worth consideration as the quality of these interactions can relate to how families decide to seek and use treatment services for ASD. Among a nationally representative sample of families of children with autism and other developmental disabilities, one study [165] found that Black parents of children with autism were more likely to report not having a personal doctor and not spending enough time with a doctor compared to White parents of children with autism; this disparity also existed when Black parents of children with autism were compared to Black and White parents of children with other developmental disabilities. Similarly, the study indicated that Latino parents of children with autism were more likely than White parents to report that their child's doctor did not listen to them. In a study conducted by the same research team among Latino and White children with ASD and other developmental disabilities, the researchers indicated that quality of provider interaction mediated the relationship between ethnicity and healthcare utilization. That is, Latino parents who reported spending enough time with their children's provider, the provider listening carefully, the provider being culturally sensitive, and the provider making the parent feel like a partner were also less likely to report difficulty using services and less problems with referrals. Racial and ethnic groups besides Latinos were not considered in the Parish, Magana, Rose, Timberlake, and Swaine study [11], yet the implications may suggest that other racial and ethnic groups whom do not have quality interactions with providers may be more likely to have difficulties accessing ASD-specific services.

Family Perspective: Beliefs About Autism Among Racial and Ethnic Groups

ASD is a condition described by how individuals lack or are deficient in certain traits that result in adverse consequences for daily functioning. The most current edition of the DSM explains that ASD is a product of "deficits in using social communication for social purposes" and "deficits [resulting] in functional limitations," among several other criteria [166]. Some have pointed out that this medical model of disability, as portrayed by its inherent deficits, is a strictly Western perspective that does not leave room to account for culturally specific modes of social communication and social interaction [155]. By proposing that the diagnosis of disabilities such as ASD relies on clinicians to identify whether an individual's behavior deviates significantly from that of his/her peers, this medical model of disability becomes progressively more difficult to implement in multicultural contexts across the USA wherein the "normative" sample may not behave in a uniform way. Likewise, differing social expectations for girls' and boys' behavior, particularly in multicultural contexts, may contribute to delayed diagnosis in girls.

Acculturation, the social and psychological change processes that take place when culturally distinct people, groups, and social influences come into contact [167], is essential to the discussion on how racial and ethnic groups in the USA—especially those that are recent immigrants—may view and accept disability. Parents learn to recognize their children's ASD by integrating it with their knowledge of child development and their own experiences, in order to construct a schema of what the diagnosis means to them and how it will impact their family life [168]. Parental experiences prior to their children's ASD diagnosis, such as those related to the how parents have merged their heritage culture with their receiving culture (i.e., dominant US culture), may thus play a role in how parents view their children's disability. Though parent perceptions of disability may not be the sole contributor to racial and ethnic disparities observed in the diagnosis and care of ASD, parent perceptions of disability do play a role in how parents decide to seek select treatment [169] and cope with the conditions themselves [170].

Conclusions and Implications for Practice and Policy

We began this chapter with an account of Maria—a Latina teenager who was noted to have social and developmental difficulties in early childhood and did not receive a formal diagnosis of ASD until age 15. Maria's father attributed the delayed diagnosis to intermittent insurance coverage and to his working long hours in Maria's childhood. There is little doubt that these two factors played a role in Maria's delayed diagnosis. However, after reviewing the various contributions to racial and ethnic disparities in ASD care in the USA, as well as barriers to female diagnosis, we can now understand that there may have been additional factors at play in Maria's situation.[2] Disparities in the diagnosis and care of ASD can occur at the healthcare system, provider, and family levels; therefore it is imperative to review how to enact change at each level in order to avoid amplifying disparities, with the ultimate goal of reducing them.

From a healthcare and larger systems perspective, encouraging policies that acknowledge the complexity of the ASD system for all families, and particularly for families of girls, children of color, and/or those who have low income, may be the first step to reducing disparities. Beginning with systems of eligibility for ASD, allocating fiscal and personnel resources to providing a seamless integration between the medical and educational systems may help reduce burden for families who may use one system but not the other or those who may be overwhelmed by the nuances of both systems and feel deterred from pursuing an initial evaluation. Incentivizing universal developmental and ASD-specific screenings among insurance companies and medical providers may additionally assist in identifying people of color with ASD who may not have thought to request a formal screening. Making

[2] There are many helpful frameworks, such as the Help-Seeking Behavior Model [171], that can be applied to understanding how the interaction between cultural factors and the healthcare system could have led to delays in Maria's being correctly diagnosed and receiving appropriate care. A comprehensive discussion and comparison of these theoretical models is beyond the scope of this chapter, but suffice it to say, there has been a long-standing interest among our colleagues in the research community about the reason(s) for observed disparities among different cultural groups seeking care for conditions like autism.

ASD services more affordable or ensuring comprehensive insurance coverage, regardless of income or immigration status, may also improve access to treatment services for families who may have previously found services to be inaccessible.

Healthcare providers, community workers, and other professionals working with individuals with families of color also need to be aware of disparities that exist in the identification and treatment of ASD. Encouraging continual trainings and education on ASD, including its differential presentation across the sexes would build clinical expertise for providers, especially those who may have been educated at a time when less was known about the condition. Moreover, healthcare organizations and providers should promote cultural competence in approaching the topic of ASD with families and in conducting screenings, evaluations, and in providing treatments. Just as autism is a spectrum, families may too have a variety of cultural beliefs and practices they bring in to interactions with providers. Finally, encouraging the cultural validation of screening tools for ASD—as opposed to simply translating a tool into another language—may be a worthwhile approach in the identification of ASD among racial and ethnic groups. Similarly, future refinement of DSM criteria and ASD diagnostic assessment instruments, including additions of female-oriented behavior examples or sex-specific algorithms, would likely support more timely referral and ASD diagnosis across sexes.[3]

Finally, reducing disparities in the diagnosis and care of ASD may take the form of disseminating more knowledge of child development and ASD. Circulating information on ASD using language that is comprehensible to different racial and ethnic groups of varying educational backgrounds is key to raising awareness on ASD that will combat stigmatized associations of the condition. Including girls and children of color in family-facing materials is crucial so that families understand that ASD affects all children. Beyond spreading awareness of ASD and tackling mental health stigma, it is necessary to educate families on potential pathways to diagnosis in their community. Fostering direct parent-to-parent communication

[3] New policies can also shift the way basic research is conducted to improve scientific understanding of ASD and support more equitable access to diagnosis and treatment. For example, as in most other biomedical fields, male animal models dominate research in ASD and related disorders like Rett syndrome. Researchers have historically avoided using female animals based on the assumption that hormonal fluctuations in females may alter results (which is precisely why female inclusion is important). Excluding females from study design to simplify experiments, decrease costs, or increase power means researchers have been missing valuable data.

In 1993, the National Institutes of Health (NIH) passed the Revitalization Act, which mandated that all of its funded research include girls and women. As a result, over half of participants in NIH-funded clinical research are now women. Similarly, recent NIH policy aims to eliminate sex and gender bias in animal and cell-based biomedical studies. Specifically, funding is reserved for experiments that equally balance male and female cells or animals unless explicitly and justifiably aiming to investigate sex-specific questions. These types of policy reforms can have potentially very powerful implications for ASD research without being financially costly. However, efforts to address the issue of sex and race inclusion across biomedical research must be multidimensional—for example, incorporating program oversight, review and policy, and educational outreach and training [172].

among communities of color and parents of girls through family support groups or parent mentors may facilitate access to resources for some parents. After attaining a diagnosis, following up with families to ensure that they seek, use, and continue using effective services for ASD (through a family navigator, for instance) may help keep families of color engaged in treatment services for ASD, thereby reducing racial and ethnic disparities in ASD care.

Editors' Note Why include a chapter on sex and racial/ethnic disparities in ASD identification in a book focused primarily on the intersection between trauma and neurodevelopmental disorder? There are two reasons. First, we wish to present an evenhanded view of the problem of diagnostic disparity. Although one focus of this book is the problem of mislabeling TSRD as ASD—both from a treatment and public health policy perspective—this is not to say that we can be complacent about early diagnosis and treatment of ASD. It has clearly been established that it is important to diagnose and treat ASD early, to improve outcomes. In no way do we wish to leave the reader with the impression that we recommend any lessening of ASD awareness or any reduction in services for children with ASD. Quite the contrary, we need to continue to strive to provide early diagnosis of ASD and more robust supports and therapies for children with ASD and their families and reserve these supports for those who truly meet criteria for ASD. At the same time, providing ASD supports for children who actually have a TSRD potentially delays their acquisition of appropriate treatments while diverting resources for those who have a true ASD and will strongly benefit from ASD-directed therapies (but see following chapter by Bear, Alverson, and Smith). As illustrated in this chapter, more work remains to be done in improving our early diagnosis and treatment of ASD, particularly in underserved racial/ethnic minority populations. It is of great concern that, as described in this chapter, children of color with ASD are more likely than White children with ASD to be misdiagnosed with adjustment disorder or conduct disorder, and girls are more likely than boys to have delays in diagnosis. So, at the risk of being redundant (as we would rather be redundant than be misunderstood on this point), we do not advocate for any less awareness of or action regarding diagnosis and treatment of ASD, even while we recommend the heightening of awareness of the differential diagnosis of ASD, including TSRD.

Second, as cogently argued in relation to girls with ASD, having an ASD diagnosis compounds the problems already faced by children from racial and ethnic minority groups with microaggressions and more overt forms of racism and discrimination. Unfortunately, ASD "puts another target on these children's backs" in terms of prejudice and bullying. Currently in Massachusetts (and many other states are beginning to follow suit), ASD is subject to special protections under the Massachusetts Anti-Bullying Law and other laws designed to protect people with disabilities from abuse and mistreatment. In the section that follows, we hope to add even further nuance to this discussion by evoking the larger policy implications of progressive educational and public health initiatives that think broadly about the needs of children with disabilities.

References

1. Autism and Developmental Disabilities Monitoring Network Surveillance Year 2008 Principal Investigators, Centers for Disease Control and Prevention. Prevalence of autism spectrum disorders--Autism and Developmental Disabilities Monitoring Network, 14 sites, United States, 2008. MMWR Surveill Summ. 2012;61(3):1–19.
2. CDC. Prevalence of autism spectrum disorders - Autism and Developmental Disabilities Monitoring Network, United States, 2006. MMWR Surveill Summ. 2009;58(10):1–20.
3. CDC. Prevalence of autism spectrum disorder among children aged 8 years - Autism and Developmental Disabilities Monitoring Network, 11 sites, United States, 2010. MMWR Surveill Summ. 2014;63(2):1–21.
4. Christensen DL, Baio J, van Naarden Braun K, Bilder D, Charles J, Constantino JN, Daniels J, Durkin MS, Fitzgerald RT, Kurzius-Spencer M, Lee LC, Pettygrove S, Robinson C, Schulz E, Wells C, Wingate MS, Zahorodny W, Yeargin-Allsopp M, Centers for Disease Control and Prevention (CDC). Prevalence and characteristics of autism spectrum disorder among children aged 8 years—Autism and Developmental Disabilities Monitoring Network, 11 sites, United States, 2012. MMWR Surveill Summ. 2016;65:1–23.
5. Hill AP, Zuckerman KE, Fombonne E. Epidemiology of autism spectrum disorder. In: Volkmar FR, editor. Handbook of autism and pervasive developmental disorders, vol. 1. 4th ed. Hoboken: Wiley; 2014. p. 57–96.
6. DeVilbiss EA, Lee BK. Brief report: trends in US national autism awareness from 2004 to 2014: the impact of national autism awareness month. J Autism Dev Disord. 2014;44(12):3271–3. https://doi.org/10.1007/s10803-014-2160-4.
7. Zahorodny W, Shenouda J, Howell S, Rosato NS, Peng B, Mehta U. Increasing autism prevalence in metropolitan New Jersey. Autism. 2014;18(2):117–26. https://doi.org/10.1177/1362361312463977.
8. Shelton JF, Hertz-Picciotto I, Pessah IN. Tipping the balance of autism risk: potential mechanisms linking pesticides and autism. Environ Health Perspect. 2012;120(7):944–51. https://doi.org/10.1289/ehp.1104553.
9. Volk HE, Lurmann F, Penfold B, Hertz-Picciotto I, McConnell R. Traffic-related air pollution, particulate matter, and autism. JAMA Psychiat. 2013;70(1):71–7. https://doi.org/10.1001/jamapsychiatry.2013.266.
10. Liptak GS, Benzoni LB, Mruzek DW, Nolan KW, Thingvoll MA, Wade CM, Fryer GE. Disparities in diagnosis and access to health services for children with autism: data from the National Survey of Children's Health. J Dev Behav Pediatr. 2008;29(3):152–60. https://doi.org/10.1097/DBP.0b013e318165c7a0.
11. Parish S, Magana S, Rose R, Timberlake M, Swaine JG. Health care of Latino children with autism and other developmental disabilities: quality of provider interaction mediates utilization. Am J Intellect Dev Disabil. 2012;117(4):304–15. https://doi.org/10.1352/1944-7558-117.4.304.
12. Mandell DS, Wiggins LD, Carpenter LA, Daniels J, DiGuiseppi C, Durkin MS, Kirby RS. Racial/ethnic disparities in the identification of children with autism spectrum disorders. Am J Public Health. 2009;99(3):493–8. https://doi.org/10.2105/ajph.2007.131243.
13. White SW, Oswald D, Ollendick T, Scahill L. Anxiety in children and adolescents with autism spectrum disorders. Clin Psychol Rev. 2009;29(3):216–29. https://doi.org/10.1016/j.cpr.2009.01.003.
14. Simonoff E, Pickles A, Charman T, Chandler S, Loucas T, Baird G. Psychiatric disorders in children with autism spectrum disorders: prevalence, comorbidity, and associated factors in a population-derived sample. J Am Acad Child Adolesc Psychiatry. 2008;47(8):921–9. https://doi.org/10.1097/CHI.0b013e318179964f.
15. Kerns CM, Newschaffer CJ, Berkowitz SJ. Traumatic childhood events and autism spectrum disorder. J Autism Dev Disord. 2015;45(11):3475–86. https://doi.org/10.1007/s10803-015-2392-y.

16. Lounds Taylor JL, Gotham KO. Cumulative life events, traumatic experiences, and psychiatric symptomatology in transition-aged youth with autism spectrum disorder. J Neurodev Disord. 2016;8:28. https://doi.org/10.1186/s11689-016-9160-y.
17. Hoover DW. The effects of psychological trauma on children with autism spectrum disorder. 2015. https://www.kennedykrieger.org/sites/default/files/patient-care-files/effects-psychological-trauma-children-autism.pdf. Retrieved 20 Jan 2018.
18. Bird G, Cook R. Mixed emotions: the contribution of alexithymia to the emotional symptoms of autism. Transl Psychiatry. 2013;3(7):e285. https://doi.org/10.1038/tp.2013.61.
19. Zeitlin SB, McNally RJ, Cassiday KL. Alexithymia in victims of sexual assault: an effect of repeated traumatization? Am J Psychiatry. 1993;150(4):661–3.
20. Gillott A, Standen PJ. Levels of anxiety and sources of stress in adults with autism. J Intellect Disabil. 2007;11(4):359–70.
21. Jansen LM, Gispen-de Wied CC, Wiegant VM, Westenberg HG, Lahuis BE, van Engeland H. Autonomic and neuroendocrine responses to a psychosocial stressor in adults with autistic spectrum disorder. J Autism Dev Disord. 2006;36(7):891–9. https://doi.org/10.1007/s10803-006-0124-z.
22. Weiss NH, Tull MT, Lavender J, Gratz KL. Role of emotion dysregulation in the relationship between childhood abuse and probable PTSD in a sample of substance abusers. Child Abuse Negl. 2013;37(11):944–54.
23. American Psychiatric Association. Diagnostic and statistical manual of mental disorders: DSM 5. 5th ed. Arlington: American Psychiatric Association; 2013.
24. Lord C, Schopler E, Revicki D. Sex differences in autism. J Autism Dev Disord. 1982;12(4):317–30.
25. Loomes R, Hull L, Mandy WPL. What Is the male-to-female ratio in autism spectrum disorder? A systematic review and meta-analysis. J Am Acad Child Adolesc Psychiatr. 2017;56(6):466–74. https://doi.org/10.1016/j.jaac.2017.03.013.
26. Blumberg SJ, Bramlett MD, Kogan MD, Schieve LA, Jones JR, Lu MC. Changes in prevalence of parent-reported autism spectrum disorder in school-aged U.S. children: 2007 to 2011–2012. (No. 65). US Department of Health and Human Services, Centers for Disease Control and Prevention, National Center for Health Statistics. 2013.
27. Kanner L. Autistic disturbances of affective contact. Nerv Child. 1943;2:217–50.
28. Asperger H. The "autistic psychopathy" in childhood. Arch Psychiatr Nervenkr. 1944;117(1):76–136.
29. Zwaigenbaum L, Bryson SE, Szatmari P, Brian J, Smith IM, Roberts W, Roncadin C. Sex differences in children with autism spectrum disorder identified within a high-risk infant cohort. J Autism Dev Disord. 2012;42(12):2585–96.
30. Mandy W, Chilvers R, Chowdhury U, Salter G, Seigal A, Skuse D. Sex differences in autism spectrum disorder: evidence from a large sample of children and adolescents. J Autism Dev Disord. 2012;42(7):1304–13.
31. Huerta M, Bishop SL, Duncan A, Hus V, Lord C. Application of DSM-5 criteria for autism spectrum disorder to three samples of children with DSM-IV diagnoses of pervasive developmental disorders. Am J Psychiatr. 2012;169(10):1056–64.
32. McPartland JC, Reichow B, Volkmar FR. Sensitivity and specificity of proposed DSM-5 diagnostic criteria for autism spectrum disorder. J Am Acad Child Adolesc Psychiatry. 2012;51(4):368–83.
33. Reinhardt VP, Wetherby AM, Schatschneider C, Lord C. Examination of sex differences in a large sample of young children with autism spectrum disorder and typical development. J Autism Dev Disord. 2014;45(3):697–706.
34. Fombonne E. The epidemiology of autism: a review. Psychol Med. 1999;29(4):769–86.
35. Volkmar FR, Szatmari P, Sparrow SS. Sex differences in pervasive developmental disorders. J Autism Dev Disord. 1993;23(4):579–91.
36. Yeargin-Allsopp M, Rice C, Karapurkar T, Doernberg N, Boyle C, Murphy C. Prevalence of autism in a US metropolitan area. JAMA. 2003;289(1):49–55.

37. Banach R, Thompson A, Szatmari P, Goldberg J, Tuff L, Zwaigenbaum L, Mahoney W. Brief report: relationship between non-verbal IQ and gender in autism. J Autism Dev Disord. 2009;39(1):188.
38. Fombonne E. Epidemiology of pervasive developmental disorders. Pediatr Res. 2009;65(6):591–8.
39. Fombonne E. Epidemiological surveys of autism and other pervasive developmental disorders: an update. J Autism Dev Disord. 2003;33(4):365–82.
40. Lai DC, Tseng YC, Hou YM, Guo HR. Gender and geographic differences in the prevalence of autism spectrum disorders in children: analysis of data from the national disability registry of Taiwan. Res Dev Disabil. 2012;33(3):909–15.
41. Mandell DS, Listerud J, Levy SE, Pinto-Martin JA. Race differences in the age at diagnosis among medicaid-eligible children with autism. J Am Acad Child Adolesc Psychiatry. 2002;41(12):1447–53.
42. Posserud MB, Lundervold AJ, Gillberg C. Autistic features in a total population of 7–9-year-old children assessed by the ASSQ (Autism Spectrum Screening Questionnaire). J Child Psychol Psychiatry. 2006;47(2):167–75.
43. Anello A, Reichenberg A, Luo X, Schmeidler J, Hollander E, Smith CJ, Silverman JM. Brief report: parental age and the sex ratio in autism. J Autism Dev Disord. 2009;39(10):1487–92.
44. Croen LA, Najjar DV, Fireman B, Grether JK. Maternal and paternal age and risk of autism spectrum disorders. Arch Pediatr Adolesc Med. 2007;161(4):334–40.
45. Reichenberg A, Gross R, Weiser M, Bresnahan M, Silverman J, Harlap S, Knobler HY. Advancing paternal age and autism. Arch Gen Psychiatry. 2006;63(9):1026–32.
46. Reich T, Cloninger CR, Guze SB. The multifactorial model of disease transmission: I. Description of the model and its use in psychiatry. Br J Psychiatry. 1975;127(1):1–10.
47. Tsai L, Stewart MA, August G. Implication of sex differences in the familial transmission of infantile autism. J Autism Dev Disord. 1981;11(2):165–73.
48. Werling DM, Geschwind DH. Sex differences in autism spectrum disorders. Curr Opin Neurol. 2013;26(2):146–53.
49. Jacquemont S, Coe BP, Hersch M, Duyzend MH, Krumm N, Bergmann S, Eichler EE. A higher mutational burden in females supports a "female protective model" in neurodevelopmental disorders. Am J Hum Genet. 2014;94(3):415–25.
50. Zhao X, Leotta A, Kustanovich V, Lajonchere C, Geschwind DH, Law K, Ye K. A unified genetic theory for sporadic and inherited autism. Proc Natl Acad Sci. 2007;104(31):12831–6.
51. Ozonoff S, Young GS, Carter A, Messinger D, Yirmiya N, Zwaigenbaum L, Hutman T. Recurrence risk for autism spectrum disorders: a Baby Siblings Research Consortium study. Pediatrics. 2011;128(3):e488–95.
52. Robinson EB, Lichtenstein P, Anckarsäter H, Happé F, Ronald A. Examining and interpreting the female protective effect against autistic behavior. Proc Natl Acad Sci. 2013;110(13):5258–62.
53. Filges I, Röthlisberger B, Blattner A, Boesch N, Demougin P, Wenzel F, Miny P. Deletion in Xp22. 11: PTCHD1 is a candidate gene for X-linked intellectual disability with or without autism. Clin Genet. 2011;79(1):79–85.
54. Celestino-Soper PB, Shaw CA, Sanders SJ, Li J, Murtha MT, Ercan-Sencicek AG, Ou Z. Use of array CGH to detect exonic copy number variants throughout the genome in autism families detects a novel deletion in TMLHE. Hum Mol Genet. 2011;20(22):4360–70.
55. Blasi F, Bacchelli E, Pesaresi G, Carone S, Bailey AJ, Maestrini E. Absence of coding mutations in the X-linked genes neuroligin 3 and neuroligin 4 in individuals with autism from the IMGSAC collection. Am J Med Genet B Neuropsychiatr Genet. 2006;141((3):220–1.
56. Lu AT, Cantor RM. Allowing for sex differences increases power in a GWAS of multiplex Autism families. Mol Psychiatry. 2012;17(2):215–22.
57. Ronald A, Happé F, Bolton P, Butcher LM, Price TS, Wheelwright S, Plomin R. Genetic heterogeneity between the three components of the autism spectrum: a twin study. J Am Acad Child Adolesc Psychiatry. 2006;45(6):691–9.

58. Auyeung B, Taylor K, Hackett G, Baron-Cohen S. Foetal testosterone and autistic traits in 18 to 24-month-old children. Mol Autism. 2010;1(1):11.
59. Dworzynski K, Ronald A, Bolton P, Happé F. How different are girls and boys above and below the diagnostic threshold for autism spectrum disorders? J Am Acad Child Adolesc Psychiatry. 2012;51(8):788–97.
60. Kopp S, Gillberg C. The Autism Spectrum Screening Questionnaire (ASSQ)-Revised Extended Version (ASSQ-REV): an instrument for better capturing the autism phenotype in girls? A preliminary study involving 191 clinical cases and community controls. Res Dev Disabil. 2011;32(6):2875–88.
61. Bargiela S, Steward R, Mandy W. The experiences of late-diagnosed women with autism spectrum conditions: an investigation of the female autism phenotype. J Autism Dev Disord. 2016;46(10):3281–94.
62. Mattila ML, Kielinen M, Linna SL, Jussila K, Ebeling H, Bloigu R, Moilanen I. Autism spectrum disorders according to DSM-IV-TR and comparison with DSM-5 draft criteria: an epidemiological study. J Am Acad Child Adolesc Psychiatry. 2011;50(6):583–92.
63. Carter AS, Black DO, Tewani S, Connolly CE, Kadlec MB, Tager-Flusberg H. Sex differences in toddlers with autism spectrum disorders. J Autism Dev Disord. 2007;37(1):86–97.
64. Hartley SL, Sikora DM. Sex differences in autism spectrum disorder: an examination of developmental functioning, autistic symptoms, and coexisting behavior problems in toddlers. J Autism Dev Disord. 2009;39(12):1715.
65. Solomon M, Miller M, Taylor SL, Hinshaw SP, Carter CS. Autism symptoms and internalizing psychopathology in girls and boys with autism spectrum disorders. J Autism Dev Disord. 2012;42(1):48–59.
66. Frazier TW, Georgiades S, Bishop SL, Hardan AY. Behavioral and cognitive characteristics of females and males with autism in the simons simplex collection. J Am Acad Child Adolesc Psychiatry. 2014;53(3):329–40.
67. Hattier MA, Matson JL, Tureck K, Horovitz M. The effects of gender and age on repetitive and/or restricted behaviors and interests in adults with autism spectrum disorders and intellectual disability. Res Dev Disabil. 2011;32(6):2346–51.
68. Szatmari P, Liu XQ, Goldberg J, Zwaigenbaum L, Paterson AD, Woodbury-Smith M, et al. Sex differences in repetitive stereotyped behaviors in autism: implications for genetic liability. Am J Med Genet B Neuropsychiatr Genet. 2012;159(1):5–12.
69. Nichols S, Moravcik G, Tetenbaum SP. Girls growing up on the autism spectrum: what parents and professionals should know about the pre-teen and teenage years. London: Jessica Kingsley; 2008.
70. Rosbrook A, Whittingham K. Autistic traits in the general population: what mediates the link with depressive and anxious symptomatology? Res Autism Spectr Disord. 2010;4(3):415–24.
71. Spencer N, Devereux E, Wallace A, Sundrum R, Shenoy M, Bacchus C, Logan S. Disabling conditions and registration for child abuse and neglect: a population-based study. Pediatrics. 2005;116(3):609–13.
72. Soler-Baillo JM, Marx BP, Sloan DM. The psychophysiological correlates of risk recognition among victims and non-victims of sexual assault. Behav Res Ther. 2005;43(2):169–81.
73. Roberts AL, Koenen KC, Lyall K, Robinson EB, Weisskopf MG. Association of autistic traits in adulthood with childhood abuse, interpersonal victimization, and posttraumatic stress. Child Abuse Negl. 2015;45:135–42.
74. Folstein SE, Rosen-Sheidley B. Genetics of autism: complex aetiology for a heterogeneous disorder. Nat Rev Genet. 2001;2(12):943–55.
75. Bhopal R, Donaldson L. White, European, Western, Caucasian, or what? Inappropriate labeling in research on race, ethnicity, and health. Am J Public Health. 1998;88(9):1303–7.
76. United States Census Bureau. About race. 2017. https://www.census.gov/topics/population/race/about.html.
77. Durkin MS, Maenner MJ, Baio J, Christensen D, Daniels J, Fitzgerald R, Yeargin-Allsopp M. Autism spectrum disorder among US children (2002-2010): socioeconomic, racial, and

ethnic disparities. Am J Public Health. 2017;107(11):1818–26. https://doi.org/10.2105/ajph.2017.304032.
78. Palmer RF, Walker T, Mandell D, Bayles B, Miller CS. Explaining low rates of autism among Hispanic school children in Texas. Am J Public Health. 2010;100(2):270–2. https://doi.org/10.2105/ajph.2008.150565.
79. Delobel-Ayoub M, Ehlinger V, Klapouszczak D, Maffre T, Raynaud JP, Delpierre C, Arnaud C. Socioeconomic disparities and prevalence of autism spectrum disorders and intellectual disability. PLoS ONE. 2015;10(11):e0141964. https://doi.org/10.1371/journal.pone.0141964.
80. Leonard H, Glasson E, Nassar N, Whitehouse A, Bebbington A, Bourke J, Stanley F. Autism and intellectual disability are differentially related to sociodemographic background at birth. PLoS ONE. 2011;6(3):e17875. https://doi.org/10.1371/journal.pone.0017875.
81. Williams E, Thomas K, Sidebotham H, Emond A. Prevalence and characteristics of autistic spectrum disorders in the ALSPAC cohort. Dev Med Child Neurol. 2008;50(9):672–7. https://doi.org/10.1111/j.1469-8749.2008.03042.x.
82. Dickerson AS, Rahbar MH, Pearson DA, Kirby RS, Bakian AV, Bilder DA, Slay Wingate M. Autism spectrum disorder reporting in lower socioeconomic neighborhoods. Autism. 2016;21(4):470–80. https://doi.org/10.1177/1362361316650091.
83. Durkin MS, Maenner MJ, Meaney FJ, Levy SE, DiGuiseppi C, Nicholas JS, Schieve LA. Socioeconomic inequality in the prevalence of autism spectrum disorder: evidence from a U.S. cross-sectional study. PLoS ONE. 2010;5(7):e11551. https://doi.org/10.1371/journal.pone.0011551.
84. Smedley A, Smedley BD. Race as biology is fiction, racism as a social problem is real: anthropological and historical perspectives on the social construction of race. Am Psychol. 2005;60(1):16.
85. Yudell M, Roberts D, DeSalle R, Tishkoff S. Taking race out of human genetics. Science. 2016;351(6273):564–5. https://doi.org/10.1126/science.aac4951.
86. Jarquin VG, Wiggins LD, Schieve LA, van Naarden-Braun K. Racial disparities in community identification of autism spectrum disorders over time; Metropolitan Atlanta, Georgia, 2000-2006. J Dev Behav Pediatr. 2011;32(3):179–87. https://doi.org/10.1097/DBP.0b013e31820b4260.
87. Pedersen A, Pettygrove S, Meaney FJ, Mancilla K, Gotschall K, Kessler DB, Cunniff C. Prevalence of autism spectrum disorders in Hispanic and non-Hispanic white children. Pediatrics. 2012;129(3):e629–35. https://doi.org/10.1542/peds.2011-1145.
88. American Psychological Association, Presidential Task Force on Education Disparities. Ethnic and racial disparities in education: psychology's contributions to understanding and reducing disparities. 2012. https://www.apa.org/ed/resources/racial-disparities.pdf.
89. American Psychological Association (APA). Ethnic and racial minorities and socioeconomic status. Resource Guide and Publications. 2018.
90. Coker TR, Elliott MN, Toomey SL, Schwebel DC, Cuccaro P, Emery ST, Schuster MA. Racial and ethnic disparities in ADHD diagnosis and treatment. Pediatrics. 2016;2016:e20160407.
91. Charman T, Taylor E, Drew A, Cockerill H, Brown JA, Baird G. Outcome at 7 years of children diagnosed with autism at age 2: predictive validity of assessments conducted at 2 and 3 years of age and pattern of symptom change over time. J Child Psychol Psychiatry. 2005;46(5):500–13. https://doi.org/10.1111/j.1469-7610.2004.00377.x.
92. Kleinman JM, Ventola PE, Pandey J, Verbalis AD, Barton M, Hodgson S, Fein D. Diagnostic stability in very young children with autism spectrum disorders. J Autism Dev Disord. 2008;38(4):606–15. https://doi.org/10.1007/s10803-007-0427-8.
93. Mandell DS, Novak MM, Zubritsky CD. Factors associated with age of diagnosis among children with autism spectrum disorders. Pediatrics. 2005;116(6):1480–6.
94. Wiggins LD, Baio J, Rice C. Examination of the time between first evaluation and first autism spectrum diagnosis in a population-based sample. J Dev Behav Pediatr. 2006;27(2 Suppl):S79–87.

95. Magaña S, Lopez K, Aguinaga A, Morton H. Access to diagnosis and treatment services among latino children with autism spectrum disorders. Intellect Dev Disabil. 2013;51(3): 141–53. https://doi.org/10.1352/1934-9556-51.3.141.
96. Magaña S, Parish SL, Rose RA, Timberlake M, Swaine JG. Racial and ethnic disparities in quality of health care among children with autism and other developmental disabilities. Intellect Dev Disabil. 2012;50(4):287–99. https://doi.org/10.1352/1934-9556-50.4.287.
97. Fountain C, King MD, Bearman PS. Age of diagnosis for autism: individual and community factors across 10 birth cohorts. J Epidemiol Community Health. 2011;65(6):503–10. https://doi.org/10.1136/jech.2009.104588.
98. Mandell DS, Morales KH, Xie M, Lawer LJ, Stahmer AC, Marcus SC. Age of diagnosis among Medicaid-enrolled children with autism, 2001-2004. Psychiatr Serv. 2010;61(8):822–9. https://doi.org/10.1176/appi.ps.61.8.822.
99. Shattuck PT, Durkin M, Maenner M, Newschaffer C, Mandell DS, Wiggins L, Cuniff C. Timing of identification among children with an autism spectrum disorder: findings from a population-based surveillance study. J Am Acad Child Adolesc Psychiatry. 2009;48(5):474–83. https://doi.org/10.1097/CHI.0b013e31819b3848.
100. Tek S, Landa RJ. Differences in autism symptoms between minority and non-minority toddlers. J Autism Dev Disord. 2012;42(9):1967–73. https://doi.org/10.1007/s10803-012-1445-8.
101. Mandell DS, Ittenbach RF, Levy SE, Pinto-Martin JA. Disparities in diagnoses received prior to a diagnosis of autism spectrum disorder. J Autism Dev Disord. 2007;37(9):1795–802. https://doi.org/10.1007/s10803-006-0314-8.
102. Magana S, Parish SL, Son E. Have racial and ethnic disparities in the quality of health care relationships changed for children with developmental disabilities and ASD? Am J Intellect Dev Disabil. 2015;120(6):504–13. https://doi.org/10.1352/1944-7558-120.6.504.
103. Magaña S, Parish SL, Son E. Functional severity and Latino ethnicity in specialty services for children with autism spectrum disorder. J Intellect Disabil Res. 2016;60(5):424–34. https://doi.org/10.1111/jir.12293.
104. Taylor JL, Henninger NA. Frequency and correlates of service access among youth with autism transitioning to adulthood. J Autism Dev Disord. 2015;45(1):179–91. https://doi.org/10.1007/s10803-014-2203-x.
105. Rogers SJ, Estes A, Lord C, Vismara L, Winter J, Fitzpatrick A, Dawson G. Effects of a brief Early Start Denver model (ESDM)-based parent intervention on toddlers at risk for autism spectrum disorders: a randomized controlled trial. J Am Acad Child Adolesc Psychiatry. 2012;51(10):1052–65. https://doi.org/10.1016/j.jaac.2012.08.003.
106. Rogers SJ, Vismara LA. Evidence-based comprehensive treatments for early autism. J Clin Child Adolesc Psychol. 2008;37(1):8–38. https://doi.org/10.1080/15374410701817808.
107. Vismara LA, Rogers SJ. Behavioral treatments in autism spectrum disorder: what do we know? Annu Rev Clin Psychol. 2010;6:447–68. https://doi.org/10.1146/annurev.clinpsy.121208.131151.
108. Myers SM, Johnson CP, American Academy of Pediatrics Council on Children With Disabilities. Management of children with autism spectrum disorders. Pediatrics. 2007;120(5):1162–82.
109. National Research Council, Committee on Educational Interventions for Children with Autism, Division of Behavioral and Social Sciences and Education. Educating children with autism. Washington, DC: Natinal Academy Press; 2001.
110. Weitlauf AS, McPheeters ML, Peters B, Sathe N, Travis R, Aiello R, Warren Z. AHRQ Comparative Effectiveness Review: therapies for children with autism spectrum disorder: behavioral interventions update. 2014. http://effectivehealthcare.ahrq.gov/ehc/products/544/1945/autism-update-report-140806.pdf.
111. Leigh JP, Grosse SD, Cassady D, Melnikow J, Hertz-Picciotto I. Spending by California's Department of Developmental Services for persons with autism across demographic and expenditure categories. PLoS ONE. 2016;11(3):e0151970. https://doi.org/10.1371/journal.pone.0151970.

112. Individuals with Disability Education Act (IDEA): Part B, Assistance for education of all children with disabilities. 2004.
113. Individuals with Disability Education Act (IDEA): Part C (birth-2 years old). 2004. http://idea.ed.gov/part-c/statutes.
114. Rosenberg RE, Landa R, Law JK, Stuart EA, Law PA. Factors affecting age at initial autism spectrum disorder diagnosis in a national survey. Autism Res Treat. 2011;2011:874619. https://doi.org/10.1155/2011/874619.
115. Zuckerman KE, Sinche B, Cobian M, Cervantes M, Mejia A, Becker T, Nicolaidis C. Conceptualization of autism in the Latino community and its relationship with early diagnosis. J Dev Behav Pediatr. 2014;35(8):522–32. https://doi.org/10.1097/DBP.0000000000000091.
116. Shavers VL. Measurement of socioeconomic status in health disparities research. J Natl Med Assoc. 2007;99(9):1013–23.
117. Thomas P, Zahorodny W, Peng B, Kim S, Jani N, Halperin W, Brimacombe M. The association of autism diagnosis with socioeconomic status. Autism. 2011;16(2):201–13.
118. Goin-Kochel RP, Mackintosh VH, Myers BJ. How many doctors does it take to make an autism spectrum diagnosis? Autism. 2006;10(5):439–51. https://doi.org/10.1177/1362361306066601.
119. Hidalgo NJ, McIntyre L, McWhirter E. Sociodemographic differences in parental satisfaction with an autism spectrum disorder diagnosis. J Intellect Develop Disabil. 2015;40(2):147–55. https://doi.org/10.3109/13668250.2014.994171.
120. Shattuck PT, Grosse S, Parish S, Bier D. Utilization of a Medicaid-funded intervention for children with autism. Psychiatr Serv. 2009;60(4):549–52. https://doi.org/10.1176/appi.ps.60.4.549.
121. Cidav Z, Marcus SC, Mandell DS. Implications of childhood autism for parental employment and earnings. Pediatrics. 2012;129(4):617–23. https://doi.org/10.1542/peds.2011-2700.
122. Vohra R, Madhavan S, Sambamoorthi U, St Peter C. Access to services, quality of care, and family impact for children with autism, other developmental disabilities, and other mental health conditions. Autism. 2014;18(7):815–26. https://doi.org/10.1177/1362361313512902.
123. Zuckerman KE, Lindly OJ, Bethell CD, Kuhlthau K. Family impacts among children with autism spectrum disorder: the role of health care quality. Acad Pediatr. 2014;14(4):398–407. https://doi.org/10.1016/j.acap.2014.03.011.
124. Schieve LA, Boulet SL, Blumberg SJ, Kogan MD, Yeargin-Allsopp M, Boyle CA, Rice C. Association between parental nativity and autism spectrum disorder among US-born non-Hispanic white and Hispanic children, 2007 National Survey of Children's Health. Disabil Health J. 2012;5(1):18–25. https://doi.org/10.1016/j.dhjo.2011.09.001.
125. Lin SC, Yu SM, Harwood RL. Autism spectrum disorders and developmental disabilities in children from immigrant families in the United States. Pediatrics. 2012;130(Suppl 2):S191–7. https://doi.org/10.1542/peds.2012-0900R.
126. Becerra TA, von Ehrenstein OS, Heck JE, Olsen J, Arah OA, Jeste SS, Ritz B. Autism spectrum disorders and race, ethnicity, and nativity: a population-based study. Pediatrics. 2014;134(1):e63–71. https://doi.org/10.1542/peds.2013-3928.
127. Elsabbagh M, Divan G, Koh YJ, Kim YS, Kauchali S, Marcin C, Fombonne E. Global prevalence of autism and other pervasive developmental disorders. Autism Res. 2012;5(3):160–79. https://doi.org/10.1002/aur.239.
128. Khan NZ, Gallo LA, Arghir A, Budisteanu B, Budisteanu M, Dobrescu I, Elsabbagh M. Autism and the grand challenges in global mental health. Autism Res. 2012;5(3):156–9. https://doi.org/10.1002/aur.1239.
129. Samms-Vaughan ME. The status of early identification and early intervention in autism spectrum disorders in lower- and middle-income countries. Int J Speech Lang Pathol. 2014;16(1):30–5. https://doi.org/10.3109/17549507.2013.866271.
130. Zeglam AM, Maound AJ. Prevalence of autistic spectrum disorders in Tripoli, Libya: the need for more research and planned services. East Mediterr Health J. 2012;18(2):184–8.

131. Pan Y, Lubkemann S. Observing census enumeration of non-english speaking households in the 2010 census: evaluation report. 2013. https://www.census.gov/srd/papers/pdf/ssm2013-02.pdf.
132. Zuckerman KE, Sinche B, Mejia A, Cobian M, Becker T, Nicolaidis C. Latino parents' perspectives on barriers to autism diagnosis. Acad Pediatr. 2014;14(3):301–8. https://doi.org/10.1016/j.acap.2013.12.004.
133. Yu B. Issues in bilingualism and heritage language maintenance: perspectives of minority-language mothers of children with autism spectrum disorders. Am J Speech Lang Pathol. 2013;22(1):10–24. https://doi.org/10.1044/1058-0360(2012/10-0078.
134. Zuckerman KE, Lindly OJ, Sinche BK. Parental concerns, provider response, and timeliness of autism spectrum disorder diagnosis. J Pediatr. 2015;166(6):1431–9. https://doi.org/10.1016/j.jpeds.2015.03.007.
135. Alegria M. The challenge of acculturation measures: what are we missing? A commentary on Thomson & Hoffman-Goetz. Soc Sci Med. 2009;69(7):996–8. https://doi.org/10.1016/j.socscimed.2009.07.006.
136. Colby SL, Ortman JM. Projections of the size and composition of the U.S. population: 2014 to 2060 [Press release]. 2015.
137. Appelbaum E, Boushey H, Schmitt J. The economic importance of women's rising hours of work. 2014. https://www.americanprogress.org/issues/economy/reports/2014/04/15/87638/the-economic-importance-of-womens-rising-hours-of-work/.
138. Smedley BD, Stith AY, Nelson AR. Unequal treatment: confronting racial and ethnic disparities in healthcare. Washington, DC: National Academies Press; 2003.
139. Shattuck PT. The contribution of diagnostic substitution to the growing administrative prevalence of autism in US special education. Pediatrics. 2006;117(4):1028–37. https://doi.org/10.1542/peds.2005-1516.
140. Barton EE, Harris B, Leech N, Stiff L, Choi G, Joel T. An analysis of state autism educational assessment practices and requirements. J Autism Dev Disord. 2016;46(3):737–48.
141. Kalkbrenner AE, Daniels JL, Emch M, Morrissey J, Poole C, Chen J-C. Geographic access to health services and diagnosis with an autism spectrum disorder. Ann Epidemiol. 2011;21(4):304–10. https://doi.org/10.1016/j.annepidem.2010.11.010.
142. Sturm R, Ringel JS, Andreyeva T. Geographic disparities in children's mental health care. Pediatrics. 2003;112(4):e308.
143. Zuckerman KE, Perrin JM, Hobrecker K, Donelan K. Barriers to specialty care and specialty referral completion in the community health center setting. J Pediatr. 2013;162(2):409.e401–14.e401. https://doi.org/10.1016/j.jpeds.2012.07.022.
144. Bethell CD, Kogan MD, Strickland BB, Schor EL, Robertson J, Newacheck PW. A national and state profile of leading health problems and health care quality for US children: key insurance disparities and across-state variations. Acad Pediatr. 2011;11(3 Suppl):S22–33. https://doi.org/10.1016/j.acap.2010.08.011.
145. Ngui EM, Flores G. Satisfaction with care and ease of using health care services among parents of children with special health care needs: the roles of race/ethnicity, insurance, language, and adequacy of family-centered care. Pediatrics. 2006;117(4):1184–96.
146. U.S. Department of Health and Human Services, Health Resources and Services Administration, Maternal and Child Health Bureau. The health and well-being of children: a portrait of states and the nation, 2011–2012. Rockville, MD: U.S. Department of Health and Human Services; 2014. http://mchb.hrsa.gov/nsch/2011-12/health/
147. National Center for Health Statistics. Preschool and kindergarten enrollment. 2016. http://nces.ed.gov/programs/coe/indicator_cfa.asp.
148. Guerrero AD, Rodriguez MA, Flores G. Disparities in provider elicitation of parents' developmental concerns for US children. Pediatrics. 2011;128(5):901–9. https://doi.org/10.1542/peds.2011-0030.
149. Herlihy LE, Brooks B, Dumont-Mathieu T, Barton ML, Fein D, Chen CM, Robins DL. Standardized screening facilitates timely diagnosis of autism spectrum disorders in a

diverse sample of low-risk toddlers. J Dev Behav Pediatr. 2014;35(2):85–92. https://doi.org/10.1097/dbp.0000000000000014.
150. Howlin P, Asgharian A. The diagnosis of autism and Asperger syndrome: findings from a survey of 770 families. Dev Med Child Neurol. 1999;41(12):834–9.
151. Ryan S, Salisbury H. You know what boys are like': pre-diagnosis experiences of parents of children with autism spectrum conditions. Br J Gen Pract. 2012;62(598):e378–83. https://doi.org/10.3399/bjgp12X641500.
152. Bornstein MH, Cote LR. Who is sitting across from me? Immigrant mothers' knowledge of parenting and children's development. Pediatrics. 2004;114(5):e557–64.
153. Norbury CF, Sparks A. Difference or disorder? Cultural issues in understanding neurodevelopmental disorders. Dev Psychol. 2013;49(1):45–58. https://doi.org/10.1037/a0027446.
154. Pachter LM, Dworkin PH. Maternal expectations about normal child development in 4 cultural groups. Arch Pediatr Adolesc Med. 1997;151(11):1144–50.
155. Ratto AB, Reznick JS, Turner-Brown L. Cultural effects on the diagnosis of autism spectrum disorder among Latinos. Focus Autism Other Dev Disabil. 2015;31:275–83. https://doi.org/10.1177/1088357615587501.
156. Magana S, Smith LE. The use of the autism diagnostic interview-revised with a Latino population of adolescents and adults with autism. J Autism Dev Disord. 2012;43(5):1098–105. https://doi.org/10.1007/s10803-012-1652-3.
157. Bornstein MH, Cote LR, Haynes OM, Hahn CS, Park Y. Parenting knowledge: experiential and sociodemographic factors in European American mothers of young children. Dev Psychol. 2010;46(6):1677–93. https://doi.org/10.1037/a0020677.
158. Johnson CP, Myers SM, American Academy of Pediatrics Council on Children With Disabilities. Identification and evaluation of children with autism spectrum disorders. Pediatrics. 2007;120(5):1183–215. https://doi.org/10.1542/peds.2007-2361.
159. Siu AL, et al. Screening for autism spectrum disorder in young children: US Preventive Services Task Force recommendation statement. JAMA. 2016;315(7):691–6.
160. Zuckerman KE, Mattox K, Donelan K, Batbayar O, Baghaee A, Bethell C. Pediatrician identification of Latino children at risk for autism spectrum disorder. Pediatrics. 2013;132(3):445–53. https://doi.org/10.1542/peds.2013-0383.
161. Horovitz M, Matson JL, Rieske RD, Kozlowski AM, Sipes M. The relationship between race and challenging behaviours in infants and toddlers with autistic disorder and pervasive developmental disorder-not otherwise specified. Dev Neurorehabil. 2011;14(4):208–14. https://doi.org/10.3109/17518423.2011.566596.
162. Sell NK, Giarelli E, Blum N, Hanlon AL, Levy SE. A comparison of autism spectrum disorder DSM-IV criteria and associated features among African American and white children in Philadelphia County. Disabil Health J. 2012;5(1):9–17. https://doi.org/10.1016/j.dhjo.2011.08.002.
163. Cuccaro ML, Brinkley J, Abramson RK, Hall A, Wright HH, Hussman JP, Pericak-Vance MA. Autism in African American families: clinical-phenotypic findings. Am J Med Genet B Neuropsychiatr Genet. 2007;144b(8):1022–6. https://doi.org/10.1002/ajmg.b.30535.
164. Rhoades RA, Scarpa A, Salley B. The importance of physician knowledge of autism spectrum disorder: results of a parent survey. BMC Pediatr. 2007;7:37. https://doi.org/10.1186/1471-2431-7-37.
165. Warfield ME, Crossman MK, Delahaye J, Der Weerd E, Kuhlthau KA. Physician perspectives on providing primary medical care to adults with autism spectrum disorders (ASD). J Autism Dev Disord. 2015;45(7):2209–17. https://doi.org/10.1007/s10803-015-2386-9.
166. Stein DJ, Phillips KA, Bolton D, Fulford KW, Sadler JZ, Kendler KS. What is a mental/psychiatric disorder? From DSM-IV to DSM-V. Psychol Med. 2010;40(11):1759–65. https://doi.org/10.1017/S0033291709992261.
167. Schwartz SJ, Unger JB, Zamboanga BL, Szapocznik J. Rethinking the concept of acculturation: implications for theory and research. Am Psychol. 2010;65(4):237–51. https://doi.org/10.1037/a0019330.

168. Avdi E, Griffin C, Brough S. Parents' constructions of professional knowledge, expertise and authority during assessment and diagnosis of their child for an autistic spectrum disorder. Br J Med Psychol. 2000;73(Pt 3):327–38.
169. Mire SS, Gealy W, Kubiszyn T, Burridge AB, Goin-Kochel RP. Parent perceptions about autism spectrum disorder influence treatment choices. Focus Autism Other Dev Disabil. 2015;32(4):305–18.
170. Hebert EB, Koulougliotі C. Parental beliefs about cause and course of their child's autism and outcomes of their beliefs: a review of the literature. Issues Compr Pediatr Nurs. 2010;33(3):149–63. https://doi.org/10.3109/01460862.2010.498331.
171. Eraldi R, et al. The help-seeking behavior model. Adm Policy Ment Health Ment Health Serv Res. 2006;33:607–22. https://doi.org/10.1007/s10488-006-0063-1.
172. Clayton JA, Collins FS. NIH to balance sex in cell and animal studies. Nature. 2014;509(7500):282–3.

Chapter 10
Challenges with Transition to Adulthood

Ami Bear, Raegan Smith, and Charlotte Alverson

Vignette

Molly initially presented to clinic at 8 years of age for comprehensive developmental behavioral assessment of impulsive and oppositional behaviors and sensory hypersensitivity. At that time, she had a previous diagnosis of ADHD, and her mother had been told that she had "autistic tendencies." Review of medical and social history revealed Molly was born at 33 and 3/7 weeks gestational age weighing 2422 g, following premature rupture of membranes and otherwise uncomplicated pregnancy. Shortly after birth, she was placed in foster care due to concerns of inability of her biological mother to meet her needs. The mother and baby were living in the same home as sex offenders, and there was significant drug and alcohol use in the home. Molly was subsequently placed in four different foster homes until 9 months of age when she was ultimately placed into the home of her current adoptive family. At that time, history was notable for the fact that she was not yet sitting up or trying to move around. She exhibited a lot of self-soothing behaviors suggesting she had spent a significant amount of time alone in her crib.

During her initial assessment at age 8, cognitive testing was average overall. Diagnostic interview did not meet criteria for autism spectrum disorder (ASD). Ratings made based on the Autism Diagnostic Observation Schedule (ADOS) Module 3 were inconclusive. Molly showed appropriate eye contact

A. Bear (✉) · R. Smith
Child Development and Rehabilitation Center, Oregon Health and Science University, Eugene, OR, USA
e-mail: bear@ohsu.edu; smithrae@ohsu.edu

C. Alverson
College of Education, University of Oregon, Eugene, OR, USA
e-mail: calverso@uoregon.edu

J. M. Fogler, R. A. Phelps (eds.), *Trauma, Autism, and Neurodevelopmental Disorders*, https://doi.org/10.1007/978-3-030-00503-0_10

and varied facial expressions, and her mood was quite variable throughout the visit. The team concluded that the diagnoses that best fit Molly were ADHD, reactive attachment disorder, and sensory hypersensitivities, not ASD. The team recommended medical and behavioral therapy for ADHD and behavioral support and counseling for Molly and her family surrounding issues of attachment. Family was receptive to this feedback and planned to pursue recommendations.

Eight years later, Molly's mother called the clinic with the following updates and concerns: shortly after her initial comprehensive diagnostic assessment, Molly was seen by another provider, who diagnosed her with ASD. With this diagnosis, Molly obtained county developmental disability support services and case management. Her behaviors became increasingly difficult at home, including fictitious claims of being pregnant, due to a fictitious rape, and self-cutting behaviors. This, in turn, led to eventual placement in a developmental disability group home at age 13. For the next 3 years, she resided in this group home and was under the specialty care of psychiatric providers. She was prescribed multiple medications, including high doses of antipsychotic medications. Unfortunately, she experienced metabolic side effects including weight gain and breast development on medications. These side effects were then treated with additional medications, unfortunately.

At age 16, Molly had a reassessment for determination of continuation of developmental disability supports by a psychologist contracted by the county Office of Developmental Disability Services. The psychologist determined that she actually did not meet criteria for ASD. Although she continued to have significant adaptive impairment, it was felt that a developmental disability was not the primary cause of this impairment. As a result, she lost all supports related to a developmental disability, including her group home, county supports, and care coordination.

Molly was abruptly returned to her home without any supports in place. There continued to be significant struggles in the home environment. She tried to attend public school but was unable to stay past 9:20 in the morning before being sent home for disruptive tantrums and meltdowns. Due to a paucity of local providers in their small community, her mother had significant difficulty finding mental health supports but eventually obtained a local therapist for her. Due to significant iatrogenic weight gain, Molly and her mother worked with her primary care provider (PCP) to attempt to wean her off her medications. Molly received consultation from an outreach psychiatric nurse practitioner once, who made adjustments to her medications, but was not able to receive ongoing psychiatric care. Although Molly was endorsing visual hallucinations, she was denied supports from a local organization specializing in emerging psychosis based on phone intake. Thus, she did not receive a comprehensive psychiatric assessment. Eventually, her behaviors were so distressing both at home and school, that her mother found placement at a residential mental health facility about 2 h from their home.

At age 17, Molly returned to clinic, this time to our transition clinic. She was currently residing at a residential facility and attending school there. She was receiving counseling but still was not receiving any psychiatric care. She continued to have daily tantrums and somatic complaints at the facility. Her mother reported that the residential treatment facility was continuing to have monthly meetings to determine whether Molly could remain at this facility as the staff there expressed concern that Molly's behaviors were becoming too disruptive to other young women at the facility. Molly and her mother presented to the transition clinic with the primary concern of obtaining for Molly adequate services to provide her the support she would continue to need during this vulnerable period of transition to adulthood. The mother reported feeling particularly hopeless: The supports Molly received from Developmental Disability Services were less than helpful and were then removed abruptly. The supports she was receiving in the mental health system were not quite effective or sufficient; and, to complicate matters, there were constant threats to discontinue even these inadequate supports.

Need for Transition Services

The above case illustrates the complexity of youth who have been affected by stress and trauma during the developmental period. Like youth with a recognized developmental disability, youth who experienced early stress and trauma need significant social supports during the vulnerable period of transition to adulthood. Unfortunately, unlike youth with developmental disabilities, youth with one or more mental health disorders are generally not eligible for county-based social supports, such as Developmental Disability Services. Mental health services are minimal in the rural area where Molly lives and do not offer the "wraparound supports" available through Developmental Disabilities Services or the Department of Mental Health services offered in major metropolitan areas. There are, at least nominally, mental health services available to support young adults like Molly with severe mental health disorders, but Molly's referral was rejected from one program, and inadequate supports were provided by an alternative program.

Transition for Youth with Developmental Disabilities

The process of transition is a challenging time for all youth with disabilities and particularly so for those who experience special healthcare needs. Transition services, usually conveyed through the public education system as part of the

Individuals with Disabilities Education Act of 2004, are defined as a coordinated set of activities that are intended to help youth move from high school to adult roles and responsibilities [1]. Transition services can encompass a wide array of coordinated activities based on the child's needs. In terms of medical transition, this is a period associated with gaps in care or delayed access to care. Decline in healthcare utilization and visits during this period is pervasive, often due to lapses in adherence, follow-up, or insurance [2]. This period may be especially difficult for youth whose special healthcare needs involve mental health or developmental disability, including intellectual disability. The 2009–2010 National Survey of Children with Special Health Care Needs indicate that the majority of young adults with special healthcare needs are not receiving needed transition preparation [3]. The consensus statement on healthcare transition for young adults with special healthcare needs [4] underscores the importance of affordable and uninterrupted service, facilitated by (a) an identified point person and (b) a written plan in place by age 14 that is easily portable between pediatric and adult healthcare system [3]. Specifically looking at ADHD, Fogler and colleagues note the problem that there is no clearly defined department for ADHD among adult specialties, as there is for other lifelong conditions such as diabetes or epilepsy. Furthermore, even when an adult care service center is identified, the transition may fail [5].

Cheak-Zamora and et al. [6] found that fewer than 15% of youth aged 12–17 received adequate healthcare transition services. McManus et al. [7] reported that only 40–41% of youth with special healthcare needs received healthcare services. Shattuck and et al. [8] found that 39% of young adults from a nationally representative sample, aged 19–23 at the time of data collection, had not received mental health, medical, speech, or case management services after leaving high school. Community supports and services are generally meant to facilitate moving individuals with disabilities into living wage jobs and acquiring other services to attain various degrees of independent living. In an analysis of the 2005–2006 National Survey of Children With Special Health Care Needs survey, Lotstein et al. [3] found that only 41% of parents of youth with special healthcare needs met all four core performance outcomes for having had a transition-related discussion about "...(a) future adult providers, (b) future adult healthcare needs, (c) changes in health insurance, and (d) encouraging their child to take responsibility for his or her care" (p. e145).

Cross-sectional studies show that there is a decline in the use of mental health services in adolescents and youth as compared to adults, despite the presence of documentation that recommends that ongoing services should be in place [9]. Moreover, adolescent transition does not only involve healthcare transition but includes transition in education, employment, residence, and community participation. Many models that provide transition services operate within their own domains (healthcare transition as a separate process as educational and vocational transition).

Transition Services for Youth with Mental Healthcare Needs

Social supports and case management play a large role in ensuring successful transition to adulthood for youth with mental healthcare needs. In 2015, Myers et al. [10] examined community participation among youths with autism spectrum disorder (ASD). The study noted a significant decline in community participation from adolescence to adulthood and that the presence of case management led to increased community and social participation in adulthood. This is particularly important information related to the above case. When diagnosed with ASD, Molly qualified for and received case management through her county's developmental disabilities office. Yet, when reevaluated and diagnosed with a mental illness, there were no similar supports offering care coordination based upon adaptive impairment due to a trauma and stressor-related disorder (TSRD) or other mental illness. This is a common theme we encounter in our clinic's transition program. Many youth affected by mental illness and/or TSRD come seeking a developmental disability diagnosis to obtain much-needed supports. Unfortunately, when a developmental disability is not identified, we find ourselves lacking resources to provide much-needed case management. In Molly's case, we referred her to an organization aimed at providing care coordination and case management for youth with symptoms of emerging psychosis, as Molly had endorsed visual and auditory hallucinations. The organization reviewed Molly's case and felt her symptoms emerge from PTSD rather than a true emerging psychotic disorder; thus, she did not qualify for their care (but see Prock and Fogler, Chap. 3, this volume).

Overview of Treatment Recommendations for Youth in Transition

In this chapter, and this book for that matter, we are proposing a model of practice that some may consider controversial: Based on clinical judgment, and well-considered hypotheses about pathophysiology, our prescribing colleagues will talk openly about "off-label" uses of medication for symptoms and conditions other than the ones they were approved for by the FDA. Due to exclusionary criteria used in efficacy studies for evidence-based psychotherapy, individuals presenting for treatment in community settings would often be excluded from outcome research on the basis of comorbidities or not quite meeting full DSM criteria for the condition(s) under study. We are thus proposing that clinicians in the field are justified in considering novel applications of evidence-based treatments and take a similar "off-label" mindset when it comes to behavioral therapies for diagnostically complex children—especially with such complicated features of both neurodevelopmental disorders *and* TSRD. In other words, depending on the presenting symptoms and contextual factors, the same psychological treatment models/practices may be indicated to address common social-emotional and behavioral problems, regardless of diagnosis (ASD vs. PTSD vs. RAD, etc.). Examples include programs with parent training or family therapy components, cognitive-behavioral therapy, and applied behavior analysis (ABA) [11–14].

Practitioners must consider the degree of structure needed around the application of learning principles to effect behavior change. One might argue that all families impacted by significant behavioral and emotional disturbances, regardless of diagnosis, could potentially benefit from interventions designed and carried out by practitioners who possess a broad knowledge of behavioral learning principles. Be that as it may, the specific skill set with which any given clinician presents may be more attuned to one diagnostic population over another; and, the qualitative aspects of implementing any approach will depend greatly on level of experience, specialized training, and adherence to professional standards of the practitioner, as well as the family's priorities.

For example, ABA is a frequently recommended intervention for addressing problem behaviors and adaptive impairments in the population of individuals with ASD (https://www.ncbi.nlm.nih.gov/pubmed/18775375). ABA involves a high level of structure (i.e., all components of treatment are data-driven; quantitative behavioral data are crucial for creation of treatment plans, adjustments to treatment components, and measuring progress). In contrast, evidence-based versions of parent management training (PMT) rely upon a relatively moderate amount of behavioral data to inform treatment planning along the way. In the context of PMT, individualized goals emphasize particular areas of strengths/weaknesses in parents' use of previously taught parenting skills (e.g., parent-child interaction therapy), whereas ABA interventions rely upon the use of highly individualized and, in some cases, more circumscribed behavioral targets. Both approaches (ABA and PMT) rely upon the use of positive reinforcement, as well as management of behavioral antecedents and consequences in general.

Thus, when there are diagnostic concerns about ASD versus TSRD, there is potential benefit from participation in any high-quality intervention based upon behavioral learning principles or cognitive theory, particularly when targeting overlapping symptom presentation of the primary or comorbid diagnoses (e.g., impaired self-regulation skills, impaired social communication, coercive parent-child interactions, obsessive-compulsive habits). Some would likely object to a possible lack of parsimony; still, we would posit that for some individuals, it is more important to prioritize treatment of behavioral symptoms and developmental skills deficits than to provide referrals and funding/coverage for potentially inadequate treatment based solely upon diagnostic label.

Somewhat paradoxically, we would also posit that misdiagnosis of ASD versus TSRD could lead to an unfortunate situation in which there is a striking mismatch between treatment approach and the needs of the patient. For example, a child who has been misdiagnosed with ASD when presenting problems are better conceptualized as a TSRD may present with reactivity that interferes with treatment effectiveness (e.g., annoyance in response to repetitive stimuli and/or otherwise poor response to the high level of structure and repetition inherent in ABA).

When families and practitioners find a lack of desirable response to a series of interventions, the temptation is to diagnose a developmental disability in order to increase access to services (see Chap. 1), but as we see in Molly's case, the harder won, but arguably better solution clinically, required a systemic appreciation for the high level of need in populations of youth presenting with complex history of adverse events. That said, Molly's response to attachment-focused treatment alone following initial evaluation was insufficient to achieve behavioral and developmental success and prevent escalation of problems. One might argue that the need for environmental support of the patient and her family was simply too great. When a youth presents with adaptive impairments attributable to TSRD, interventions must be planned across many levels of the system, just as with youths whose adaptive impairments are primarily attributable to ASD [15]. At least some youths with trauma history require a full-time (or nearly full-time) therapeutic environment to improve psychological functioning, with interventions implemented at an intensity level similar to the treatments warranted for at least some youths with ASD (http://www.tricountywomenscentre.org/uploads/5/7/6/6/5766610/courtois_-_complex_trauma_complex_reactions.pdf; https://link.springer.com/article/10.1080%2F19361520903120467). Thus, it is a social injustice that some families are expected to meet their youths' needs without additional environmental support.

Another consideration with regard to efforts to find effective interventions for complex youth is that misdiagnosing ASD may result in referral to group services, such as social skills training [16] or group residential placements, as in the above vignette. When considering how interventions and placements are structured, providers, educators, and community support workers must consider the impact of homogeneity versus heterogeneity in group settings. For example, with the Program for the Education and Enrichment of Relational Skills [17] (PEERS), an evidence-based, ecologically valid model of social skills intervention designed for adolescents and young adults with ASD, treatment groups are constructed with a preference for homogeneity dependent upon the level of internalizing vs. externalizing behaviors with which patients present, in addition to specific diagnosis. We would agree with this sentiment and urge providers to also consider differences in social-cognitive and social-emotional development when determining appropriate referrals/interventions. For example, individuals presenting with attachment and/or trauma-related disorders may benefit from ABA but would likely fit poorly into group settings where the predominant population served has low-functioning ASD or intellectual disability. Conversely, due to the higher level of anticipated emotional reactivity and dysregulation, that same adolescent with TSRD should likely not be placed into a social skills group with adolescents with simple phobias, social anxiety, or uncomplicated ADHD.

Furthermore, treatment plans are greatly impacted by the individual's need for supports during and between treatment sessions [18]. This is particularly salient for older youth who are able to participate in verbally mediated interventions (i.e., talk therapy). Youth who present for cognitive-behavioral therapy (CBT) to address obsessive-compulsive symptoms or social anxiety without the presence of neurodevelopmental disorder are more likely to present with the adaptive resources needed to support generalization of skills as long as parents remain involved and are able to provide between-session support.

In contrast, individuals with ASD may require an even higher level of environmental support for the generalization of cognitive-behavioral coping skills [18]. When adaptive impairment is clearly attributable to ASD, it is possible to secure additional environmental support via community-based programs to implement interventions targeting comorbid anxiety and/or disruptive behavior disorders. However, when the adaptive impairment is primarily attributable to TSRD, the community standard does not match the science. As discussed elsewhere in this book, there are neurological/physiological bases for developmental impairment in individuals with mental health injuries sustained in childhood (https://www-cambridge-org.liboff.ohsu.edu/core/services/aop-cambridge-core/content/view/C6AB7D5DFD218B267BD642BE5B6618DA/S0954579401003078a.pdf/developmental_traumatology_the_psychobiological_development_of_maltreated_children_and_its_implications_for_research_treatment_and_policy.pdf). Both populations (ASD and TSRD) may benefit from CBT targeting anxiety and/or mood-related symptoms; and both may present with neurodevelopmental differences and disorders necessitating adaptations. In other words, the level of support needed to achieve treatment goals will need to be individually tailored to the child's presenting problem and level of functioning, regardless of diagnosis.

At the same time, misdiagnosing a TSRD as ASD will almost certainly perpetuate avoidance symptoms and/or disrupted attachment processes and would, therefore, preclude opportunity for fully informed consent regarding an individual's choices of appropriate treatment options. For example, families may be misdirected to ABA services when what is actually indicated as a primary intervention is trauma-focused CBT (TF-CBT) or attachment-based therapy. Attempts to process adverse events or increase positive parent-child interactions via behavioral or cognitive-behavioral intervention will not be made if the assessment, diagnosis, and treatment recommendations do not identify the need for it. Over time, neglecting appropriate treatment targets will further complicate the overall clinical presentation.

The Fundamental Problem Revisited

Molly's story highlights one of the fundamental problems associated with transition services for young adults: *diagnosis-specific services*. In transition clinic, we work hard to appropriately diagnose, regardless of the availability of services, or lack thereof. Whereas many developmental disabilities have specific testing criteria (e.g., intellectual disability), or rely on historical and exam data (e.g., fetal alcohol spectrum disorder) for diagnosis, we often find that ASD is invoked by diagnosticians trying to be helpful, as the structured observations and interview which form the core of the ASD diagnostic assessment are relatively subjective. As in Molly's case, the ASD diagnosis was given by outside providers presumably to help Molly access services only available for those with a developmental disability diagnosis.

However, when this inaccurate diagnosis was eventually questioned, Molly abruptly lost services. Equally concerning as this abrupt loss of services, the interventions that Molly was receiving—intended to target a misapplied diagnosis of ASD—were inappropriate and thus ineffective.

To develop evidence-based interventions for specific conditions and then to allocate funds to provide these services to individuals who need them is, of course, crucial. But, to refer children to the wrong services not only undermines the whole system but also potentially causes additional harm due to the delay in receipt of appropriate services. Specifically, treating children with TSRD with only rigidly applied behavioral treatments for ASD, or vice versa, is counterproductive at best, and at worst, contraindicated and harmful. As noted, some off-label behavioral strategies may be helpful for both of these disorders; however, if one is not mindful of co-occurring conditions, these can be missed or at least not prioritized, which can potentially be harmful to the individual.

Transition to adulthood is a vulnerable time for all individuals. Typically, this period is supported by multiple systems, including the home and family environment, educational systems, community programs and participation, and medical care. For individuals who experience TSRDs, these systems are particularly crucial. Even if these systems are all currently in place for an individual—and as in Molly's case, often they are not—it takes a great deal of sophistication to smoothly coordinate these systems. Furthermore, due to the existence of a TSRD, these individuals require much more intensive supports as they emerge as young adults. Various professional groups have created guidelines highlighting the importance of thoughtful, comprehensive, and coordinated transition planning, but, all too often, these guidelines are not met. We seek to achieve a high standard level of care for youths with either or both mental health disorders and neurodevelopmental disabilities. This standard applies to a minimum level of community support, care coordination, and psychosocial intervention needed for successful transition, whether the challenges arise from TSRD or ASD or other mental health or developmental disorders. Integrated treatments are needed in order to appropriately serve the needs of individuals with complex clinical presentations. Regardless of whether challenges are attributable to trauma-inflicted injuries or genetically predisposed biological anomalies, treatment plans and supports should include an individually tailored array of evidence-based and "off-label" practices, tailored to functional assessment of the individual. This theme will be further developed in the concluding chapter of this book.

References

1. US Department of Education. Topic: secondary transition. http://idea.ed.gov/explore/view/p/,root,dynamic,TopicalBrief,17,.html. Accessed 12 Mar 2017.
2. Prior M, McManus M, White P, Davidson L. Measuring the "triple aim" in transition care: a systematic review. Pediatrics. 2014;134(6):e1648–61.

3. Lotstein DS, Ghandour R, Cash A, McGuire E, Strickland B, Newacheck P. Planning for health care transitions: results from the 2005–2006 National Survey of Children With Special Health Care Needs. Pediatrics. 2009;123:e145–52.
4. A Consensus Statement on Health Care Transitions for Young Adults With Special Health Care Needs American Academy of Pediatrics. American Academy of Family Physicians. American College of Physicians-American Society of Internal Medicine Pediatrics. Dec 2002; 110(3):1304–1306.
5. Fogler JM, Burke D, Lynch J, Barbaresi WJ, Chan E. Topical review: transitional services for teens and young adults with attention deficit and hyperactivity disorder: a process map and proposed model to overcoming barriers to care. J Pediatr Psychol. 2017;42(10):1108–13.
6. Cheak-Zamora NC, Farmer JE, Mayfield WA, Clark MJ, Marvin AR, Law JK, Law PA. Health care transition services for youth with autism spectrum disorders. Rehabil Psychol. 2014; 59(3):340–8.
7. McManus MA, Pollack LR, Cooley WC, McAllister JW, Lotstein D, Strickland B, Mann MY. Current status of transition preparation among youth with special needs in the United States. Pediatrics. 2013;131:1090–7. https://doi.org/10.1542/peds.2012-3050.
8. Shattuck PT, Wagner M, Narendorf S, Sterzing P, Hensley M. Post-high school service use among young adults with an autism spectrum disorder. Arch Pediatr Adolesc Med. 2011;165: 141–6.
9. Reale L, et al. Mental disorders and transition to adult mental health services: a scoping review. Eur Psychiatry. 2015;30(8):932–42.
10. Myers E, Davis BE, Stobbe G, et al. Community and social participation among individuals with autism spectrum disorder transitioning to adulthood. J Autism Dev Disord. 2015;45:2373. https://doi.org/10.1007/s10803-015-2403-z.
11. Open trial pilot of PCIT for children with ASD. http://www.tandfonline.com/doi/full/10.1080/07317107.2016.1267999?scroll=top&needAccess=true&.
12. Preventing maltreatment with a community-based implementation of PCIT. https://link.springer.com/article/10.1007/s10826-012-9708-8.
13. Lang R, Regester A, Lauderdale S, Ashbaugh K, Haring A. Treatment of anxiety in autism spectrum disorders using cognitive behavior therapy: a systematic review. Dev Neurorehabil. 2010;13(1):53–63.
14. Danial JT, Wood JJ. Cognitive behavioral therapy for children with autism: review and considerations for future research. J Dev Behav Pediatr. 2013;34(9):702–15. http://www.ncbi.nlm.nih.gov/pubmed/23917373. Retrieved 17 Aug 2016.
15. Saxe GN, Ellis BH, Kaplow JB. Collaborative treatment of traumatized children and teens. New York: Guilford; 2006.
16. Olsson NC, Flygare O, Coco C, Gorling A, Rade A, Chen Q, Lindstedt K, Berggren S, Serlachius E, Jonsson U, Tammimies K, Kjellin L, Bolte S. Social skills training for children and adolescents with autism spectrum disorder: a randomized controlled trial. J Am Acad Child Adolesc Psychiatry. 2017;56(7):585–92.
17. PEERS. Treatment planning for person-centered care: the road to mental health and addiction recovery. San Diego, CA: Elsevier Academic Press; 2005. xxi, 291 pp.
18. Wood J, Drahota A, Sze K, Har K, Chiu A, Langer DA. Cognitive behavioral therapy for anxiety in children with autism spectrum disorders: a randomized, controlled trial. J Child Psychol Psychiatry. 2009;50(3):224–34. Sofronoff et al. (2005) in the same journal (pp. 1152–1160).

Chapter 11
Trauma and Neurodevelopmental Disorders from a Public Health Perspective

Sarah R. Lowe, Kate L. Walsh, Emma Opthof, and Petty Tineo

Vignette

Mrs. T presents to a mental health clinic in the Northeastern region of the United States with her 8-year-old son J, whom she adopted from foster care 3 months prior. Mrs. T reports that she has noticed some behaviors in her son that she finds troubling. She says that he seems distracted and "dazed," and startles easily when she tries to "wake him from his trance." Furthermore, he has not yet slept through the night, frequently awakening with great distress and unable to be comforted. During the day, J engages in what Mrs. T describes as "repetitive play," sitting alone with his action figures and endlessly enacting "battle scenes" with them. Most distressing to Mrs. T is that she perceives J as not "properly attaching" to her. He avoids physical contact with Mrs. T and physically pushes her away when she tries to embrace him. He is also socially withdrawn at home and at school, not initiating or responding to interactions with his parents, siblings, teachers, and peers.

Mrs. T reports that she has some preliminary ideas about her son's condition based on information she has seen on television and read about online. Specifically, she surmises that her son might have either autism spectrum disorder (ASD) based on his social withdrawal and repetitive play or reactive attachment disorder (RAD) based on his "dazed" demeanor and resistance to affection and physical contact.

S. R. Lowe (✉) · E. Opthof · P. Tineo
Department of Psychology, Montclair State University, Montclair, NJ, USA
e-mail: lowes@mail.montclair.edu; opthofe1@mail.montclair.edu; tineop1@mail.montclair.edu

K. L. Walsh
Ferkauf Graduate School of Psychology, Bronx, NY, USA
e-mail: kate.walsh@einstein.yu.edu

J. M. Fogler, R. A. Phelps (eds.), *Trauma, Autism, and Neurodevelopmental Disorders*, https://doi.org/10.1007/978-3-030-00503-0_11

The clinician meets with J three times, and while he is initially reticent and does not answer questions, he eventually discloses that he was frequently punched, spanked, and hit with hard objects at one of his foster homes. Based on his observations of J, J's disclosure, and information from J's parents and teacher, the clinician comes to a diagnosis of post-traumatic stress disorder (PTSD).

Mrs. T is initially very surprised to hear of her son's diagnosis, commenting that she thought PTSD was something that "only affects veterans and rape victims" and that she had "no idea that kids could have PTSD!" She is comforted, however, hearing about the many empirically supported treatments for children with PTSD.

Still, Mrs. T has several questions about her son's conditions. She asks the following questions:

- *How common is child abuse and other forms of trauma in children?*
- *What factors increase and decrease risk for trauma exposure?*
- *How common is PTSD among children in the United States?*
- *Other than trauma exposure, what factors put children at risk of PTSD? What factors might protect trauma-exposed children from suffering from PTSD?*
- *Do children who have experienced trauma suffer from other disorders, such as RAD? How common are these disorders, and what are risk factors for them?*
- *What about neurodevelopmental disorders that might "look" similar but do not include trauma exposure in their diagnostic criteria—like ASD? What is the prevalence of these disorders?*
- *What are risk and protective factors for neurodevelopmental disorders?*
- *Do children who have experienced trauma ever develop neurodevelopmental disorders as well? Do trauma-related and neurodevelopmental disorders ever co-occur?*
- *What can we as a society do to prevent the occurrence and persistence of PTSD and these other disorders?*

Being familiar with the public health literature on trauma-related and neurodevelopmental disorders, the clinician is able to provide some answers to Mrs. T's questions. However, he is also careful to warn her about some of the limitations of the literature, advising her that there is "a lot that we have left to learn."

As the clinician in the above scenario notes, the questions that the client is asking can be answered from a public health perspective. More specifically, Mrs. T's questions about how common, or *prevalent*, different disorders are, and predictors of those disorders are addressed in the public health subfield of *epidemiology*. Epidemiology focuses on the distribution and causes of disease in human populations and on developing and testing means for the prevention and control of disease and is considered the cornerstone of public health. In this chapter, we will review the epidemiologic research on the prevalence and predictors of trauma-related and neurodevelopmental disorders, with attention to limitations to the extant literature that render conclusions tentative at best. Finally, we will conclude with an overview of public health approaches to addressing trauma, and trauma-related and neurodevelopmental disorders.

Children's Exposure to Traumatic Events

Prevalence

Table 11.1 provides a summary of epidemiologic studies exploring the prevalence of *potentially traumatic events* (PTEs). According to the fifth edition of the *Diagnostic and Statistical Manual of Mental Disorders* [27], events that could trigger PTSD involve exposure to actual or threatened death, serious injury, or sexual violation and can occur in scenarios in which the individual directly experiences the event, witnesses the event in person, learns that the event occurred to a friend or close family member (or, if the child is 6 years old or younger, to a parent or caregiving figure), or experiences repeated exposure of aversive details of an event (but not through media, photographs, television, or movies, unless such exposure is work-related). A notable change to *DSM-5*, relative to the *DSM-IV* [28, 29], is that an event no longer requires an immediate emotional response to the event, such as intense fear, helplessness, or horror, for it to qualify as traumatic [27]. With few exceptions (e.g., [5]), the vast majority of epidemiologic studies assess trauma in a manner consistent with *DSM-5* in that they have participants indicate whether they have experienced any events on a checklist and then assess PTSD symptoms irrespective of whether the participant experienced an emotional response during the event.

The epidemiologic studies covered in Table 11.1 are those that included either nationally or regionally representative samples of children and adolescents. In addition to the United States, countries represented in these studies include those in East Asia (e.g., China: [1]), the Middle East (e.g., Israel: [7]), Europe (e.g., Denmark: [3]; Iceland: [6]), as well as Mexico [10] and South Africa [11]. Although most studies focused on the general child and/or adolescent population within a given region or country, a few included representative samples of high-risk child or adolescent populations, such as refugees in a given area [8, 26]. The youngest children represented across the reviewed studies were 18 months old [25], and the oldest were in their early 20s (e.g., [24]), although any study that exclusively focused on participants ages 18 and older were excluded from the review. The prevalence of exposure to one or more PTEs is listed for the full sample when available, and subsamples if not. In addition, we highlight the prevalence of some events that might be

Table 11.1 Summary of epidemiologic studies on the prevalence of potentially traumatic events

Reference	County	*N*; Study description	# of PTEs assessed	Prevalence of PTEs
[1]	China (regional)	3175; students ages 15–17 in Xi'an	1 (bullying victimization)	*Any PTE (specifically, bullying victimization):* Lifetime, 54.9%; past year, 44.6%
[2]	Cyprus (regional)	1645; elementary and high school students (ages unspecified) in rural, urban, and suburban areas	1 (bullying victimization)	*Any PTE (specifically moderate and severe bullying victimization)*: 11.3%
[3]	Denmark (national)	390; eighth graders ages 13–15	20	*Any PTE*: 87% of girls, 78% of boys; *physical abuse*, 3.6% (4.2% of girls, 3.1% of boys); *sexual abuse*, 1.5% (2.6% of girls, 0.5% of boys); *physical assault*, 4.6% (4.2% of girls, 5.1% of boys); *rape*, 1.8% (2.6% of girls, 1.0% of boys); *bereavement*, 51.8% (58.9% of girls, 44.6% of boys)
[4]	East Jerusalem/ West Bank (regional and high-risk group)	1000; Palestinian school children ages 12–16 in East Jerusalem and the West Bank	10	*Any PTE*: 54.7%; *physical abuse or assault*, 14.8%; *sexual assault*, 0.7%
[5]	Germany (regional)	2548; Early Developmental Stages of Psychopathology (EDSP) study; adolescents and young adults ages 14–24 in Munich; assessed at baseline (T0), and an average of 19.7 and 42 months thereafter (T1, T2)	11 (*included DSM-IV A2 criterion*)	*Any PTE*: Lifetime, 16.7% at T0; past 42 months (i.e., between T0 and T2): 20.3%

(continued)

Table 11.1 (continued)

Reference	County	*N*; Study description	# of PTEs assessed	Prevalence of PTEs
[6]	Iceland (national)	206; 9th grade students ages 13–15	20	*Any PTE*: 74% of girls; 79% of boys; *physical abuse*, 2.9% (3.9% girls, 2.0% boys); *sexual abuse*, 3.9% (5.8% girls, 2.0% boys); *physical assault*, 7.8% (6.8% girls, 9.0% boys); *rape*, 3.3% (5.8% girls, 1.0% boys); *bereavement*, 42.7% (44.7% girls, 41.0% boys)
[7]	Israel (national)	4151; Jewish and Arab Israeli students ages 13–17	24 (14 war-related events; 10 other events)	*Sexual abuse*, 7.9% *(asked of Jewish participants only)*; *physical assault*, 4.0%; *bereavement*, 32.0%
[8]	Iraq (regional and high-risk group)	201; Kurdistanian children ages 6–18 living in Duhok City in Iraqi Kurdistan	30	*Sexual abuse*: 0.0%
[9]	Lithuania (national)	183; adolescents ages 13–17	20	*Any PTE*: 80.2% (79.8% of girls, 80.7% of boys); *physical abuse*, 3.8% (6.1% of girls, 1.2% of boys); *sexual abuse*, 4.4% (8.1% of girls, 0.0% of boys); *physical assault*, 4.4% (4.0% of girls, 4.8% of boys); *rape*, 1.6% (3.0% of girls, 0.0% of boys); *bereavement*, 24.2% (25.3% of girls, 22.9% of boys)
[10]	Mexico (regional)	3005; Mexican Adolescent Mental Health Survey; adolescents ages 12–17 in the Mexico City metropolitan area	23	*Any PTE*: 68.9%; *physical abuse*, 13.2% (14.2% of girls, 12.2% of boys); *rape*, 1.3% (2.0% of girls, 0.6% of boys); *bereavement*, 25.8% (28.7% of girls, 22.9% of boys)

(continued)

Table 11.1 (continued)

Reference	County	*N*; Study description	# of PTEs assessed	Prevalence of PTEs
[11]	South Africa (regional)	148; ethnically Northern Sotho children ages 6–10 from the rural community of Dikgale	7	*Any PTE*: 67%; *sexual abuse or rape (by a relative or friend)*: 8.0%
[12]	Sri Lanka (regional)	420; school children ages 10–14 from provinces affected by armed conflict	Not specified	**Any PTE:** 92%
[8]	Sweden (regional and high-risk group)	111; Kurdistanian children ages 6–18 living in the Uppsala City in Sweden	30	*Sexual abuse*: 2.7%
[13]	Switzerland (national)	6787; 9th graders (97% ages 14.0–16.9)	13	*Any PTE*: 56.1% (56.6% of girls, 55.7% of boys); *physical abuse*, 6.9% (8.9% of girls, 4.9% of boys); *sexual abuse*, 3.1% (4.4% of girls, 2.0% of boys)
[14]	Taiwan (national)	6233; 4th graders (ages unspecified)	5 (all forms of child maltreatment)	*Physical abuse*: Paternal, 15.0%; maternal, 14.7%; *sexual violence*, 9.2%
[15]	United States (national)	1763; adolescent girls ages 12–17	1 (sexual assault, assessed by 4 items)	*Sexual assault*: 11.8%
[16]	United States (national)	1443; National Youth Victimization Prevention Study; two-wave representative study of children ages 10–16; Time 2 (T2) occurred an average of 15 months after Time 1 (T1)	12 (all related to victimization)	*Any PTE*: 38.4% before T1; 21% between T1 and T2
[17]	United States (national)	2000; children ages 10–16	12	*Any PTE (excluding "corporal punishment"):* Lifetime, 35.1%, past year, 25.4%; *physical abuse ("corporal punishment"):* lifetime, 74.5%, past year, 28.5%

(continued)

Table 11.1 (continued)

Reference	County	*N*; Study description	# of PTEs assessed	Prevalence of PTEs
[18, 19]	United States (national)	1467; Developmental Victimization Survey; children ages 2–17, assessed at T1 (baseline) and T2 (1-year follow-up)	34 events, covering 5 categories of victimization (e.g., physical assault, sexual victimization)	*Any PTE*: Past year: 70% at T2; *physical assault*, past year, 55% at T1, 49% at T2; *sexual victimization*, past year, 8% at T1, 8% at T2
[20]; [21]	United States (national)	4023; National Survey of Adolescents; adolescents ages 12–17	4 categories (each assessed with multiple items)	*Any PTE (excluding bereavement)*: 48% (44.1% of girls, 51.3% of boys); *physical assault*, 22.5% (26.1% of boys, 18.8% of girls); *sexual assault*, 8.2% (13.2% of girls, 3.5% of boys); *bereavement*, 48.2%
[22]	United States (national)	6483; National Comorbidity Survey-Adolescent Replication; adolescents ages 13–17	19	*Any PTE*: 61.8%; *physical abuse*, 2.0%; *sexual assault*, 3.8%; *rape*, 2.5%; *bereavement*, 28.2%
[23]	United States (regional)	1420; Great Smoky Mountains Study; children ages 9, 11, and 13 in Western North Carolina, followed until age 16	17	*Any PTE*: Lifetime, 68.2% (68.4% of girls, 52.0% of boys); past 3 months, 5.9% (6.0% of girls, 5.9% of boys)
[24]	United States (regional)	490; second wave of a longitudinal epidemiologic study of public school students in a South Carolina district; adolescents ages 16–22	4	*Any PTE*: White boys, 11.6%, White girls, 16.6%, Black boys, 15.8%, Black girls, 25.2%; *rape or sexual abuse*, White boys, 1.5%, White girls, 9.4%, Black boys, 0.0%, Black girls, 12.9%
[25]	United States (regional)	917; 18- to 36-month-olds from the Greater New Haven area	9	*Any PTE* (experienced between 6 and 36 months): 23.4%
[26]	United States (regional and high-risk group)	194; Cambodian refugees ages 13–25 living in either Portland, OR, or Salt Lake City, UT	Not specified	*Any PTE*: 92.8%

Note. PTE potentially traumatic event. Lifetime prevalence rates of events are listed unless otherwise specified. Prevalence rates of selected PTE types (e.g., physical abuse, sexual abuse, rape, bereavement) are included. Prevalence rates of other events (e.g., natural disasters, motor vehicle accidents) can be found in the original sources, if available of particular importance, such as physical abuse and assault, sexual assault and rape, and bereavement, when reported in studies.

Lifetime exposure to PTEs across these studies ranged from 11.6% among White male public school students ages 16–22 in South Carolina [24] to 92.8% among Cambodian refugees ages 13–25 living in Portland, Oregon, and Salt Lake City, Utah. Focusing on regionally or nationally representative studies in the United States that did not focus on high-risk populations or report on subsamples only, the prevalence of lifetime PTE exposure ranged from 23.4% in a sample of 18- to 36-month-olds in the Greater New Haven, Connecticut area, to 68.2% among 16-year-olds in Western North Carolina [23].

The overall trends in PTE exposure across the studies therefore suggest that lifetime trauma exposure increased markedly from childhood to adolescence and that additional factors influencing exposure are gender, race and ethnicity, and refugee status. At the same time, the variation in these factors across studies limits the extent to which the prevalence of PTEs across regions and nations can be compared. An additional consideration is the number of PTEs assessed across studies, with some studies focusing on one specific PTE (e.g., bullying victimization: [2]; sexual assault: [15]), and others assessing 20 or more PTEs (e.g., [9, 10]). For the purposes of our case study, we might therefore recommend that the clinician review the results of the one nationally representative study in the United States, published in the past decade, in which 10 or more lifetime PTEs were assessed, and the lifetime prevalence of any PTE exposure was reported: the National Comorbidity Study-Adolescent Replication (NCS-A: [22]). In this study of adolescents ages 13–17, 61.8% reported lifetime exposure to one or more of 19 PTEs.

Another notable trend in Table 11.1 is variation in the prevalence of selected traumatic events. A consistent cross-national finding among studies that comprehensively assessed trauma exposure is that bereavement, typically defined as the unexpected death of a close friend or family member, is among the most commonly experience PTEs, with prevalence ranging from 28.2% to 48.2% in nationally representative US samples [21, 22] and 24.2% to 51.8% in nationally representative studies abroad [3, 9]. Other selected forms of trauma are relatively less common; for example, in the national survey of adolescents in Iceland, 42.7% had experienced bereavement, whereas 2.9% experienced physical abuse, 7.8% physical assault, 3.9% sexual abuse, and 3.3% rape [6]. Similar patterns of relative prevalence were observed in national studies in Denmark [3], Lithuania [9], Mexico [10], and the United States (e.g., [22]). Despite consistency in trends, there was nonetheless variation in prevalence of specific PTE cross national, such that, for example, the prevalence of physical abuse in nationally representative US studies was as low as 2.0% in the NCS-A [22] and as high as 74.5% in a study of adolescents two decades prior, wherein children reported on "corporal punishment" [17]. This example shows how prevalence can vary dramatically depending on how items are worded, as well as potential variability in trends of exposure over time.

Q: How common is child abuse and other forms of trauma in children?

A: Although the prevalence of child abuse and other forms of trauma in children varies across studies, a recent large nationally representative study of children ages

13–17 found that the majority of participants (61.8%) had experienced at least 1 of 19 potentially traumatic events. The prevalence of physical abuse in the study was 2.0%.

Predictors of Trauma Exposure

Research to date has documented a range of factors that are associated with risk for PTE exposure. These can be roughly divided into four categories: (1) demographic characteristics, (2) other exposures, (3) mental health, and (4) familial and peer relationships.

Demographic Characteristics Several demographic characteristics have been found to shape risk for PTE exposure. First, child gender is differentially associated with risk, depending on the type of PTE. Across epidemiologic studies, girls are at greater risk for PTEs related to sexual contact and intimate partnership, including sexual abuse, sexual assault, rape, physically assault by an intimate partner, and stalking (e.g., [9]; [22]). Girls are also more likely than boys to report bereavement (e.g., [22]; [10]), as well as indirect exposure (i.e., hearing that a close friend or family member was exposed) to a variety of events, such as bereavement or sexual abuse, perhaps reflecting girls' greater interpersonal orientation or more extensive social networks ([9]; [3]). In contrast, boys are generally more likely to be exposed to PTEs related to nonsexual physical violence (e.g., being beaten, shot, physically assaulted, or threats of physical violence) ([9]; [13]), to witness violence (e.g., [3]; [13]) and to be involved in serious accidents (e.g., [22]; [10]).

Second, and similarly, the relationship between child age and PTE exposure depends on the type of traumatic event. For example, in the NCS-A, younger age was associated with increased risk for PTEs such as physical abuse by a caregiver and kidnapping, whereas older age was associated with increased risk for intimate partner violence and car accidents [22]. Further studies have shown that adolescents are at increased risk for PTEs such as drug-/alcohol-facilitated or incapacitated sexual assault [15] and experiencing the death of a close friend [21], as well as *polyvictimization*, or being the victim of multiple types of PTEs [18].

Third, a handful of studies have reported variation in PTE exposure by child race or ethnicity. Non-Hispanic Black children have been found to report more incidences of bereavement (e.g., [21, 22]) and exposure to a greater overall number of PTEs [24]. The NCS-A further found that non-Hispanic Black children were at increased risk for stalking, accidents, and witnessing violence and Hispanic children for intimate partner violence, stalking, accidents, and witnessing violence, relative to non-Hispanic White children [22]. Outside of the United States, children of non-Swiss nationality living in Switzerland were found at be at increased risk for more extensive PTE exposure [13]. In contrast, another investigation found that Jewish children in Israel were at increased risk of exposure to a greater number of war-related PTEs and for some war-related PTEs specifically (e.g., being present at the scene of a fallen missile) but at decreased risk for other war-related PTEs (e.g., having a friend or family member hurt or killed by a missile), relative to their Arab counterparts [7].

Fourth, indicators of lower socioeconomic status have been consistently associated with increased PTE risk, including lower household income [21], poverty status [25], lower parental education, and parental unemployment (e.g., [3, 13]). One conflicting finding was that, among a nationally representative sample of Icelandic youth, higher parental education was associated with events in which a child came close to being injured or killed, and higher maternal education was associated with increased risk for robbery or theft [6]. Children not living with both biological parents have also been found to be at increased risk for exposure across several investigations (e.g., [6, 22, 25]).

Finally, studies have documented regional differences in PTE risk (e.g. [10, 17]). The NCS-A found that living in an urban environment was associated with increased risk for physical abuse by a caregiver, and with reporting that a loved one had experienced a PTE, but lower risk for car accidents [22].

Other Exposures A few epidemiologic studies have explored the co-occurrence of different types of PTEs. For example, Finkelhor and Dziuba-Leatherman [17] reported that, with the exception of family assaults, each form of victimization was associated with an increased likelihood of having experienced another form of victimization and that children who had experienced violence to the genitals (e.g., via hitting or kicking) or attempted kidnapping were especially likely to have had experienced other victimization events. In a further longitudinal study, Finkelhor et al. [19] found that having experienced one form of victimization (e.g., physical assault) was associated with increased risk of experiencing the same form of victimization a year later. Furthermore, each form of victimization increased risk for experiencing other forms of victimization in the following year, such that, for example, physical assault was associated with increased risk of six other forms of victimization (e.g., sexual victimization, property crime), as well as *polyvictimization*, that is, the experience of multiple forms of victimization. The only exception to this pattern was that sexual victimization was not prospectively associated with increased risk for physical assault or peer/sibling victimization.

Mental Health Other epidemiologic research has explored mental health indices as prospective predictors of PTE exposure. For example, in the Great Smoky Mountain Study, which has followed a representative sample of children in Western North Carolina, having a history of depressive disorders was predictive of a child's first PTE exposure [23]. Depressive disorders were not associated with subsequent trauma exposure among a representative sample of adolescents in Munich, Germany, however, whereas anxiety disorders were predictive of any subsequent PTEs), and anxiety disorders, illicit drug dependence, and nicotine dependence was associated with increased risk for subsequent sexual and assaultive trauma, specifically [5]. Similarly, McLaughlin et al. [22] found variability in associations between four classes of preexisting disorders (behavior disorders, fear and distress disorders, substance use disorders, and bipolar disaster) and the 19 PTEs assessed in the NCS-A.

Family and Peer Relationships Researchers have also identified that a number of family problems, including familial alcohol and drug abuse, are associated with increased risk for PTE exposure (e.g., [30]) and for polyvictimization [18]. Conversely, in a study of Palestinian children living in the Gaza Strip, children who reported greater perceived support from their parents were less likely to have had experienced PTEs [31]. Although largely unexplored in the epidemiologic literature, peer relationships are also likely related to PTE exposure. For example, Finkelhor et al. [19] found that, among adolescents who have been polyvictimized at baseline, those who reported more good friends were less likely to have been polyvictimized in the following year.

Q: What factors increase and decrease risk for trauma exposure?

A: Research has shown that the risk for trauma exposure is not uniform across children. Girls are at greater risk of some events (e.g., sexual abuse and assault), whereas boys are at greater risk of others (e.g., experiences physical violence or threats thereof). Similarly, younger children are at increased risk of some events (e.g., physical abuse by a caregiver), whereas older children are at increased risk of others (e.g., death of a close friend). Children who are racial or ethnic minorities also seem to be at greater risk of some, but not all, potentially traumatic events. More consistently, children of lower socioeconomic status or who do not live with two biological parents are at heightened risk of exposure. Living in an urban environment also increases risk of some events (e.g., physical abuse by a caregiver), but decreases risk of others (e.g., car accidents). Other risk factors for trauma exposure include prior exposure to trauma, mental health problems (with psychiatric disorders acting as risk factors for some, but not all, forms of trauma), and family problems (e.g., familial alcohol and drug abuse). Conversely, support from parents and peers seem to protect against exposure.

Trauma- and Stressor-Related Disorders

Although trauma exposure is associated with a range of mental and behavioral health conditions, we define trauma- and stressor-related disorders in the current chapter as disorders in which trauma exposure is a diagnostic criterion, and, as such, all individuals diagnosed with the disorder will have been exposed to at least one PTE. Trauma- and stressor-related disorders under this definition include PTSD, acute stress disorder, bereavement-related disorder (BRD), reactive attachment disorder (RAD), and disinhibited social engagement disorder (DSED). Several epidemiologic studies have explored the prevalence and predictors of PTSD among children and adolescents. In contrast, very few studies have explored the other trauma- and stressor-related disorders, contributing to uncertainty about how many young people have these disorders and who might be at particular risk.

PTSD

Prevalence of PTSD Table 11.2 summarizes the methods and findings of studies focused on the prevalence of PTSD in nationally or regionally representative samples of children and adolescents worldwide, with some studies focused on high-risk samples such as disaster survivors (e.g., [40]) and refugees (e.g., [37]). Many, but not all, of these studies overlap with those exploring trauma exposure. Again, in addition to the United States, the studies include samples from East Asia (China: [32]), the Middle East (e.g., Israel: [7]; Lebanon: [35]), Europe (e.g., Iceland: [6]; Switzerland: [13]), as well as Mexico [10] and South Africa [11]. The youngest children sampled across these studies were 6-year-olds ([8]; [11]; [33]), and the oldest were in their early 20s (e.g., [38]; [37]). Again, studies focused on youth ages 18 and older were excluded from the review, and the prevalence of PTSD is listed for the full sample when available and subsamples if not.

As shown in Table 11.2, there was variation across the studies in the time period since the PTE for which participants were to report on symptoms, ranging from the prior 2 weeks [32] to one's lifetime (e.g., [3]). The most commonly reported timeframes were the past month, to discern a current PTSD diagnosis consistent with *DSM* criteria, and lifetime. The prevalence of past-month PTSD ranged from 0.1% among White male public school students ages 16–22 in South Carolina [24] to 34.1% among Palestinian children ages 12–16 living in East Jerusalem and the West Bank [4]. Lifetime prevalence of PTSD ranged from 1.3% among adolescents and young adults ages 14–24 in Munich, Germany, to 21.5% in the study of Cambodian refugees ages 13–25 living in Portland or Salt Lake City [37]. These minimum and maximum rates of PTSD, in combination with those on PTE, suggest the influence of risk status and population-level PTE exposure on PTSD prevalence.

No nationally representative studies within the United States have used a past-month timeframe. The National Survey of Adolescents (NSA) and NSA-Replication, both including adolescents aging 12–17, assessed PTSD in reference to a past 6 months' timeframe and documented prevalence rates of 5.0% and 3.9%, respectively [21, 36]. The NCS-A assessed lifetime PTSD and reported a prevalence of 4.7% [22].

In addition to the reference time period, four additional sources of variation that could influence prevalence rates are evident in comparing the NSA and NSA-R to the NCS-A, as well as in examining the full set of studies. First, studies differ in their "reference event," that is, the PTE in which participants are to connect, or "anchor," any PTSD symptoms. Some studies do not anchor PTSD symptoms to any event in particular (e.g., [36]), whereas others use a "worst" event method in which participants anchor their symptoms to the event they identify as having been most distressing or upsetting (e.g., [3, 22]), and still others have all participants utilize the same reference event such as a natural or human-made disaster (e.g., [32, 38]). It is possible that disaster survivors are experiencing more severe symptoms stemming from another PTE or that participants' self-reported "worst" events might

Table 11.2 Summary of epidemiology studies on the prevalence of post-traumatic stress disorder

Reference	Country	*N*; study description	Measure; classification system	PTSD prevalence; time period; reference event
[32]	China (regional and high-risk group)	3052; students ages 8–19 from the counties of Wenchuan and Maoxian, 2 areas most severely affected by the 2008 Wenchuan earthquake, survey 1-year post-earthquake	CPSS; *DSM-IV*	8.6%; past 2 weeks; Wenchuan earthquake
[2]	Cyprus (regional)	1645; elementary and high school students (ages unspecified) in rural, urban, and suburban areas	Posttraumatic Stress Questionnaire; classification system unspecified	"Serious or very serious" symptoms, 10.0%; timing unspecified; bullying victimization
[3]	Denmark (national)	390; eight graders ages 13–15	HTQ Part IV; *DSM-IV*	9.0%; lifetime; "worst" event
[4]	East Jerusalem/ West Bank (regional and high-risk group)	1000; Palestinian children ages 12–16 in East Jerusalem and the West Bank	SCID-IV PTSD module; *DSM-IV*	34.1%; past month; reference event unspecified
[33]	Gaza Strip (regional and high-risk group)	239; Palestinian children ages 6–11 in the Gaza Strip	CPTS-RI; *DSM-III-R*	72.8%, PTSD reactions of at least mild severity (31.8% mild, 35.6% moderate, 5.4% severe); timing unspecified; reference event unspecified
[31]	Gaza Strip (regional and high-risk group)	412; Palestinian children ages 12–16 in the Gaza Strip	SCID-IV PTSD module; *DSM-IV*	30.8%; past month; reference event unspecified
[34]; [5]	Germany (regional)	2548; Early Developmental Stages study; longitudinal study of adolescents and young adults ages 14–24 in Munich assessed at baseline and a 34–50-month follow-up	Munich-CIDI; *DSM-IV*	Baseline, 1.3% full PTSD, 5.6% either full or subthreshold PTSD; lifetime; "worst" event; follow-up, 5.0% either full or subthreshold PTSD; cumulative incidence; "worst" event

(continued)

Table 11.2 (continued)

Reference	Country	*N*; study description	Measure; classification system	PTSD prevalence; time period; reference event
[8]	Iraq (regional and high-risk group)	201; Kurdistanian children ages 6–18 living in Duhok City in Iraqi Kurdistan	PSS-C; *DSM-IV*	32.3%; timing unspecified; "worst" event
[7]	Israel (national)	4151; Jewish and Arab Israeli students ages 13–17	UCLA-RI; *DSM-IV*	6.9%; past month; reference event unspecified
[35]	Lebanon (regional)	386; children and adolescents (average age 11.5; maximum age 19) from South Lebanon and Southwest Bekaa assessed 3 weeks after war exposure (Phase 1); random subsample (n = 143) reassessed a year later (Phase 2)	DICA-R; *DSM-III-R*	Phase 1, 26.0%; Phase 2, 1.4%; past month; reference event unspecified
[9]	Lithuania (national)	183; adolescents ages 13–17	HTQ Part IV; *DSM-IV*	6.1%; lifetime; "worst" event
[10]	Mexico (regional)	3005; Mexican Adolescent Mental Health Survey; adolescents ages 12–17 in the Mexico City metropolitan area	CIDI; *DSM-IV*	1.8%; lifetime; "worst" event
[11]	South Africa (regional)	148; ethnically Northern Sotho children ages 6–10 from the rural community of Dikgale	CPTSDI; *DSM-III*	8.4%; timing unspecified; reference event unspecified
[12]	Sri Lanka (regional)	420; school children ages 10–14 from provinces affected by armed conflict	UCLA-RI; *DSM-IV*	23%; past month; reference event unspecified
[8]	Sweden (regional and high-risk group)	111; Kurdistanian children ages 6–18 living in the Uppsala City in Sweden	PSS-C; *DSM-IV*	11.0%; timing unspecified; "worst" event
[13]	Switzerland (national)	6787; 9th graders (97% ages 14.0–16.9)	UCLA-RI, adolescent version; *DSM-IV-TR*	4.2%; past month; reference event unspecified

(continued)

Table 11.2 (continued)

Reference	Country	*N*; study description	Measure; classification system	PTSD prevalence; time period; reference event
[22]	United States (national)	6483; National Comorbidity Survey-Adolescent Replication; adolescents ages 13–17	CIDI; *DSM-IV*	4.7%; lifetime; "worst" event
[21]	United States (national)	4023; National Survey of Adolescents; adolescents ages 12–17	Modified version of the National Women's Study PTSD module; *DSM-IV*	5.0%; past 6 months; reference event unspecified
[36]	United States (national)	3614; National Survey of Adolescents-Replication; adolescents ages 12–17 at baseline	PTSD module from the National Survey of Adolescents and National Women's Study; *DSM-IV*	3.9%; past 6 months; symptoms not anchored to a specific reference event
[23]	United States (regional)	1420; Great Smoky Mountains Study; children ages 9, 11, and 13 in Western North Carolina, followed until age 16	CAPA; *DSM-IV*	0.5%; past 3 months at age 16 assessment; "worst" event
[24]	United States (regional)	490; second wave of a longitudinal epidemiologic study of public school students in a South Carolina district; adolescents ages 16–22	Novel measure for study; *DSM-IV*	White boys, 0.1%; White girls, 3.5%; Black boys, 0.8%; Black girls, 2.9%; past month; reference event unspecified
[37]	United States (regional and high-risk group)	209; Cambodian refugees ages 13–25 living in either Portland, OR, or Salt Lake City, UT	K-SADS-E; *DSM-III-R*	21.5% , lifetime; and 18.2%, current; reference event unspecified
[38]	United States (regional and high-risk group)	8236 New York City public school students ages 9–21 sampled 6 months after the September 11, 2011, World Trade Center (WTC) attacks	DPS; *DSM-IV*	10.6%; current; WTC attacks (as specified in [39])

(continued)

Table 11.2 (continued)

Reference	Country	*N*; study description	Measure; classification system	PTSD prevalence; time period; reference event
[40]	United States (regional and high-risk group)	2000; adolescents ages 12–17 areas affected by the 2011 tornados in Alabama and Joplin, Missouri sampled approximately 4–5 to 13–14 months post-tornado	PTSD module from the National Survey of Adolescents and other large-scale epidemiologic studies; *DSM-IV*	6.7%; since the tornado; reference event unspecified

Note. *CAPA* child and adolescent psychiatric assessment, *CIDI* composite international diagnostic interview, *CPSS* child PTSD symptom scale, *CPTS-RI* child post-traumatic stress reaction index, *CPTSDI* children's PTSD inventory, *DICA-R* diagnostic interview for children and adolescents revised, *DPS* diagnostic interview schedule for children predictive scales, *HTQ* Harvard trauma questionnaire, *K-SADS-E* schedule of affective disorders and schizophrenia for school-age children-epidemiologic version, *PSS-C* posttraumatic stress symptoms for children, *PTSD* post-traumatic stress disorder, *SCID-IV* structured clinical interview for DSM-IV, *UCLA-RI* UCLA PTSD reaction index

not be the source of their PTSD symptomatology, thereby leading to underestimated prevalence rates. Second, several measures were used to classify participants as having probable PTSD across studies, and variability in the sensitivity and specificity of these measures could be a further source of variation in prevalence rates. Third, and relatedly, classification systems used to determine PTSD caseness across studies range from *DSM-III* (e.g., [11]) to *DSM-IV-TR* (e.g., [13]), further limiting cross-study comparisons (for a historical review of PTSD in the *DSM*, see Friedman [41]). None of the studies reviewed assessed for *DSM-5* PTSD, although two notable studies of adolescent and young adult disaster survivors have reported marked consistency between *DSM-5* and *DSM-IV-TR* PTSD cases [42, 43]. Finally, in the majority of studies, assessment of PTSD symptoms is contingent upon a child reporting one or more PTEs, and, as such, PTSD prevalence is inherently tied to the number of PTEs assessed.

Q: How common is PTSD among children in the United States and elsewhere?

A: The prevalence of PTSD among children in the United States and elsewhere varies substantially across studies including nationally and regionally representative samples. In the United States, a nationally representative study of children ages 13–17 found a lifetime PTSD prevalence of 4.7%. Two nationally representative studies of children ages 12–17 found that 3.9% and 5.0% of participants had suffered from PTSD in the past month. It is important to note that no epidemiologic studies to date have assessed PTSD as defined in the most recent version of the DSM (DSM-5), and therefore further research is needed.

Predictors of PTSD The same categories of factors that were explored as predictors of PTEs have also been included in epidemiologic studies predicting

PTSD. While of the trends for PTEs and PTSD are consistent, there are some notable exceptions, including gender differences.

Demographics A relatively consistent pattern in the literature is that girls are at greater risk for PTSD than boys, a finding that has been demonstrated both among general population samples (e.g., [13]; [22]; [7]), and among child and adolescent survivors of disasters (e.g., [40]; [38]). Inconsistent with this pattern, boys were at increased risk of PTSD relative to girls in a nationally representative sample of fourth graders in Taiwan and among Palestinian adolescents living in East Jerusalem and the West Bank [4]. Similarly, whereas several studies have found older children, or children who experience PTEs later in childhood, to be at greater risk for PTSD (e.g., [23]; [44]), others have found younger children to be at greater risk [45], particularly for hyperarousal symptoms ([9]; [3]).

No studies to our knowledge have shown race or ethnic minority status to be predictive of PTSD in the United States. The NCS-A found that children who were born in the United States versus elsewhere were less likely to recovery from PTSD [22]. Additionally, Arab students in Israel were at increased risk, relative to their Jewish counterparts [7]. Finally, in the study of Palestinian children living in the Gaza Strip, those residing north of Gaza City, which the investigators argue is proxy for refugee status, were at higher risk [33]. This finding is consistent with the particularly high prevalence of PTSD among Cambodian refugees in the United States reported previously [37].

Various markers of low socioeconomic status have been associated with increased risk of PTSD onset, including low parental education, living in a single-parent household, financial hardship, and receipt of government assistance [4, 8, 9, 31], as well as PTSD non-recovery [22].

Trauma Exposure Characteristics Various factors related to trauma exposure have been associated with risk for PTSD. First, exposure to PTEs prior to the reference event increases risk for PTSD (e.g., [23]; [22]); for example, adolescent disaster survivors who had experienced a pre-disaster PTE were more likely to experience disaster-related PTSD [40]. Similarly, having experienced PTEs since the reference event is associated with increased risk for PTSD and PTSD non-recovery (e.g., [9]; [22]).

Other epidemiologic research has investigated which PTEs are associated with the highest conditional risk for developing PTSD, and consistently the PTEs with the highest risk are those involving interpersonal violence, including sexual assault, rape, physical assault, and child physical abuse (e.g., [3, 9, 23]). Among child and adolescent survivors of the same reference event, those with more severe exposure or whose exposure was followed by greater life disruption have been found to be at greater risk, for example, earthquake survivors who experienced bereavement or who had to relocate post-disaster [32] and children in New York City who lost a friend or loved one in the September 11 terrorist attacks [45] or whose parents had lost their job in the aftermath of the attacks [39]. Among adolescent survivors of sexual assault in the NSA, those who were injured during the event or whose perpetrator was a family member, acquaintance, or recognized non-acquaintance (versus a stranger) were at increased risk [46, 47].

Finally, a consistent finding is that children and adolescents who have experienced a higher number of PTEs are at increased risk for PTSD, whether symptoms were reported in reference to their "worst" event or not (e.g., [9, 13, 48]).

Mental Health A few epidemiologic studies have documented that children with preexisting mental health conditions, including fear and distress disorders, substance use disorders, and bipolar disorder are at increased risk of PTSD following PTE exposure (e.g., [35]; [22]). Other studies have shown PTSD to be comorbid with a range of conditions, such as depression, suicidality, somatic symptoms, separation anxiety, substance use, attention deficit hyperactivity disorder (ADHD), and conduct problems, although patterns of comorbidity have varied across investigations (e.g., [40]; [23]).

Family Factors As for PTEs, family factors have been shown to be both risk and protective factors for PTSD. On the one hand, mental health symptoms in family members, including anxiety, PTSD symptoms, and alcohol problems, have been associated with increased risk ([44]; [4]; [37]). On the other, youth who report better relationships with their parents and more parental support were protected against PTSD ([16]; [31]).

Q: Other than trauma exposure, what factors put children at risk of PTSD? What factors might protect trauma-exposed children from suffering from PTSD?

A: Consistent risk factors for PTSD are female sex, low socioeconomic status, prior trauma exposure, exposure to multiple or more severe traumatic events, preexisting or co-occurring mental health problems, and family mental health problems. Some traumatic events, versus others, are also associated with greater risk, including events involving interpersonal violence, such as sexual assault, rape, physical assault, and physical abuse by a caretaker. Age has been inconsistently associated with PTSD, with some studies showing older children to be at greater risk and others showing younger children to be at greater risk. Younger children seem to be more likely than their older counterparts to suffer from symptoms of hyperarousal, including exaggerated startle responses, poor concentration, and sleep disturbances. Higher quality and more supportive relationships with parents are protective against PTSD. Again, it is important to note that epidemiologic research today is based on previous version of the DSM and further studies are needed that use PTSD as defined in the DSM-5.

Acute Stress Disorder

Relative to PTSD, the epidemiologic literature has provided less information about the prevalence and predictors of acute stress disorder, likely due to the temporal nature of the disorder, that is, that it can only occur within the first month of trauma exposure. As discussed elsewhere [49], several challenges face researchers seeking to understand acute stress disorder among representative samples, including the likelihood that only a few participants would have experienced a traumatic event during the prior month in general population samples, potential retrospective bias in having trauma-exposed participants report on their initial post-trauma symptoms, and difficulty securing funding and resources to assess a representative sample of survivors of the same mass traumatic event (i.e., an event that affects members of an entire community).

An alternative approach to examining acute stress disorder is to assess consecutively admitted patients in the aftermath of a mass traumatic event. Notably, this approach does not capture representative samples, as survivors who present to the hospital are likely to have faced higher levels of exposure than those who do not, but does allow for explorations of the prevalence and predictors of acute stress disorder symptoms in the population of hospital admits. Liu et al. [50] conducted a study using this approach in the aftermath of the Wenchuan earthquake. Participants ($N = 118$) were consecutive admissions ages 5–18 at a local pediatric surgery department, and, among them, 54.3% screened positive for acute stress disorder. Prevalence estimates were significantly higher among girls versus boys. In a multivariable model, indicators of more severe exposure and injuries (whether the participant was buried in the earthquake, whether the participant had a parent or relatives who was injured or killed during the earthquake, and whether the participants' injuries necessitated amputation or operation) were associated with more severe acute stress disorder symptoms.

Other researchers have drawn on consecutive hospital admissions in a normative context—that is, not in the aftermath of a mass traumatic event—to estimate the prevalence and predictors of acute stress disorder. Again, such studies are not representative of all trauma survivors, including survivors of trauma-related injuries that do not require immediate care and survivors of PTEs that generally do not result in injuries (e.g., bereavement, witnessing violence), but nonetheless provide insight into this topic. At least studies to our knowledge have taken this approach. First, Kassam-Adams and Winston [51] drew on a cohort of children, ages 8–17, who were hospital at a level I pediatric trauma center for injuries sustained as a pedestrian, bicyclist, or motor vehicle passenger. Among this sample, 8% met criteria for acute stress disorder and 14% for subsyndromal acute stress disorder. Age was a significant predictor of acute stress disorder status, such that children ages 8–11 were significantly more likely to meet criteria for either full or subsyndromal acute stress disorder than those ages 12–17. Second, a study of consecutive admissions of children ages 5–16 to an accident and emergency department found that, depending on the criteria used, 11–15% suffered from probable acute stress disorder [52]. Third, among children ages 7–13 consecutively admitted to a major trauma hospital, 10% met criteria for full and 18% for subsyndromal acute stress disorder [53]. Notably, two of these studies found in longitudinal analyses that subsyndromal acute stress disorder was a better predictor of subsequent PTSD than full ASD [51, 53].

Bereavement-Related Disorder

Bereavement-related disorder (BRD) was introduced to the DSM-5 based on literature exploring how normal grief after the death of a loved one becomes pathological, including research on complicated grief (CG). No epidemiologic studies to our knowledge have explored the prevalence and predictors of BRD, and none focused on CG among children and adolescents specifically. A population-based study of persons aged 14–95 in Germany found the prevalence of CG to be 3.7% in the full sample, 6.7% among bereaved participants, and 4.4% among bereaved participants ages 14–20 [54]. Risk factors for developing CG included female gender, cancer as the cause of death, being age 61 or older, and having lost a child or spouse. Relative bereaved participants ages 61 and older, those ages 14–20 had .28 the odds reporting CG.

Reactive Attachment Disorder and Disinhibited Social Engagement Disorder

The distinction between reactive attachment disorder (RAD) and disinhibited social engagement disorder (DSED) is also new to the DSM-5, and no epidemiologic studies to our knowledge have explored their prevalence as currently defined or the prevalence of RAD in prior versions of the DSM. Three epidemiologic studies, however, have explored the phenomenology of these disorders using factor analytic methods.

First, Kay and Green [55] assessed RAD and DSED symptoms among sequential referrals of youth ages 10–16 at risk of multiple breakdowns of out-of-home care placements in England. Using the Development and Well-Being Assessment-Reactive Attachment Disorder (DAWBA-RAD), the investigators used exploratory factor analysis (EFA) and found support for a model consisting of four factors: (1) disinhibited indiscriminate, (2) attention seeking, (3) superficial relationships, and (4) unpredictability. Caseness for total symptoms and each factor subscale were defined as being greater than two standard deviations above the mean for a low-risk comparison group of low socioeconomic youth who had never been in out-of-home care. Over half (63%) of participants met this criterion for total RAD symptoms, 58% for disinhibited indiscriminate, 52% for attention seeking, 56% for superficial relationships, and 20% for unpredictability. Several predictors of total scale and factor subscale were explored, and significant associations included higher total scores and superficial relationships factor scores among children with earlier entry into out-of-home care; history of multiple maltreatments with higher attention-seeking factor scores; antisocial behavior and alcohol and substance misuse with superficial relationships factor scores; emotional problems with superficial relationships and attention-seeking factor scores; attention and overactivity and self-harm and suicide with attention-seeking factor scores; and peer relationship problems with disinhibited indiscriminate factor scores.

A study of all Norwegian children ages 6–10 in long-term foster care also used the DAWBA-RAD but, unlike the prior study, used a confirmatory factor analytic approach that provided support for a two-factor model with RAD symptom loading on one factor and DSED symptoms loading on the other [56]. Descriptively, the sample reported higher DSED symptoms than RAD symptoms, indicating that the latter are less common in this population. RAD and DSED factors were significantly and positively correlated, and both were associated with functional impairment and help-seeking behaviors.

Finally, a study of all internationally adopted children ages 6–15 in Finland used EFA on a different measure of attachment behaviors—the Disturbances of Attachment Interview—and found support for a three-factor model consisting of disinhibited, inhibited, and "clingy" behaviors [57]. After establishing this model, the investigators categorized participants into those with disinhibited symptoms only (19%), inhibited symptoms only (18%), mixed symptoms (25%), and no symptoms (41%). Relative to those with no symptoms, participants in all other groups reported significantly higher internalizing, externalizing and ADHD symptoms, with the highest levels observed in the mixed symptom group.

Taken together, the results of these three studies suggest that RAD and DSED symptoms are elevated among children in foster care relative to children of similar socioeconomic status, that RAD and DSED symptoms are distinct from each other but highly correlated, and that they also co-occur with symptoms of other psychiatric disorders. The extant research, however, does not provide information about the prevalence of these disorders, as no study to our knowledge has employed DSM-5 criteria to identify probable cases. Likewise, none of the reviewed studies assessed children's PTE exposure and therefore it is unknown what percentage of children with RAD and DSED symptoms have experienced trauma.

Q: Do children who have experienced trauma suffer from other disorders, such as RAD? How common are these disorders, and what are risk factors for them?

A: Yes, children who have experienced trauma can have acute stress disorder, a condition with symptoms similar to PTSD, but that is diagnosed only in the first month after a traumatic event. Although no studies have explored the prevalence among children in representative samples, studies drawing on data from consecutively admitted to the hospital following a traumatic event have found prevalence rates ranging from 8% to over 50%, and female gender, younger age, and more severe trauma exposure have been identified as risk factors. Another disorder that can specifically follow the trauma of bereavement is bereavement-related disorder (BRD). Although no studies have explored the prevalence of BRD, one study explored a similar construct, complicated grief (CG), and found its prevalence to be 4.4% among bereaved youth ages 14–20. No known studies have explored predictors of BRD or CG among children and adolescents using representative samples. Finally, it is presumed that childhood trauma (e.g., physical abuse, neglect) can lead to reactive attachment disorder (RAD) and disinhibited social engagement disorder (DSED), two outcomes that are distinct yet have been found to co-occur both with each other and other mental health conditions. No known studies have documented the prevalence and predictors of RAD and DSED as defined in the DSM-5.

Neurodevelopmental Disorders Often Confused with Trauma-Related Disorders

Other disorders diagnosed in childhood share some similarities with trauma and stressor-related disorders, although the causes and treatments for such conditions vary substantially. As noted in other chapters, differential diagnosis can be somewhat challenging, especially because there is significant comorbidity between trauma and stressor-related disorders and neurodevelopmental disorders. Below, we review the prevalence of neurodevelopmental disorders, with particular attention to attention deficit hyperactivity disorder (ADHD) and autism spectrum disorder (ASD), as well as the comorbidity between neurodevelopmental disorders and trauma- and stressor-related disorders.

Attention Deficit Hyperactivity Disorder

Symptoms of ADHD and PTSD are both characterized by difficulties concentrating and with impulsivity and irritability. Unlike PTSD, however, the symptoms of ADHD must be persistent across settings; however, this diagnostic criterion is not consistently applied (e.g., [58]), which can complicate differential diagnosis. Meta-analyses of studies of non-referred children suggest that the worldwide prevalence of ADHD in childhood/adolescence ranges from 5.3% to 7.1% depending on the source of information (e.g., parent/teacher/child; [59, 60]). These meta-analyses have included data from representative samples as well as from convenience samples drawn from schools and communities. As described in the paragraphs below, there is significant heterogeneity in these prevalence estimates that can be attributed to a number of methodological differences across studies.

Table 11.3 presents the results of 12 studies using representative samples of children and adolescents to report on the prevalence of *DSM-IV* ADHD. In the United States, current prevalence of ADHD among 6–17-year-olds is 8.2% [67], 12-month prevalence of ADHD among 8–15-year-olds is 8.6% [71], and lifetime prevalence of ADHD among 13–18-year-olds is 8.7% [70]. Among 4-year-olds, past 3-month prevalence rates are 8.8% when impairment is required for the diagnosis [68]. Internationally, rates of ADHD vary such that representative samples from Germany have yielded a prevalence estimate of 4.8–5.0% [63, 66], while data from Brazil, Australia, Taiwan, and Puerto Rico suggest that the prevalence of ADHD is approximately 7.5% [61, 64, 65, 72]. The lone study from Qatar found a slightly higher current prevalence rate of 9.4% [62]; this study is also the only study in the table that relied solely on teacher reports, which may yield higher prevalence rates than either parent or child/adolescent reports alone (for a review, see [73]).

Although the studies presented in Table 11.3 use *DSM-IV* definitions of ADHD, numerous studies have used *DSM-III* and *DSM-III-R* criteria (for review of these studies, see [73]). Studies show significant variability in prevalence based on the

Table 11.3 Summary of epidemiology studies on the prevalence of attention deficit hyperactivity disorder

Reference	Country	N; study description	Classification system; instrument	Reporter	ADHD prevalence (time period)
[61]	Puerto Rico	1896; 4–17 year old children	DSM-IV; interview	Parent and youth	7.5% (12 month)
[62]	Qatar	1541; 6–12 year old children recruited from primary schools	DSM-IV; Conners	Teacher	9.4% (current)
[63]	Germany	2452; 7–17 year old children/ adolescents	DSM-IV; symptom checklist	Parent	5.0% (current)
[64]	Taiwan	1070; 7th grade students	DSM-IV; interview and symptom checklist	Adolescent and teacher	7.5% (3 month)
[65]	Australia	3597; 6–17 year old children/ adolescents	DSM-IV; interview	Parent	7.5% (12 month)
[66]	Germany	17,461; 3–17 year old children/ adolescents	DSM-IV; report of medical diagnosis	Parent	4.8% (lifetime)
[67]	United States	61,779 6–17 year old children	DSM-IV; report of medical diagnosis	Parent	8.2% (current)
[68]	United States	796; 4 year old children recruited from schools and primary care	DSM-IV; interview and questionnaire	Parent	8.8% (3 month) w/ impairment
[69]	France	1012; 6–12 year old children from a household sample	DSM-IV; interview	Parent	3.5% (current)
[70]	United States	10,123; 13–18 year old adolescents	DSM-IV; interview	Parent and adolescent	8.7% (lifetime)
[71]	United States	3042; 8–15 year old children/ adolescents	DSM-IV; interview	Parent	8.6% (12 month)
[72]	Brazil	485; 14–17 year old adolescents from representative household sample	DSM-IV; self-report screener	Adolescent	7.6% (12 month)

diagnostic classification system (e.g., *DSM-IV* vs. *DSM-IIIR*) employed [59]. Specifically, lower prevalence estimates have been obtained for studies using *DSM-III-R* or ICD-10 criteria relative to those using *DSM-IV* criteria [59, 73, 74].

There also is significant variability in prevalence based on source of information (e.g., parent/teacher/patient report), type of assessment (interview vs. rating scale), and algorithm for determining diagnosis including whether or not impairment is required. In a meta-analysis of 86 studies of children and adolescents that used *DSM-IV* criteria only, prevalence estimates ranged from 5.9 to 7.1% depending on the source of information [60]. Some studies have asked parents whether a doctor or medical professional ever diagnosed their child with ADHD (e.g., [66, 67]), while others have asked for parent, teacher, and adolescent to report on current symptoms and calculated prevalence based on various rules (e.g., all reporters must indicate symptoms vs. only one reporter must indicate symptoms) (e.g., [64, 70, 71]). Finally, studies have varied in whether they have required impairment to be present for a diagnosis. Specifically, studies that do not require impairment have been shown to yield higher prevalence estimates compared to studies that do require impairment (for review, see [74]).

Country/region of assessment has been associated with significant variability in ADHD prevalence in non-referred children and adolescents [59]. Lower prevalence of ADHD has been found in Africa and the Middle East compared to North America [59]. Another review concluded that Iceland, Australia, Italy, and Sweden may have lower prevalence of ADHD than the United States, while Columbia, Brazil, Germany, and Ukraine may have somewhat higher prevalence of ADHD compared to the United States [60]. In the only study that directly compared international children to an age-matched sample of US children, Ukrainian children evacuated from Chernobyl had significantly higher prevalence of ADHD relative to US children (19.8% vs. 9.7%; [75]). The authors hypothesized that the environmental adversity and trauma of dislocation may have been associated with the higher prevalence rates [75]. The majority of more recent meta-analyses suggest that there are few, if any, cross-national differences in ADHD prevalence after accounting for methodological differences such as source of information, diagnostic criterion, and impairment requirement, between studies [60, 74].

Predictors of ADHD Demographic characteristics such as gender and age have been differentially associated with ADHD prevalence. Meta-analyses indicate a significantly higher pooled prevalence of ADHD for boy compared to girls (10% vs. 4%) and a higher pooled prevalence for children compared to adolescents (7% vs. 3%; [59]). At least one study has found that Hispanic children are less likely than White children to meet criteria for ADHD [67], and one review concluded that African-American children had more ADHD symptoms but were diagnosed with ADHD less frequently than White children even after controlling for socioeconomic status [76]. The authors suggested that parental knowledge and beliefs about ADHD and treatment for ADHD may partially explain this discrepancy; however, they also noted that ADHD instruments might not adequately capture ADHD symptoms in African-American youth [76]. Multiple studies have found that children from lower-income families are more likely to meet criteria for ADHD compared to children from higher-income families [61, 67, 77]. One prospective longitudinal study using a cohort of 811,803 children born in Sweden between 1992 and 2000 found that youth exposed to lower income in early childhood were at increased risk for developing ADHD [78].

Other correlates of ADHD include parental history of ADHD [24, 61], and twin and family studies indicate ADHD has a heritability estimate of 0.76 [79]. One of the candidate genes (i.e., the cannabinoid receptor CNR1) that has been explored in relation to ADHD has also been implicated in risk for PTSD [80]. Twin studies also indicate that parental alcohol dependence and maternal heavy drinking during pregnancy are associated with increased risk for childhood ADHD in girls [81], and nonrepresentative studies have linked exposure to adversity, including childhood abuse, to risk for ADHD [82, 83].

Autism Spectrum Disorder

Autism spectrum disorder (ASD) is characterized by deficits in social communication and social interaction as well as restricted repetitive behaviors, interests, and activities. PTSD can manifest in social withdrawal and/or repetition of the trauma that could mimic ASD symptoms and complicate differential diagnosis in children. Representative studies on the prevalence of ASD are presented in Table 11.4 and suggest that 0.6–2.0% of children and adolescents meet criteria for ASD, depending on the type of assessment (records review vs. screener and interview) and timeframe. Analyzing 5 years of CDC data on the prevalence of ASD, Blumberg and colleagues documented an increase in parent report of ASD from 1.16% in 2007 to 2.0% in 2011–2012 [84]. For reviews on the prevalence of specific forms of ASD, such as pervasive developmental disorders, see Faraone et al. [73].

Predictors of ASD Several demographic characteristics have been associated with ASD. For example, boys are more likely than girls to be diagnosed with ASD [84].

Table 11.4 Summary of epidemiology studies on the prevalence of autism spectrum disorder

Reference	Country	*N*; study description	Classification system; instrument	Reporter	ASD prevalence (time period)
[85]	UK	3373; 5–9 year old school children	DSM-IV; screener and interview	Parent	1.6% (current)
[84]	United States	65,556; 6–17 year old children	DSM-IV; report of medical diagnosis	Parent	2.0% (current)
[86]	United States	337,093; 8 year old children	DSM-IV; records review	N/A	1.1% (lifetime)
[87]	South Korea	55,266; 7–12 year old children	DSM-IV; screener and interview	Parent	1.9% (lifetime)
[88]	United States	78,037; 3–17 year old children	DSM-IV; report of medical diagnosis	Parent	1.1% (current)
[89]	England	14,062; children followed from birth to 11	DSM-IV; records review	N/A	0.6% (lifetime)

Some studies have found higher rates of autism is Hispanic children whose parents were both born in the United States compared to Hispanic children whose parents were both foreign-born [90]. Additionally, there appear to be racial differences in the age of autism diagnosis, with White children being diagnosed at a younger age relative to Black children (6.3 years vs. 7.9 years; [91]). Interestingly, higher socio-economic status (indexed by higher maternal education and higher median family income) has been associated with a higher prevalence of ASD, which may reflect increased awareness of the syndrome and greater resources available to engagement in the assessment process for ASD [92].

Several studies suggest a link between childhood adversity and ASD, although the directionality of these relationships is not entirely clear. In a representative sample, 46% of children with an ASD had experienced peer bullying [93]. In a nonrepresentative clinical sample of children with ASD, a significant proportion (26%) of patients had a trauma history, and 17% of the sample also met criteria for PTSD [94].

Q: What is the prevalence of neurodevelopmental disorders that might "look" similar to trauma-related disorders, but do not include trauma exposure in their diagnostic criteria?

A: Attention deficit hyperactivity disorder, which shares symptoms of impulsivity, irritability, and difficulties concentrating, with PTSD has a prevalence of 5.3–7.1% in non-referred samples and a prevalence of approximately 8% in representative samples of US children and adolescents, although the assessment timeframe, source of information, and age ranges assessed vary significantly. Autism spectrum disorders, which may share symptoms of social deficits and repetitive behaviors, have a prevalence of 0.6–2.0% in representative samples.

Q: What are the risk factors for these neurodevelopmental disorders?

A: Unlike PTSD, males are more likely to meet criteria for both ADHD and ASD. Race has been inconsistently linked with prevalence of ADHD and ASD, but as many studies rely on parent reports of a medical diagnosis, discrepancies may actually reflect racial disparities in screening, assessment, and treatment rather than true prevalence differences. Children and adolescents with ADHD and ASD also are more likely to have experienced childhood adversity, including maltreatment or abuse when compared to children without these conditions, and there are some indications that there may be shared genetic susceptibility for ADHD and PTSD.

Comorbidity of Trauma-Related Disorders and Neurodevelopmental Disorders

Data from representative samples reveal that PTSD and trauma-related disorders are highly comorbid with other internalizing and externalizing conditions [23, 95, 96]. In a representative national sample of adolescents in the United States, 47% and

30% of boys with PTSD also met criteria for a major depressive episode and substance abuse/dependence, respectively, while 71% and 24% of girls with PTSD also met criteria for a major depressive episode and substance abuse/dependence, respectively [96]. In a representative sample of youth from the Southwestern United States, children with subclinical symptoms of PTSD had significantly higher rates of comorbidity compared to children with fewer symptoms [23]. Indeed, 43% and 37% of children with PTSD symptoms met criteria for any anxiety or depressive disorder, respectively [23]. Furthermore, 13% of children with PTSD symptoms met criteria for a separation anxiety disorder, and 10% of children with PTSD also met criteria for ADHD [23]. In a random sample of detained youth, 93% of those with PTSD had at least one other comorbid disorder; substance use disorders were most common (79%), followed by ADHD and behavioral disorders (43%), and anxiety disorders (38%) [95].

Data from representative samples also reveal that ADHD is highly comorbid with a wide range of disorders including learning disorders, conduct disorder, anxiety, depression, and ASD [61, 67, 70]. Representative studies have typically focused on comorbidity between ADHD and particular classes of disorders, rather than individual disorders like PTSD. For example, in a representative sample from the United States, 17.8% of children with ADHD also met criteria for an anxiety disorder, 13.9% also met criteria for depression, and 6.0% also met criteria for ASD [67]. In a representative sample from Puerto Rico, 24.4% of children with ADHD met criteria for an anxiety disorder, and 9.3% met criteria for any depressive disorder [61]. In the NCS-A, ADHD and PTSD were both measured, but comorbidity was reported according to disorder class rather than by individual disorder; findings indicated that 20% of the sample met criteria for at least two classes of disorders [70].

Data from representative samples also indicate that ASD is highly comorbid with a wide variety of other disorders. In a subsample of children from a population-derived cohort, 70% of those with ASD had at least one other past 3-month diagnosis and 41% had two or more other diagnoses; the most common comorbid conditions were social anxiety disorder, ADHD, and oppositional defiant disorder [97].

Q: Are PTSD and neurodevelopmental disorders ever comorbid?

A: Epidemiologic data indicate that PTSD is highly comorbid with anxiety, depression, and substance use disorders, and a substantial minority of youth with PTSD (~10%) also meet criteria for ADHD or an attachment disorder. Few, if any, epidemiologic studies have specifically examined comorbidity between PTSD and ASD in youth despite high rates of bullying and peer victimization among children with ASD.

Prevention of Trauma Exposure and PTSD in Children

To reduce the incidence and prevalence of trauma-related disorders, primary, secondary, and tertiary prevention programs need to be more widely implemented. Primary prevention of trauma exposure such as child abuse in children could involve

(1) media campaigns designed to increase awareness of the prevalence and impact of childhood adversity and change the cultural acceptance of violence against children; (2) making information including crisis and referral services more widely available; (3) increasing social networks at the community and neighborhood levels; (4) enhancing competency within families by increasing parenting and coping skills; and (5) providing therapeutic intervention for high-risk groups (e.g., low socioeconomic families, single parents, and those who have experienced complicated pregnancies) [98].

Secondary prevention of trauma exposure in children could involve encouraging members of the public to identify signs of trauma and intervene to mitigate risk. For example, mandated reporter laws require child health, primary care, mental health, school, social service, and law-enforcement professionals to be aware of the signs of child abuse and neglect and to report suspected incidents to local authorities for investigation; however, there are significant discrepancies in the proportion of substantiated abuse and neglect cases and the prevalence of abuse and neglect reported to authorities, suggesting that majority of abuse cases are not reported [99]. Secondary prevention of psychiatric outcomes, including PTSD and related disorders, could involve identifying children who had already experienced trauma and delivering an early intervention to prevent the onset of symptoms. For example, information provision web-based early interventions for children and parents following pediatric accidents and unintentional injury have been associated with reduced anxiety and PTSD symptoms over a 6-month follow-up compared to children in a control condition [100, 101]. However, not all secondary prevention efforts have proven effective at reducing PTSD symptoms: a two-session brief intervention for hospitalized injured children at risk for developing PTSD was not associated with a reduction in PTSD over follow-up [51].

Tertiary prevention programs could focus on reducing risk for re-traumatization or new onset of psychiatric difficulties among children who had already been exposed to trauma or developed trauma-related psychiatric symptoms. For example, treatment approaches for trauma-related disorders such as trauma-focused cognitive behavioral therapy typically focus the final sessions on preventing revictimization and the re-emergence or worsening of symptoms (e.g., [102]).

Q: What can society do to prevent to prevent the occurrence and persistence of PTSD and these other disorders?

A: Primary, secondary, and tertiary prevention efforts are all important in reducing risk for initial and subsequent trauma exposure and mitigating risk for the onset of psychopathology in the event that exposure does occur. Media campaigns and providing parent support to at risk families are examples of important primary prevention approaches, while brief interventions following trauma exposure and trainings to prevent revictimization are examples of secondary and tertiary prevention approaches, respectively.

Conclusion

In this chapter, we have examined trauma exposure and trauma-related and neurodevelopmental disorders from a public health perspective, focusing primary on epidemiologic studies exploring the prevalence and predictors of these conditions, as well as comorbidities between them, with the goal of helping clinicians address questions that clients might have about such issues. The extant research suggests that a significant proportion of children and adolescents have been exposed to trauma, and a substantial minority develops trauma-related sequelae, including PTSD, acute stress disorder, BRD, RAD, and DSED. Neurodevelopmental disorders, such as ADHD and ASD, share some symptoms with PTSD and are somewhat more common in youth exposed to trauma. PTSD and ADHD appear to be highly comorbid, whereas the comorbidity between PTSD and ASD, as well as between other trauma-related disorders and neurodevelopmental disorders, has been largely unexplored.

In reviewing the literature, we have also highlighted some of the methodological issues that make provision of information regarding the prevalence and predictors of trauma and trauma-related and neurodevelopmental disorders difficult. These include variation in the diagnostic systems and instruments to measure conditions, the person who is reporting on the child's symptoms, and the time period in which study participants report on symptoms and highlight the need for additional epidemiologic research using consistent methodology. Nonetheless, we have aimed to provide a useful summary of the extant literature.

Finally, we have noted examples of primary, secondary, and tertiary prevention programs that would reduce the likelihood that children are exposed to traumatic life events and that they develop mental health conditions in their aftermath. Further research that sheds additional light on the extent to which children experience traumatic events and suffer from trauma-related and neurodevelopmental disorders, as well as on the factors the increase children's risk, will undoubtedly refine such prevention efforts.

References

1. Zhu Y, Chan KL. Prevalence and correlates of school bullying victimization in Xi'an, China. Violence Vict. 2015;30:714–32. https://doi.org/10.1891/0886-6708.VV-D-14-00006.
2. Papacosta ES, Paradeisioti A, Lazarou C. Bullying phenomenon and preventive programs in Cyprus's school system. Int J Ment Health Promot. 2014;16:67–80. https://doi.org/10.1080/14623730.2014.888894.
3. Elklit A. Victimization and PTSD in a Danish national youth probability sample. J Am Acad Child Adolesc Psychiatry. 2002;41:174–81. https://doi.org/10.1097/00004583-200202000-00011.
4. Khamis V. Post-traumatic stress disorder among school age Palestinian children. Child Abuse Negl. 2005;29:81–95. https://doi.org/10.1016/j.chiabu.2004.06.013.
5. Stein MB, Höfler M, Perkonigg A, Lieb R, Pfister H, Maercker A, Wittchen H. Patterns of incidence and psychiatric risk factors for traumatic events. Int J Methods Psychiatr Res. 2002;11:143–53. https://doi.org/10.1002/mpr.132.

6. Bödvarsdóttir Í, Elklit A. Victimization and PTSD-like states in an Icelandic youth probability sample. BMC Psychiatry. 2007;7:51. https://doi.org/10.1186/1471-244X-7-51.
7. Schiff M, Pat-Horenczyk R, Benbenishty R, Brom D, Baum N, Astor RA. High school students' posttraumatic symptoms, substance abuse and involvement in violence in the aftermath of war. Soc Sci Med. 2012;75:1321–8. https://doi.org/10.1016/j.socscimed.2012.05.010.
8. Ahmad A, von Knorring A, Sundelin-Wahlsten V. Traumatic experiences and post-traumatic stress disorder in Kurdistanian children and their parents in homeland and exile: an epidemiological approach. Nord J Psychiatry. 2008;62:457–63. https://doi.org/10.1080/08039480801984305.
9. Domanskaitė-Gota V, Elklit A, Christiansen DM. Victimization and PTSD in a Lithuanian national youth probability sample. Nord Psychol. 2009;61:66–81. https://doi.org/10.1027/1901-2276.61.3.66.
10. Orozco R, Borges G, Benjet C, Medina-Mora ME, Lopez-Carillo L. Traumatic life events and posttraumatic stress disorder among Mexican adolescents: results from a survey. Salud Publica Mex. 2008;50:S29–37. https://doi.org/10.1590/s0036-36342008000700006.
11. Peltzer K. Posttraumatic stress symptoms in a population of rural children in South Africa. Psychol Rep. 1999;85:646–50. https://doi.org/10.2466/PR0.85.6.646-650.
12. Elbert T, Schauer M, Schauer E, Huschka B, Hirth M, Neuner F. Trauma-related impairment in children—a survey in Sri Lankan provinces affected by armed conflict. Child Abuse Negl. 2009;33:238–46. https://doi.org/10.1016/j.chiabu.2008.02.008.
13. Landolt MA, Schnyder U, Maier T, Schoenbucher V, Mohler-Kuo M. Trauma exposure and posttraumatic stress disorder in adolescents: a national survey in Switzerland. J Trauma Stress. 2013;26:209–16. https://doi.org/10.1002/jts.21794.
14. Hsieh Y, Shen AC, Wei H, Feng J, Huang SC, Hwa H. Associations between child maltreatment, PTSD, and internet addiction among Taiwanese students. Comput Hum Behav. 2016;56:209–14. https://doi.org/10.1016/j.chb.2015.11.048.
15. McCauley JL, Conoscenti LM, Ruggiero KJ, Resnick HS, Saunders BE, Kilpatrick DG. Prevalence and correlates of drug/alcohol-facilitated and incapacitated sexual assault in a nationally representative sample of adolescent girls. J Clin Child Adolesc Psychol. 2009;38:295–300. https://doi.org/10.1080/15374410802698453.
16. Boney-McCoy S, Finkelhor D. Is youth victimization related to trauma symptoms and depression after controlling for prior symptoms and family relationships? A longitudinal, prospective study. J Consult Clin Psychol. 1996;64:1406–16. https://doi.org/10.1037/0022-006X.64.6.1406.
17. Finkelhor D, Dziuba-Leatherman J. Children as victims of violence: a national survey. Pediatrics. 1994;94:413–20. https://doi.org/10.1016/0278-2391(95)90744-0.
18. Finkelhor D, Ormrod RK, Turner HA. Polyvictimization and trauma in a national longitudinal cohort. Dev Psychopathol. 2007a;19:149–66. https://doi.org/10.1017/S0954579407070083.
19. Finkelhor D, Ormrod RK, Turner HA. Re-victimization patterns in a national longitudinal sample of children and youth. Child Abuse Negl. 2007b;31:479–502. https://doi.org/10.1016/j.chiabu.2006.03.012.
20. Hanson RF, Borntrager C, Self-Brown S, Kilpatrick DG, Saunders BE, Resnick HS, Amstadter A. Relations among gender, violence exposure, and mental health: the national survey of adolescents. Am J Orthopsychiatry. 2008;78:313–21. https://doi.org/10.1037/a0014056.
21. Rheingold AA, Smith DW, Ruggiero KJ, Saunders BE, Kilpatrick DG, Resnick HS. Loss, trauma exposure, and mental health in a representative sample of 12-17-year-old youth: data from the national survey of adolescents. J Loss Trauma. 2004;9:1–19. https://doi.org/10.1080/15325020490890598.
22. McLaughlin KA, Koenen KC, Hill ED, Petukhova M, Sampson NA, Zaslavsky AM, Kessler RC. Trauma exposure and posttraumatic stress disorder in a national sample of adolescents. J Am Acad Child Adolesc Psychiatry. 2013;52:815–30. https://doi.org/10.1016/j.jaac.2013.05.011.
23. Copeland WE, Keeler G, Angold A, Costello EJ. Traumatic events and posttraumatic stress in childhood. Arch Gen Psychiatry. 2007;64:577–84. https://doi.org/10.1001/archpsyc.64.5.577.

24. Cuffe SP, Addy CL, Garrison CZ, Waller JL, Jackson KL, McKeown RE, Chilappagari S. Prevalence of PTSD in a community sample of older adolescents. J Am Acad Child Adolesc Psychiatry. 1998;37:147–54. https://doi.org/10.1097/00004583-199802000-00006.
25. Mongillo EA, Briggs-Gowan M, Ford JD, Carter AS. Impact of traumatic life events in a community sample of toddlers. J Abnorm Child Psychol. 2009;37:455–68. https://doi.org/10.1007/s10802-008-9283-z.
26. Sack WH, Seeley JR, Clarke GN. Does PTSD transcend cultural barriers? A study from the Khmer adolescent refugee project. J Am Acad Child Adolesc Psychiatry. 1997;36:49–54. https://doi.org/10.1097/00004583-199701000-00017.
27. American Psychiatric Association. Diagnostic and statistical manual of mental disorders. 5th ed. Washington, DC: Author; 2013.
28. American Psychiatric Association. Diagnostic and statistical manual of mental disorders: DSM-IV-TR. 4th ed. Washington, DC: Author; 2000.
29. American Psychiatric Association. Diagnostic and statistical manual of mental disorders. 4th ed. Washington, DC: Author; 1994.
30. Acierno R, Kilpatrick DG, Resnick H, Saunders B, De Arellano M, Best C. Assault, PTSD, family substance use, and depression as risk factors for cigarette use in youth: findings from the national survey of adolescents. J Trauma Stress. 2000;13:381–96. https://doi.org/10.1023/A:1007772905696.
31. Thabet AA, Ibraheem AN, Shivram R, Winter EA, Vostanis P. Parenting support and PTSD in children of a war zone. Int J Soc Psychiatry. 2009;55:226–37. https://doi.org/10.1177/0020764008096100.
32. Ying L, Wu X, Lin C, Chen C. Prevalence and predictors of posttraumatic stress disorder and depressive symptoms among child survivors 1 year following the Wenchuan earthquake in China. Eur Child Adolesc Psychiatry. 2013;22:567–75. https://doi.org/10.1007/s00787-013-0400-3.
33. Thabet AM, Vostanis P. Post-traumatic stress reactions in children of war. J Child Psychol Psychiatry. 1999;40:385–91. https://doi.org/10.1111/1469-7610.00456.
34. Perkonigg A, Pfister H, Stein MB, Höfler M, Lieb R, Maercker A, Wittchen H. Longitudinal course of posttraumatic stress disorder and posttraumatic stress disorder symptoms in a community sample of adolescents and young adults. Am J Psychiatr. 2005;162:1320–7. https://doi.org/10.1176/appi.ajp.162.7.1320.
35. Karam EG, Fayyad J, Karam AN, Melhem N, Mneimneh Z, Dimassi H, Tabet CC. Outcome of depression and anxiety after war: a prospective epidemiologic study of children and adolescents. J Trauma Stress. 2014;27:192–9. https://doi.org/10.1002/jts.21895.
36. Cisler JM, Amstadter AB, Begle AM, Resnick HS, Danielson CK, Saunders BE, Kilpatrick DG. A prospective examination of the relationships between PTSD, exposure to assaultive violence, and cigarette smoking among a national sample of adolescents. Addict Behav. 2011;36:994–1000. https://doi.org/10.1016/j.addbeh.2011.05.014.
37. Sack WH, Clarke GN, Seeley J. Posttraumatic stress disorder across two generations of Cambodian refugees. J Am Acad Child Adolesc Psychiatry. 1995;34:1160–6. https://doi.org/10.1097/00004583-199509000-00013.
38. Hoven CW, Duarte CS, Wu P, Erickson EA, Musa GJ, Mandell DJ. Exposure to trauma and separation anxiety in children after the WTC attack. Appl Dev Sci. 2004;8:172–83. https://doi.org/10.1207/s1532480xads0804_1.
39. Comer JS, Fan B, Duarte CS, Wu P, Musa GJ, Mandell DJ, Hoven CW. Attack-related life disruption and child psychopathology in New York City public school children 6-months post-9/11. J Clin Child Adolesc Psychol. 2010;39:460–9. https://doi.org/10.1080/15374416.2010.486314.
40. Adams ZW, Sumner JA, Danielson CK, McCauley JL, Resnick HS, Grös K, Ruggiero KJ. Prevalence and predictors of PTSD and depression among adolescent victims of the Spring 2011 tornado outbreak. J Child Psychol Psychiatry. 2014;55:1047–55. https://doi.org/10.1111/jcpp.12220.

41. Friedman MJ. PTSD history and overview. 2016. https://www.ptsd.va.gov/professional/ptsd-overview/ptsd-overview.asp. Retrieved 8 July 2016.
42. Carmassi C, Akiskal HS, Yong SS, Stratta P, Calderani E, Massimetti E, Akisal KK, Rossi A, Dell'Osso L. Post-traumatic stress disorder in DSM-5: Estimates of prevalence and criteria comparison versus DSM-IV-TR in a non-clinical sample of earthquake survivors. J Affect Disord. 2013;151:843–8. https://doi.org/10.1016/j.jad.2013.07.020.
43. Hafstad GS, Dyb G, Jensen TK, Steinberg AM, Pynoos RS. PTSD prevalence and symptom structure of DSM-5 criteria in adolescents and young adults surviving the 2011 shooting in Norway. J Affect Disord. 2014;169:40–6. https://doi.org/10.1016/j.jad.2014.06.055.
44. Hanson RF, Self-Brown S, Fricker-Elhai A, Kilpatrick DG, Saunders BE, Resnick H. Relations among parental substance use, violence exposure and mental health: the national survey of adolescents. Addict Behav. 2006;31:1988–2001. https://doi.org/10.1016/j.addbeh.2006.01.012.
45. Rosen CS, Cohen M. Subgroups of New York City children at high risk of PTSD after the September 11 attacks: a signal detection analysis. Psychiatr Serv. 2010;61:64–9. https://doi.org/10.1176/appi.ps.61.1.64.
46. Broman-Fulks JJ, Ruggiero KJ, Hanson RF, Smith DW, Resnick HS, Kilpatrick DG, Saunders BE. Sexual assault disclosure in relation to adolescent mental health: Results from the national survey of adolescents. J Clin Child Adolesc Psychol. 2007;36:260–6. https://doi.org/10.1080/15374410701279701.
47. Lawyer SR, Ruggiero KJ, Resnick HS, Kilpatrick DG, Saunders BE. Mental health correlates of the victim-perpetrator relationship among interpersonally victimized adolescents. J Interpers Violence. 2006;21:1333–53. https://doi.org/10.1177/0886260506291654.
48. Macdonald A, Danielson CK, Resnick HS, Saunders BE, Kilpatrick DG. PTSD and comorbid disorders in a representative sample of adolescents: the risk associated with multiple exposures to potentially traumatic events. Child Abuse Negl. 2010;34:773–83. https://doi.org/10.1016/j.chiabu.2010.03.006.
49. Lowe SR, Blachman-Forshay J, Koenen KC. Epidemiology of trauma and trauma-related disorders: trauma as a public health issue. In: Schnyder U, Cloitre M, editors. Evidence-based treatments for trauma-related psychological disorders: A practical guide for clinicians. New York: Springer; 2015. p. 11–40.
50. Liu K, Liang X, Guo L, Li Y, Li X, Xin B, Huang M, Li Y. Acute stress disorder in the paediatric surgical children and adolescents injured during the Wenchuan earthquake in China. Stress Health. 2009;26:262–9. https://doi.org/10.1002/smi.1288.
51. Kassam-Adams N, Winston FK. Predicting child PTSD: the relationship between acute stress disorder and PTSD in injured children. J Am Acad Child Adolesc Psychiatry. 2004;43:403–11. https://doi.org/10.1097/01.chi.0000112486.08386.c2.
52. Bryant B, Mayou R, Wiggs L, Ehlers A, Stores G. Psychological consequences of road traffic accidents for children and their mothers. Psychol Med. 2004;34:335–46. https://doi.org/10.1017/S0033291703001053.
53. Bryant RA, Salmon K, Sinclair E, Davidson P. The relationship between acute stress disorder and posttraumatic stress disorder in injured children. J Trauma Stress. 2007;20:1075–9. https://doi.org/10.1002/jts.20282.
54. Kersting A, Brahler E, Glaesmer H, Wagner B. Prevalence of complicated grief in a representative population-based sample. J Affect Disord. 2011;131:339–43. https://doi.org/10.1016/j.jad.2010.11.032.
55. Kay C, Green J. Reactive attachment disorder following early maltreatment: systematic evidence beyond the institution. J Abnorm Child Psychol. 2013;41:571–81. https://doi.org/10.1007/s10802-012-9705-9.
56. Lehmann S, Breivik K, Heiervang ER, Havik T, Havik OE. Reactive attachment disorder and disinhibited social engagement disorder in school-aged foster children – a confirmatory approach to dimensional measures. J Abnorm Child Psychol. 2016;44:445–57. https://doi.org/10.1007/s10802-015-0045-4.

57. Elovainio M, Raaska H, Sinkkonen J, Mäkipää S, Lapinleimu H. Associations between attachment-related symptoms and later psychological problems among international adoptees: results from the FinAdo study. Scand J Psychol. 2015;56:53–61. https://doi.org/10.1111/sjop.12174.
58. Magnusson P, Smari J, Gretarsdottir H, Þrandardottir H. Attention-deficit/hyperactivity symptoms in Icelandic schoolchildren: assessment with the attention deficit/hyperactivity rating scale-IV. Scand J Psychol. 1999;40:301–6. https://doi.org/10.1111/1467-9450.404130.
59. Polanczyk G, de Lima MS, Horta BL, Biederman J, Rohde LA. The worldwide prevalence of ADHD: a systematic review and metaregression analysis. Am J Psychiatr. 2007;164:942–8. https://doi.org/10.1176/appi.ajp.164.6.942.
60. Willcutt EG. The prevalence of DSM-IV attention-deficit/hyperactivity disorder: a meta-analytic review. Neurotherapeutics. 2012;9:490–9. https://doi.org/10.1007/s13311-012-0135-8.
61. Bauermeister JJ, Shrout PE, Ramírez R, Bravo M, Alegría M, Martínez-Taboas A, Chávez L, Rubio-Stipec M, García P, Ribera JC, Canino G. ADHD correlates, comorbidity, and impairment in community and treated samples of children and adolescents. J Abnorm Child Psychol. 2007;35:883–98. https://doi.org/10.1007/s10802-007-9141-4.
62. Bener A, Al Qahtani R, Abdelaal I. The prevalence of ADHD among primary school children in an Arabian society. J Atten Disord. 2006;10(1):77–82.
63. Döpfner M, Breuer D, Wille DPN, Erhart M, Ravens-Sieberer U, Bella Study Group. How often do children meet ICD-10/DSM-IV criteria of attention deficit-/hyperactivity disorder and hyperkinetic disorder? Parent-based prevalence rates in a national sample–results of the BELLA study. Eur Child Adolesc Psychiatry. 2008;17:59–70. https://doi.org/10.1007/s00787-008-1007-y.
64. Gau SS, Chong MY, Chen TH, Cheng AT. A 3-year panel study of mental disorders among adolescents in Taiwan. Am J Psychiatr. 2005;162:1344–50. https://doi.org/10.1176/appi.ajp.162.7.1344.
65. Graetz BW, Sawyer MG, Hazell PL, Arney F, Baghurst P. Validity of DSM-IV ADHD subtypes in a nationally representative sample of Australian children and adolescents. J Am Acad Child Adolesc Psychiatry. 2001;40:1410–7. https://doi.org/10.1097/00004583-200112000-00011.
66. Huss M, Hölling H, Kurth BM, Schlack R. How often are German children and adolescents diagnosed with ADHD? Prevalence based on the judgment of health care professionals: Results of the German health and examination survey (KiGGS). Eur Child Adolesc Psychiatry. 2008;17:52–8. https://doi.org/10.1007/s00787-008-1006-z.
67. Larson K, Russ SA, Kahn RS, Halfon N. Patterns of comorbidity, functioning, and service use for US children with ADHD, 2007. Pediatrics. 2011;127(3):462–70. https://doi.org/10.1542/peds.2010-0165d.
68. Lavigne JV, LeBailly SA, Hopkins J, Gouze KR, Binns HJ. The prevalence of ADHD, ODD, depression, and anxiety in a community sample of 4-year-olds. J Clin Child Adolesc Psychol. 2009;38:315–28. https://doi.org/10.1080/15374410902851382.
69. Lecendreux M, Konofal E, Faraone SV. Prevalence of attention deficit hyperactivity disorder and associated features among children in France. J Atten Disord. 2011;15:516–24. https://doi.org/10.1177/1087054710372491.
70. Merikangas KR, He JP, Burstein M, Swanson SA, Avenevoli S, Cui L, Benjet C, Georgiades K, Swendsen J. Lifetime prevalence of mental disorders in U.S. adolescents: results from the National Comorbidity Survey Replication - Adolescent Supplement (NCS-A). J Am Acad Child Adolesc Psychiatry. 2010b;49:980–9. https://doi.org/10.1016/j.yped.2011.04.014.
71. Merikangas KR, He JP, Brody D, Fisher PW, Bourdon K, Koretz DS. Prevalence and treatment of mental disorders among US children in the 2001-2004 NHANES. Pediatrics. 2010a;125:75–81. https://doi.org/10.1016/j.ypsy.2010.09.035.
72. Polanczyk G, Laranjeira R, Zaleski M, Pinsky I, Caetano R, Rohde LA. ADHD in a representative sample of the Brazilian population: estimated prevalence and comparative adequacy of criteria between adolescents and adults according to the item response theory. Int J Methods Psychiatr Res. 2010;19:177–84. https://doi.org/10.1002/mpr.319.

73. Faraone SV, Sergeant J, Gillberg C, Biederman J. The worldwide prevalence of ADHD: is it an American condition? World Psychiatry. 2003;2:104–13. https://doi.org/10.1176/appi.ajp.164.6.942.
74. Polanczyk GV, Willcutt EG, Salum GA, Kieling C, Rohde LA. ADHD prevalence estimates across three decades: an updated systematic review and meta-regression analysis. Int J Epidemiol. 2014;43:434–42. https://doi.org/10.1093/ije/dyt261.
75. Gadow KD, Nolan EE, Litcher L, Carlson GA, Panina N, Golovakha E, Sprafkin J, Bromet EJ. Comparison of attention-deficit/hyperactivity disorder symptoms subtypes in Ukrainian schoolchildren. J Am Acad Child Adolesc Psychiatry. 2000;39(12):1520–7. https://www.jaacap.org/article/S0890-8567(09)60419-6/abstract.
76. Miller TW, Nigg JT, Miller RL. Attention deficit hyperactivity disorder in African American children: what can be concluded from the past ten years? Clin Psychol Rev. 2009;29:77–86. https://doi.org/10.1016/j.cpr.2008.10.001.
77. Froehlich TE, Lanphear BP, Epstein JN, Barbaresi WJ, Katusic SK, Kahn RS. Prevalence, recognition, and treatment of attention-deficit/hyperactivity disorder in a national sample of US children. Arch Pediatr Adolesc Med. 2007;161:857–64. https://doi.org/10.1001/archpedi.161.9.857.
78. Larsson H, Sariaslan A, Långström N, D'Onofrio B, Lichtenstein P. Family income in early childhood and subsequent attention deficit/hyperactivity disorder: a quasi-experimental study. J Child Psychol Psychiatry. 2014;55:428–35. https://doi.org/10.1111/jcpp.12140.
79. Faraone SV, Perlis RH, Doyle AE, Smoller JW, Goralnick JJ, Holmgren MA, Sklar P. Molecular genetics of attention deficit hyperactivity disorder. Biol Psychiatry. 2005;57:1313–23. https://doi.org/10.1016/j.biopsych.2004.11.024.
80. Lu AT, Ogdie MN, Järvelin MR, Moilanen IK, Loo SK, McCracken JT, Cantor RM. Association of the cannabinoid receptor gene (CNR1) with ADHD and post-traumatic stress disorder. Am J Med Genet B Neuropsychiatr Genet. 2008;147:1488–94. https://doi.org/10.1002/ajmg.b.30693.
81. Knopik VS, Sparrow EP, Madden PA, Bucholz KK, Hudziak JJ, Reich W, Todd RD. Contributions of parental alcoholism, prenatal substance exposure, and genetic transmission to child ADHD risk: a female twin study. Psychol Med. 2005;35:625–35. https://doi.org/10.1017/s0033291704004155.
82. Briscoe-Smith AM, Hinshaw SP. Linkages between child abuse and attention-deficit/hyperactivity disorder in girls: behavioral and social correlates. Child Abuse Negl. 2006;30:1239–55. https://doi.org/10.1016/j.chiabu.2006.04.008.
83. Ford JD, Racusin R, Ellis CG, Daviss WB, Reiser J, Fleischer A, Thomas J. Child maltreatment, other trauma exposure, and posttraumatic symptomatology among children with oppositional defiant and attention deficit hyperactivity disorders. Child Maltreat. 2000;5:205–17. https://doi.org/10.1177/1077559500005003001.
84. Blumberg SJ, Bramlett MD, Kogan MD, Schieve LA, Jones JR, Lu MC. Changes in prevalence of parent-reported autism spectrum disorder in school-aged U.S. children: 2007 to 2011–2012. Natl Health Stat Report. 2013;65:1–11. https://www.cdc.gov/nchs/data/nhsr/nhsr065.pdf.
85. Baron-Cohen S, Scott FJ, Allison C, Williams J, Bolton P, Matthews FE, Brayne C. Prevalence of autism-spectrum conditions: UK school-based population study. Br J Psychiatry. 2009;194:500–9. https://doi.org/10.1192/bjp.bp.108.059345.
86. Autism and Developmental Disabilities Monitoring Network Principal Investigators, Centers for Disease Control and Prevention (CDC). Prevalence of autism spectrum disorders—autism and developmental disabilities monitoring network, 14 sites, United States, 2008. MMWR Surveill Summ. 2012;61:1–19. https://www.cdc.gov/mmwr/preview/mmwrhtml/ss6103a1.htm.
87. Kim YS, Leventhal BL, Koh YJ, Fombonne E, Laska E, Lim EC, Cheon KA, Kim YK, Lee H, Song DH, Grinker RR. Prevalence of autism spectrum disorders in a total population sample. Am J Psychiatry. 2011;168:904–12. https://doi.org/10.1176/appi.ajp.2011.10101532.

88. Kogan MD, Blumberg SJ, Schieve LA, Boyle CA, Perrin JM, Ghandour RM, Singh GK, Strickland BB, Trevathan E, van Dyck PC. Prevalence of parent-reported diagnosis of autism spectrum disorder among children in the US, 2007. Pediatrics. 2009;124:1395–403. https://doi.org/10.1542/peds.2009-1522.
89. Williams E, Thomas K, Sidebotham H, Emond A. Prevalence and characteristics of autism spectrum disorders in the ALSPAC cohort. Dev Med Child Neurol. 2008;50:672–7. https://doi.org/10.1111/j.1469-8749.2008.03042.x.
90. Schieve LA, Boulet SL, Blumberg SJ, Kogan MD, Yeargin-Allsopp M, Boyle CA, Rice C. Association between parental nativity and autism spectrum disorder among US-born non-Hispanic white and Hispanic children, 2007 National Survey of Children's Health. Disabil Health J. 2012;5:18–25. https://doi.org/10.1016/j.dhjo.2011.09.001.
91. Mandell DS, Listerud J, Levy SE, Pinto-Martin JA. Race differences in the age at diagnosis among Medicaid-eligible children with autism. J Am Acad Child Adolesc Psychiatry. 2002;41:1447–53. https://doi.org/10.1097/00004583-200212000-00016.
92. Bhasin TK, Schendel D. Sociodemographic risk factors for autism in a US metropolitan area. J Autism Dev Disord. 2007;37:667–77. https://doi.org/10.1007/s10803-006-0194-y.
93. Sterzing PR, Shattuck PT, Narendorf SC, Wagner M, Cooper BP. Bullying involvement and autism spectrum disorders: Prevalence and correlates of bullying involvement among adolescents with autism spectrum disorder. Arch Pediatr Adolesc Med. 2012;166:1058–64. https://doi.org/10.1001/archpediatrics.2012.790.
94. Mehtar M, Mukaddes NM. Posttraumatic stress disorder in individuals with diagnosis of autistic spectrum disorders. Res Autism Spectr Disord. 2011;5:539–46. https://doi.org/10.1016/j.rasd.2010.06.020.
95. Abram KM, Washburn JJ, Teplin LA, Emanuel KM, Romero EG, McClelland GM. Posttraumatic stress disorder and psychiatric comorbidity among detained youths. Psychiatr Serv. 2007;58:1311–6. https://doi.org/10.1176/appi.ps.58.10.1311.
96. Kilpatrick DG, Ruggiero KJ, Acierno R, Saunders BE, Resnick HS, Best CL. Violence and risk of PTSD, major depression, substance abuse/dependence, and comorbidity: results from the National Survey of Adolescents. J Consult Clin Psychol. 2003;71:692–700. https://doi.org/10.1037/0022-006x.71.4.692.
97. Simonoff E, Pickles A, Charman T, Chandler S, Loucas T, Baird G. Psychiatric disorders in children with autism spectrum disorders: prevalence, comorbidity, and associated factors in a population-derived sample. J Am Acad Child Adolesc Psychiatry. 2008;47:921–9. https://doi.org/10.1097/chi.0b013e318179964f.
98. Rosenberg MS, Reppucci ND. Primary prevention of child abuse. J Consult Clin Psychol. 1985;53:576–85. https://doi.org/10.1037//0022-006x.53.5.576.
99. Gilbert R, Kemp A, Thoburn J, Sidebotham P, Radford L, Glaser D, MacMillan HL. Recognising and responding to child abuse. Lancet. 2009;373:10–6. https://doi.org/10.1016/S0140-6736(08)61707-9.
100. Cox CM, Kenardy JA, Hendrikz JK. A randomized controlled trial of a web-based early intervention for children and their parents following unintentional injury. J Pediatr Psychol. 2010;35:581–92. https://doi.org/10.1093/jpepsy/jsp095.
101. Kenardy J, Thompson K, Le Brocque R, Olsson K. Information-provision intervention for children and their parents following pediatric accidental injury. Eur Child Adolesc Psychiatry. 2008;17:316–25. https://doi.org/10.1007/s00787-007-0673-5.
102. Cohen JA, Mannarino AP, Berliner L, Deblinger E. Trauma-focused cognitive behavioral therapy for children and adolescents: an empirical update. J Interpers Violence. 2000;15:1202–23. https://doi.org/10.1177/088626000015011007.

Chapter 12
From the Outside In: Using a Whole-School Paradigm to Improve the Educational Success of Students with Trauma Histories and/or Neurodevelopmental Disabilities

Michael Gregory and Emily Nichols

Introduction

All students need schools that provide safe and supportive educational environments if they are to maximize their learning and achieve at high levels. On its face, this seems an obvious and uncontroversial assertion, and yet education reform efforts are really only just beginning to take seriously concepts like school climate and school culture. Many of the most celebrated legal reforms of the last 50 years—including desegregation, special education, and, more recently, modifications to punitive school discipline laws—have largely centered on the *individual rights* students possess. Resulting remedies have accordingly focused on providing access, offering services, or safeguarding due process for individual students, but rarely have they tackled in a straightforward way the challenge of defining and guaranteeing a whole-school learning environment in which all students feel safe and cared for and enjoy a sense of belonging and connectedness ([1], p. 1). While educators have long known, both intuitively and on the basis of research and their own practice, that such environments are critically important for learning, law and policy have been slow to catch up to this understanding.

This lag is unfortunate for all students, but there are certain groups whose learning is particularly undermined when we fail to prioritize the creation of supportive school contexts. Students suffering the traumatic effects of exposure to violence and other childhood adversities are one such group. For nearly two decades, the Trauma

M. Gregory (✉)
Harvard Graduate School of Education, Cambridge, MA, USA
e-mail: mgregory@law.harvard.edu

E. Nichols
Medstar Georgetown Center for Wellbeing in School Environments (WISE Center), Child and Adolescent Program, Department of Psychiatry, Medstar Georgetown University Hospital, Washington, DC, USA

J. M. Fogler, R. A. Phelps (eds.), *Trauma, Autism, and Neurodevelopmental Disorders*, https://doi.org/10.1007/978-3-030-00503-0_12

and Learning Policy Initiative (TLPI), a collaboration between Massachusetts Advocates for Children (MAC) and Harvard Law School for which one of the authors works, has studied the educational consequences of childhood trauma and explored policy solutions for addressing these impacts.[1] Through an Education Law Clinic that it operates at Harvard Law School, TLPI has provided legal representation to individual families of traumatized students in the special education system. It has also partnered with educators in schools across Massachusetts to create trauma-sensitive schools. And it has advocated in the policy arena for laws, policies, and funding streams designed to meet the needs of students, families, and educators. The second author of this chapter has trained and worked in the Developmental Medicine Center (DMC) and the Advocating Success for Kids (ASK) program at Boston Children's Hospital, providing clinical services and consultation for another group particularly impacted by the lack of supportive school environments: children with neurodevelopmental disabilities. The ASK program specifically works to advocate for students from Boston Public Schools, who have neurodevelopmental disabilities and live in high poverty areas of the city, where many students are exposed to chronic stress and traumatic experiences.

In this chapter, we will describe what we have learned about the critical role that safe and supportive school cultures play in the educational success of these two groups of students. Centering on the stories of several real students and their families, the chapter will explain how individual supports and services provided to these students, typically through the special education system—while an *essential* ingredient for supporting their progress—often fail to achieve desired results when not delivered in the context of a supportive school environment. Based on the experiences of these students, as well as important insights from research, we will argue for an educational approach that shifts perspective—that moves from the outside in—by first paying close attention to the educational context that surrounds the student and then analyzing carefully the individualized services the student needs to succeed within that broader context. We will describe a process that TLPI has developed for helping educators create safe and supportive, trauma-sensitive school cultures and will argue that this process can also support the creation of inclusive school cultures that research suggests are critical for students

[1] The authors would like to express a special thank you to Susan Cole, Anne Eisner, Joel Ristuccia, Marissa Del Rosario, and Katie Ryan, the members of the TLPI team. All of the ideas expressed in this chapter related to the education of students who have experienced traumatic events and the creation of whole-school trauma-sensitive school cultures are derived from the ongoing, collective work of the TLPI team. More information about TLPI's work is available on the project's website, http://traumasensitiveshools.org. We would also like to thank all of the law students in Harvard Law School's Education Law Clinic over the years for their work representing highly vulnerable families, including those whose stories are recounted in this chapter. Additionally, we would like to thank our colleagues at Massachusetts Advocates for Children's (MAC) groundbreaking autism center (including a special thank you to Johanne Pino, Leslie Hughes, and Catherine Mayes for their very helpful feedback on this chapter), from whom we have learned a great deal about the educational needs of students on the autism spectrum and how to support their families. Finally, and most importantly, we would like to thank the many caregivers and students whose courageous journeys we have been privileged to share. Of course, all errors or omissions are attributable solely to the two present authors.

with neurodevelopmental disabilities. Throughout this chapter, the term "neurodevelopmental disability" will be used instead of "neurodevelopmental disorder," and the term "autism" will be used instead of "autism spectrum disorder" or "ASD." This usage reflects the view of some in the autism community that the term "disorder," even if clinically appropriate under the terms of the DSM-5, can nonetheless entail an unwanted and unnecessary stigma. The chapter will conclude with implications for policy.

Trauma and the Importance of Context and Culture: Embracing a New Paradigm

There is no question that special education laws provide a powerful set of tools for improving the educational experience of many students who are struggling with the consequences of trauma. Over the past 13 years, TLPI's Education Law Clinic at Harvard Law School has assisted over 250 families in the special education process and helped caregivers advocate for the specialized instruction, related services, accommodations, and placements their children have needed to be successful at school. While not all students who have endured traumatic experiences either go on to develop a trauma response or qualify as a "child with a disability,"[2] there are certainly many who do, and the federal Individuals with Disabilities Education Act (IDEA) and associated state laws are an indispensable source of support for these students and their caregivers. Nevertheless, the experience of providing legal representation to a large number of families over more than a decade has also afforded some sobering lessons about the limits of individual representation in special education for effecting a *systemic* change in the educational experiences and outcomes of traumatized students.

Consider the following real-life case examples.[3]

Marguerite

Marguerite, a Haitian-American student in the 10th grade who had a history of sexual abuse and who had also been diagnosed with an intellectual impairment and anxiety, was floundering in a large, urban high school with minimal supports in her Individualized Education Program (IEP). Through legal advocacy, Marguerite was

[2] In order to qualify for special education and related services, a student must be found eligible as a "child with a disability," which the IDEA defines as "a child (i) with intellectual disabilities, hearing impairments (including deafness), speech or language impairments, visual impairments (including blindness), serious emotional disturbance … orthopedic impairments, autism, traumatic brain injury, other health impairments, or specific learning disabilities; and (ii) who, by reason thereof, needs special education and related services" U.S.C. § 1401 (3)(A).

[3] To protect students' privacy, all names used in this chapter are pseudonyms.

offered placement in a substantially separate, therapeutic classroom for "fragile" students. The teachers in this classroom were highly skilled, the setting was small and intimate, and the presence of an appropriate peer group allowed her to start forming real friendships for the first time. However, this self-contained classroom was part of a larger therapeutic school where many of the students struggled with serious behavioral and psychiatric disabilities. The hallways and common spaces were chaotic. Physical restraints occurred on a regular basis, in full view of other students. Fights were not uncommon. While Marguerite's own classroom felt safe and supportive to her, and while her devoted teachers worked very hard to teach her the skills she was lacking, her progress stalled because she was severely triggered by the threats she perceived in the larger school community. Ultimately, her mother had to pursue placement in an out-of-district school where a calmer environment could allow Marguerite to manage her anxieties and focus on her learning.

José

José was a middle school student diagnosed with ADHD and mild learning disabilities. As a small child, he had witnessed his mother beaten nearly to death by his father. He ran next door, at 4 years old, to get help from a neighbor, while his mom lay bleeding and unconscious on the kitchen floor. Though his father was incarcerated shortly thereafter, the effects on José of having witnessed this terrifying scene were lasting and significant. He became preoccupied with the safety of his mother and three younger sisters. As José entered 8th grade, his sister Cecilia, a new sixth grader, joined him at the same middle school. Seeing himself as her protector, José got into several physical altercations with boys in her grade. When his mother would come to school for discipline proceedings, the administrators, who did not speak Spanish, failed to offer translation services. She grew confused and frustrated, and school officials blamed her for not being able to control her son's behavior. Sensing this rift between the school and his parent, José pulled away from the adults at school, even from the special educators who were providing him individualized support to improve his reading. As his fear and anger grew, so did the instances of aggressive behavior and the number of suspensions. Adding a behavior intervention plan to his IEP did not change the perception of his school principal, which was that José was a troublemaker who needed "tough love" and consequences to learn self-control. Each week, José's dream of making it to a competitive vocational high school for 9th grade, where he could learn to be an electrician, slipped further and further away.

While each of these stories is unique in its own way, both of them illustrate a similar underlying pattern: the special education system was effectively providing each of these students with much-needed individualized supports for their learning and social challenges, and yet these supports were not enough to enable these students to make effective educational progress. Marguerite was provided a new, supportive, self-contained classroom. José received one-on-one instruction to improve his reading, as well as executive functioning supports for his ADHD. However, *the lack of a safe and supportive school environment* thwarted the efficacy of these critical educational supports, and each of these students continued to struggle. The chaotic student behavior in the hallways and common areas undermined the sense of safety Marguerite felt in her specialized classroom. His principal's unwillingness to rethink the underlying reasons for José's aggression, and the lack of understanding about how to include his mom as a respected partner, led to rigid application of punitive discipline policies and an escalating cycle of disengagement. Working with both of these students—among so many others with similar stories—and having seen up close the efforts of well-meaning, diligent, highly professional regular and special educators ultimately come to little avail has taught a hard but important lesson: without a *trauma-sensitive context* within which to deliver individual services, the best efforts of special education may not result in success for traumatized students.

This critical lesson—that context is just as important as services—will be unsurprising to anyone who is familiar with the work of Mary Harvey and other pioneers in the field of community psychology. Stemming from work in the Victims of Violence program in Cambridge, MA, Harvey and others made groundbreaking contributions to our understanding of trauma by explaining the essential role that supportive communities can play in helping individuals overcome the debilitating symptoms often associated with the trauma response [34]. Particularly important is Harvey's concept of "ecological fit," which describes "the quality and helpfulness of the relationship existing between the individual and his or her social context" ([2], p. 7). As she explains, "Interventions that achieve ecological fit are those that enhance the environment-person relationship—i.e., that reduce isolation, foster social competence, support positive coping, and promote belongingness in relevant social contexts" ([2], p. 7). For children, of course, school is the primary "relevant social context" outside of their families, giving the educational setting a tremendously important role to play in mitigating the negative effects of traumatic experience [3].

In fact, we might even consider the school a special kind of social context with the potential to have a sort of "multiplier" effect on the progress of children who have been impacted by traumatic events: not only do school environments that "reduce isolation, foster social competence, support positive coping, and promote belongingness" make it possible for students to *learn effectively* notwithstanding the adverse experiences in their lives, but the learning students experience in such schools in turn can also play a major role in helping them *heal from their trauma*. Where "ecological fit" exists between the student and her school environment, there can be a reciprocal relationship between learning and healing, in which both are inextricably intertwined and where each can boost the other in powerful ways [4].[4] Of course, for students like Marguerite and José, where "ecological fit" is lacking, the opposite effect is all too common: both learning and healing can stagnate or,

[4] "Competency"—at school, a synonym for learning—has been recognized as one of three essential pillars of trauma treatment in an intervention model pioneered by these authors.

even worse, be doubly undermined in a sort of mutually reinforcing, downward spiral.

What we have seen over and over again in our special education advocacy is confusion and frustration among educators, who kindly offer students the very best treasures from their pedagogical "bags of tricks"—services, accommodations, and specialized instructional approaches—but encounter disappointment as these interventions fail to produce meaningful or sustained results. Something is wrong in these scenarios, but it is not ineffective teachers, inappropriate services, incorrigible students, or unsupportive caregivers. What is wrong is the operating paradigm that presumes services alone should be able to win the day. On the contrary, as essential as they are for student success, it is very difficult for services on their own to create an "ecological fit" where one does not already exist. Services are indeed indispensable for helping students build the skills necessary to effectively *access and benefit from* the larger school community. But expecting individualized services alone to *create* or engender a whole-school environment that is safe and supportive in the way Harvey describes is like expecting the tail to wag the dog. This helps explain the enigma of why so many students struggling in school with the traumatic effects of exposure to violence and other adversities can often seem beyond the reach of even the most state-of-the-art and sophisticated special education interventions. The interventions themselves may be phenomenal, but the context in which they are provided is often one in which students' trauma-related educational needs are misunderstood, resulting in a poor "fit" between student and environment and less-than-hoped-for progress in learning, behavior regulation, and relationships.

"Moving to Action": Putting the New Paradigm to Work in Schools[5]

Embracing the importance of context in supporting the educational success of students impacted by traumatic experience (whether or not they also have disabilities) is an essential first step to overcoming the barriers illustrated above, but it begs several important questions. What does embracing this new paradigm actually "look like" on the ground in schools? What concrete steps can educators take to create safe and supportive, trauma-sensitive learning communities that allow students like Marguerite and José to benefit from their special education services and truly flourish? How can educators embark on a process to transform the larger cultures of their schools for all students while still remaining committed to delivering on the promises of special education and providing appropriate, high-quality,

[5]All of the ideas discussed in this section come directly from Cole et al. [5]. *Helping Traumatized Children Learn, Vol. 2: Creating and Advocating for Trauma-Sensitive Schools*, Boston, MA: Massachusetts Advocates for Children (of which Michael Gregory is a co-author). Where we quote this work directly, we will offer a particular citation with page number; otherwise, we will let this general citation suffice and will not distract the reader with additional citations.

individualized services to particular students who are eligible for them? To summarize, how can educators translate this new and different way of thinking into real action?

To begin to provide answers to these questions and help educators "move to action," TLPI has spent the better part of the last two decades developing a process and a set of tools that educators in any school can use to create a trauma-sensitive learning environment. First, we have offered a definition of a "trauma-sensitive school" as a target or touchstone for educators' thinking and action: at the end of the day, what kind of school-wide context should we all be aiming for? What is a vision that can guide our collective efforts? We say "a trauma-sensitive school is one in which all students feel safe, welcomed, and supported and where addressing trauma's impact on learning on a school-wide basis is at the center of its educational mission" ([5], p. 17).

While simple enough on its surface, there are some important commitments embedded within this definition that bear highlighting, particularly in light of the present volume's focus. For one, the definition recognizes that trauma-sensitive schools are for *everyone*. Prevalence data reveal that traumatic childhood events are an all-too-ubiquitous feature of the human experience [6–10]. While it may be that only a subset of us develops traumatic symptoms that interfere substantially with our development, we all face adversities of various types throughout our childhoods, and we all have a neural architecture that depends heavily on safety and calm for optimal learning and growth [11–13]. (This generalization applies equally to students with neurodevelopmental challenges, a topic which we take up directly in later sections.) Therefore, we find it important to emphasize that "every student will learn more, build better relationships with teachers and classmates, experience greater self-esteem, and become more engaged in the life of the school when he or she is surrounded by a safe and welcoming trauma-sensitive environment" ([5], p. 88). While students like Marguerite and José may have particular trauma-related challenges that *require* a trauma-sensitive environment to enable meaningful educational progress, these environments benefit *all students*. Trauma sensitivity is not about *identifying and labeling* those students with traumatic backgrounds; rather, it is more like a universal design approach, taking for granted that all students stand to gain from school environments that help them feel safe and supported.

A second important idea embodied in the definition is that trauma sensitivity involves *the whole school*. If we accept Harvey's notion that the "ecology" or environment surrounding a person plays an important role in their healing (and for children, in the school context, their learning), then we must also accept the reality that *everyone in the school* is implicated in creating the conditions that will allow for student success. Creating a trauma-sensitive school is about transforming the culture of the school, weaving an understanding of trauma into every single thing the school does. This involves *everyone*. A strong leader who understands how to motivate her staff is critical, as is the presence of informed clinical expertise in the building. But in addition to these important components, trauma sensitivity also entails input and commitment from classroom teachers, paraprofessionals, student support staff, cafeteria workers, custodial staff, bus drivers, administrative support staff, and everyone who has a presence in the school. So important is this idea—the idea that everyone must be involved—that TLPI made the difficult decision years ago only to offer our limited professional development resources to schools that would commit to having *all leadership and staff* attend our presentations. We learned after many years of doing it the other way that efforts not inclusive of everyone in the school cannot be effective at transforming the school's culture—which means they cannot result in a trauma-sensitive school.

The third critical idea contained in the definition of a trauma-sensitive school is that trauma sensitivity must be part of the *core educational mission of the school.* This is simply another way of saying that trauma sensitivity is about *learning itself,* the central task of schools. It is about understanding the way students' brains develop, about the way they process language and information, about the way they organize themselves and get work done [3].[6] Trauma sensitivity is not an ancillary initiative, an appendage to the school's primary function, and an add-on that is there to support a small subset of struggling students. Rather, it must be seen as a fundamental facet of the teaching and learning transaction. It represents a key ingredient in the effort to overcome achievement gaps and maximize the learning of all students.

This definition of a trauma-sensitive school—and the foundational ideas embodied within it—is meant to be helpful in articulating a broad vision to which educators can aspire. But like most visions, it is lofty and can be hard to grab ahold of when it comes time to figure out how to take action. We have found it useful to flesh out the definition by operationalizing some of the observable attributes that tend to characterize those schools that are trauma-sensitive. More specifically, TLPI has identified the following six characteristics that such schools seem to have in common—these are, as we call them, the six "attributes of a trauma-sensitive school":

1. Leadership and staff *share an understanding* of trauma's impacts on learning and the need for a school-wide approach.
2. The school *supports all students to feel safe* physically, socially, emotionally, and academically.
3. The school *addresses students' needs in holistic ways*, taking into account their relationships, self-regulation, academic competence, and physical and emotional well-being.[7]
4. The school *explicitly connects students to the school community* and provides multiple opportunities to practice newly developing skills.
5. The school *embraces teamwork* and staff share responsibility for all students.
6. Leadership and staff *anticipate and adapt* to the ever changing needs of students ([5], pp. 18–26).

[6] See Chap. 1 of *Helping Traumatized Children Learn, Volume 1* for a thorough summary of the ways in which traumatic experience can impact students' learning.

[7] As this attribute makes clear, and as we wish to emphasize, appropriate, high-quality services are an integral part of a whole-school trauma-sensitive environment. In making the case for the importance of the surrounding context, we do not mean to suggest that such services are not important.

Taken together, these six attributes are a way of describing the kind of *culture* that exists in a school that is trauma-sensitive. They are a way of summarizing the *values and norms* that guide decision-making in such schools, both decision-making about individual students and about the direction and welfare of the school as a whole.

One way to translate these values and norms into concrete actions in a school is for educators to put each of the attributes into the form of a question and then ask the six questions of any action or initiative the school plans to undertake. For example, *will this action deepen our shared understanding of trauma's impacts on learning and the need for a school-wide approach?* Or *will this action help support all students to feel safe physically, socially, emotionally, and academically?* And so on. In question form, we refer to these attributes as the "Trauma-Sensitive Vision Questions." The purpose of the questions is to "encourage active reflection and thoughtful inquiry on ways to achieve the vision of a trauma-sensitive school. They serve as a touchstone or reminder to keep the vision in clear view as schools identify priorities and plan, implement, and evaluate their [actions]" ([5], p. 26). Schools we have worked with have found the questions helpful for keeping them on course as they plan actions to make their schools more trauma-sensitive. Educators in one school had the six attributes printed on lanyards that the adults could wear around their necks to keep the values in the forefront of everyone's consciousness as they carried out their work on a daily basis. In another school, educators used the questions as a sort of "screening tool" for evaluating the trauma sensitivity of actions brainstormed by colleagues in school-wide planning meetings. Given strong foundational concepts, educators are endlessly creative at devising ways to put them into practice.

In addition to the importance of a strong vision guiding educators' planning and action, there is another critical dimension to translating the "new paradigm" about safe and supportive contexts into practice. The way an organizational culture gets created is through the behaviors and actions of the people in the organization as they do their work [14]. Therefore, if educators in a school desire to transform their culture, it makes sense to engage in reflection about all the *operational functions* of the school—all the things the adults in the building do each day—and consider how each of these activities can be done in a way that is consistent with the values and norms described above. After years of working with educators in numerous schools, TLPI has learned that there are six core operational functions that characterize the daily work that goes on in virtually every school building. Together, we call these six core functions a "Flexible Framework" for analyzing the operations in a school:

1. Leadership
2. Professional development
3. Access to resources and services
4. Academic and nonacademic (classroom) strategies
5. Policies, procedures, and protocols
6. Collaboration with families ([5], p. 27; [3], p. 47)

As is probably obvious, there is nothing about these six functions that is unique to trauma sensitivity. These are six basic aspects of schools' work that would need to be considered as part of any effort to implement some change or initiative on a *school-wide basis*.

Just as with the six attributes of trauma sensitivity, TLPI has found that putting the six elements of the Flexible Framework in the form of questions can turn them into a useful planning tool as educators work to translate their understanding about the importance of a safe and supportive whole-school culture into reality. So, for example, educators can ask *what role does school and/or district leadership play in implementing this action?* Or *what professional development is necessary for staff in order to implement this action?* And so forth. Asking these questions helps ensure that all the operations of the school are consistent with trauma-sensitive values and are working to support the creation of a culture that embodies those values. They help ensure that no part of the school is "left out" of the effort to become trauma-sensitive. Educators can also use them as a way to identify potential barriers that might get in the way of culture change if not addressed proactively—for example, a district leader who may not be on board or a group of active caregivers who might be taken by surprise if not engaged early on. Where the Vision Questions, by definition, are aspirational and somewhat subjective, the Flexible Framework Questions are more structural and highly pragmatic. While the role of the Vision Questions is to help everyone remain clear on *the desired direction* to move in, the role of the Flexible Framework Questions is to help get *all the oars* of the school *laboring in that same direction*.

Taken together these two lists of questions are a set of tools that educators have found very helpful in their work to change the cultures of their schools. But these tools are not self-executing. On their own they contain no information that would help educators know how or when to use them. The tools become helpful when used as part of a *whole-school, inquiry-based action planning process* focused on the creation of a trauma-sensitive school culture. Adapting powerful theories from organizational change literature to the context of schools, TLPI has outlined a process of change any school can use to structure its journey to become trauma-sensitive. The process is built upon several foundational concepts: learning together as a whole staff, team building, asking hard questions, identifying common priorities, action planning, ongoing reflection, and data-based self-evaluation. It revolves around four iterative questions educators can use to guide their thinking and planning:

1. Why do we feel an urgency to become a trauma-sensitive school?
2. How do we know we are ready to create a trauma-sensitive action plan?
3. What actions will address staff priorities and help us become a trauma-sensitive school?
4. How do we know we are becoming a trauma-sensitive school? ([5], p. 32)

Moving through the four phases embedded in these questions (urgency, readiness, action, reflection); doing so in a recurring, cyclical way; and utilizing the Trauma-Sensitive Vision Questions and Flexible Framework Questions along the way as tools to help guide and concretize efforts—doing all of this—constitutes a process that can empower educators to create "trauma-sensitive learning communities where new ideas and expansive thinking are nurtured and where synergy and teamwork make it possible for complex issues to be explored" ([5], p. 31). When the adults in a school are part of this kind of professional learning community, they are able to generate a school culture that results in a nurturing, supportive whole-school learning environment for all their students.

The movement to create trauma-sensitive schools is still relatively new, though its momentum is quickly growing. There is still much to be learned about how the process described above might look different in different kinds of schools and communities. We also need to understand more about the barriers that can get in the way of the process and about the role external constituencies—families, community agencies, other service systems—can play in supporting (or undermining) the efforts of the educators within a school building. But even at this early stage, many educators have experienced success using this process and set of tools to translate the new paradigm about the importance of context and environment into concrete actions and real, effective, observable changes in the cultures of their schools.

Notwithstanding the promise of this new paradigm, and the hope it can inspire for a rejuvenated and more humane education system, it seems important to pause for a moment and acknowledge that it can also provoke some doubts and questions. Effectuating the transformation of a school's culture takes a substantial commitment and a fair amount of time and effort. The work to do this can feel very distant from the needs of particular students like Marguerite and José. It might also seem too protracted when staring at the crisis of the moment. This is part of what makes embracing the new paradigm so hard. When confronted with the everyday, urgent needs of students who are struggling, and the harsh realities faced by so many schools and districts, engaging in an inquiry-based process to create a trauma-sensitive whole-school culture can feel like a luxury some schools and students simply cannot afford.

However, as the stories shared earlier reveal, doing it the other way—prioritizing individual planning but neglecting the intransigent barriers and sometimes toxic effects of the larger school culture—is failing far too many students. Neither the law nor sound ethical or pedagogical judgment would allow us to set aside the obligation to provide services that meet these students' unique educational needs in favor of a school-wide initiative—this is certainly not our argument. Rather, the way forward seems to be embracing an approach that balances doing the best we can for individual students in the immediate-term while, alongside this effort, embarking on a long-term, ongoing process of transforming and replenishing the culture of the whole school. Over time, as the culture evolves, little by little, the individualized supports will become more effective. Students who were previously getting lost in the shuffle despite intensive interventions will start to become more engaged in their schools and classrooms and spend more time on productive learning. Staff who were feeling burned out, ineffectual, or underappreciated will start to reinvest in the professional mission that called them to education in the first place. At least these are the changes TLPI has witnessed unfold in schools time and time again. Looking back over their shoulders after working to create trauma-sensitive learning environments amidst a host of contemporaneous challenges, so many educators have shared the exact same sentiment with us: *Why did we wait so long to do this? We cannot go back to the way things were before.*

Students with Neurodevelopmental Disabilities and Inclusive School Cultures

Which brings us to the second population of students who are a subject of the present volume: *students with neurodevelopmental disabilities* (hereafter, abbreviated for convenience to SWND). Are the new paradigm described above and TLPI's process for translating it into observable changes in school culture relevant to this group of students? Not surprisingly, we believe the answer is *yes*. While Mary Harvey's work on "ecological fit" described the need traumatized individuals have for supportive social contexts, we do not have to stretch far to imagine the potential that safe and supportive school environments also hold for advancing the educational progress of SWND. In fact, there has been a robust discussion in the academic literature—not to mention in faculty meetings and teachers' lounges across the country—about the importance of supportive school-wide contexts for the success of these students as well. This discussion is closely linked to the disability-rights community's broader conversation about the importance of a "culture of inclusion." The vision of this inclusive culture parallels substantially Harvey's vision for social contexts that "fit" the needs of traumatized students: environments that "reduce isolation, foster social competence, support positive coping, and promote belongingness." When you step back and look at them side by side, it is easy to see that these two visions are essentially one and the same.

To provide a brief background on the history of inclusion, beginning in the mid-1990s, the UNESCO's Salamanca Statement [15] established inclusive education for all students, regardless of disability, as a basic human right. During this same period, educational practice slowly began to shift in the United States, as educators started to consider SWND not just the responsibility of special education staff, but of the whole school. For the first time, doors were opened to include them in the general education population. Since then, the percentage of students with an identified disability educated in mainstream classes has doubled [16]. Simultaneously, the prevalence of children diagnosed with autism has grown. One in 68 children is diagnosed with autism, and one in six children has a developmental disability [17]. Currently, 39% of students identified with autism, and more than half of students identified with any developmental disability (e.g., intellectual disability, speech and language impairment, attention deficit hyperactivity disorder) are educated in mainstream classrooms [16].

This dramatic shift in education has led to a larger discussion as to how to provide a true "inclusion" experience while still meeting the unique needs of such a neurodiverse population. Similar to students who have experienced trauma, most schools initially focused on how to help these students fit into the existing general school environment, through providing individualized service plans, instead of focusing on how to change the school environment to fit a more neurodiverse population. While there is no question that students benefit from classroom accommodations and individualized special education services, many SWND with the best services available still struggle to thrive in the general education environment. Individualized service plans provide little structure to inform how students should be supported in other areas of the school, such as school buses, cafeterias, and locker rooms [18]. School staff members are often left underprepared and undersupported for addressing the social and behavioral challenges that occur outside of academic instruction, including peer relationships, participation in extracurricular activities, and managing disruptive behaviors. SWND continue to be vulnerable to feeling disconnected from their school, while teachers and administrators scramble to assemble the right mix of pullout and push-in supports that will ensure the school remains compliant with "inclusion" policies. In fact, researchers have found that when schools only focus on individualized interventions while attempting inclusion, the overlooked environmental characteristics of the school often contribute to negative outcomes for SWND, such as bullying and exclusion from the school community [19]. The best efforts of school staff fall short, and at times actually create more harm, when they are not provided within the larger context of a school-wide "culture of inclusion." Essentially, SWND are facing the same lack of "ecological fit" as their peers who have experienced trauma albeit perhaps for different reasons. This is why we believe TLPI's work to support the creation of safe and supportive school cultures is so relevant to this growing population.

The driving vision for the inclusion of SWND is to have a school culture in which every student is accepted and supported by the entire school community [20, 21]. This culture is necessary for SWND to succeed socially and academically in a general education setting [22]. How to operationalize such a culture in order to make meaningful change is now the great challenge that faces educators and the disability-rights community. Progress has been made to translate this vision into on-the-ground change. While it is beyond the scope of this chapter to summarize fully this important work, we hope to highlight what we believe are some essential components, and roadblocks, to shaping a school culture of inclusion.

Schools must help students feel they belong in the community in order to see improvement in a variety of areas of development within the general education population [23]. So how do schools successfully help students feel less isolated and more connected throughout the school day? First, the school must have a *shared vision* of inclusion that is agreed upon by all school staff and communicated and modeled to the student body. Everyone must understand and agree that their school is better with SWND in the general population then without them. Successful inclusion of SWND in the general education population has the potential to create a better learning environment for SWND, their typically developing peers, and school staff [24]. When a school has truly developed such a culture, teachers feel more supported and respected, students gain important social skills and empathy, and SWND make academic, developmental, and social gains [24, 25].

Second, every member of the school community must prioritize learning about and from SWND and must receive *high-quality professional development* that supports them to do so. SWND, like their traumatized peers, are often misunderstood and, as a result, can be highly isolated in traditional general education settings. Students with autism, for example, have reported that staff often do not understand how even aspects of the physical school environment, such as crowding, noise, and last-minute changes in routine, prevent them from fully engaging in school [24]. It is widely agreed that general educators' understanding of autism and training in effective strategies for supporting students with autism is a key factor in successful inclusion efforts [24]. Despite agreeing on the value of inclusion, many teachers and principals report feeling unprepared to actually implement inclusion practices [22, 26, 27]. For example, principals without training and experience with SWND are less likely to place them in a general education classroom [24]. This trickles down to teachers feeling hesitant about asking for support in learning how to educate and manage behaviors of the SWND that are placed in their classrooms [22]. Caregivers of SWND feel less connected to and trusting of schools when principals and teachers are not perceived as being invested in the daily actions of supporting and including their children [28]. Additionally, when caregivers of typically developing students perceive teachers spending disproportionate amounts of time with SWND, or being unable to manage behavioral disruptions, they are less supportive of having their children educated in inclusion environments [29]. Prioritizing trainings about working with SWND not only changes how members of the school community interact with SWND but also how they interact with each other, drawing together the whole school community to feel more united and supported.

In addition, research indicates that creating a *safe environment* free from bullying is essential for the success of SWND. Bullying is prevalent within the population of SWND, especially those with autism. Students with autism are also more likely to be bullied when educated in a general education classroom [30], in part because such classrooms often do not exist within a larger school-wide culture of inclusion. Many characteristics of an inclusive culture, such as positive relationships between peers and parent engagement, are protective factors against bullying [30]. Another pathway to creating a safe, bully-free environment is to reduce the number of problematic behaviors that SWND exhibit. The more disruptive students are to a classroom, the more vulnerable they become to being singled out by peers [30]. Research has shown that schools can reduce the frequency of both problematic behaviors and incidents of bullying of SWND when collaboration and frequent communication with caregivers, consistent response to behaviors across settings, and appropriate staff understanding of the behavioral symptoms associated with certain disabilities are all a part of the school culture [24, 30].

Positive relationships with school staff and peers are another crucial element of an inclusive school culture for both protecting SWND against bullying and helping them feel connected to the school community [30]. Students who are in inclusion classrooms or a school with an inclusive culture are more empathic and understanding of other's differences and have greater social skills [24, 29]. Additionally, inclusion classrooms have healthier emotional climates [29]. These are prime conditions to foster meaningful social engagement between students and in which bullying is rarely accepted as a social norm. In this environment, SWND have more opportunities to learn social skills from their peers and build social competency. Paraprofessionals may be less necessary to scaffold social interactions as students are more capable of supporting one another [24].

Overall, school factors that facilitate the improvement of academic, communication, social, and self-determination skills in students with severe neurodevelopmental disabilities include school staff collaboration, staff fostering a sense of belonging, and opportunities for meaningful engagement between SWND and their typically developing peers [23]. As we take a step back, the characteristics of a school that has successfully developed such a "culture of inclusion" echo the attributes of a trauma-sensitive school. All school staff have a *shared understanding* and value the differences among their students, which allows them to collaborate and *work as a team* to meet students' needs. Students feel they belong and are *connected* to the school environment, as the school has policies and a culture in place that help *all students feel safe*. Through collaborating with parents and professional development, school staff can *adapt* to meet students' *holistic needs* and encourage their development as a whole person.

As SWND make up a relatively small percentage of the general student body, it may seem costly to commit to such a large systemic change. However, we would point out that a "culture of inclusion," similar to a trauma-sensitive school, is beneficial for all students. A recent meta-analysis of inclusion research identified benefits to all students ranging from accepting diversity to developing new social skills [24]. Teachers and school staff observed that when supporting SWND, collaboration and respect across service providers and administrators were necessary for them to feel supported and valued in working with SWND [22]. This culture is needed for staff to feel free to ask questions, request more training and support, and prevent burnout. A positive and inclusive school culture was also a "ubiquitous factor" in increasing effective family-school partnerships for all students across a variety of schools implementing a school-wide inclusion framework ([28], p. 229).

Despite the well-documented benefits of positive school culture and inclusion, students with autism are not benefiting in the same way as students with other developmental and learning needs [24]. Identified roadblocks to successful inclusion experiences for this particular group of students include school staff's lack of education about the autism spectrum, unhelpful attitudes toward autism from school administrators, a school environment that is unsupportive to students with autism, and inappropriate approaches to managing disruptive behavior by students with autism. Caregivers reported the need for more collaborative support from the school and outside resources. Multitiered approaches to behavior change, such as response to intervention and school-wide positive behavior support, often exclude SWND (including students with autism) in universal interventions, reinforcing the separation of SWND and a sense of isolation from the school community [31]. It is possible that this population may be better served by utilizing TLPI's paradigm and process for creating safe and supportive school environments.

Indeed, as we have said, one of the foundational principles of the trauma-sensitive schools movement is that trauma sensitivity is *good for all students*. Like other powerful examples of universal design—curb cuts in sidewalks, closed captioning on televisions—trauma-sensitive whole-school cultures may be *required* in order for a distinct (though not small) subset of the population to access a mainstream institution, but they also improve educational opportunities for the *whole community* [32]. It is therefore not surprising—although it is quite affirming—to observe the degree of consistency between the research on inclusive cultures for SWND and the theories that underlie trauma-sensitive schools. It is almost like these two populations of students—students suffering the impacts of trauma and SWND—are two distinct groups of canaries in the same coal mine, alerting us all to the inadvertent toxicity of many schools' cultures through the often protracted educational struggles they endure. There is an important fix that will help make the air breathable again for both groups of students: whole-school safe, supportive, and inclusive cultures that engender compassionate relationships between adults and children, that ensure every member of the community feels safe and enjoys a sense of belonging, that contain high-quality services that effectively teach skills for how to engage with and navigate that community, and where no one encounters shame or scorn for learning, talking, thinking, or feeling unique or different. The shift in mindset we have described—from *individual services and supports* to *whole-school culture transformation* (that includes but goes far beyond individual services and supports)—is equally necessary for improving educational (and life) outcomes for both groups of vulnerable students.

The Interface Between Trauma and Neurodevelopmental Disabilities

Even before the academic conversation began to demonstrate the convergence of the needs of these two groups of students, TLPI knew intuitively that the overlap existed because we had witnessed it up close through the experiences of our individual clients. While it is the contention of this chapter that a whole-school safe and supportive environment is equally an educational linchpin for students experiencing trauma *and* for SWND (i.e., in circumstances where a student experiences *one* of these challenges), it is also true that *the same student* often experiences impacts from *both* conditions. A very wise clinician, attempting to help us understand the complex and independent comorbidity of trauma with a host of other childhood impairments, once crystallized this truth very succinctly: "Remember, it is possible to have both a broken arm *and* a broken leg." We have represented numerous families in our Education Law Clinic over the years whose children have both endured traumatic experiences and received a diagnosis on the autism spectrum.

The experiences of these students are particularly instructive for teaching us about the importance of whole-school safe, supportive, and inclusive cultures. They help us see how the impacts of trauma and the symptoms of neurodevelopmental disabilities often become inextricably intertwined, such that it is hard to know where one ends and the other begins. These students often confound educators because the services and placements available for them (and the professionals trained to provide these services and teach in these classrooms) are often highly specialized, developed to respond to just one of these sets of challenges. As a result, IEPs for these students are often assembled as if it were possible to address their complicated needs as separate parts, each remediable by applying a discrete solution: Here is some ABA to address your autism diagnosis, and here is some cognitive behavioral therapy for your trauma. In fact, the whole child is greater than the sum of her parts, and often neither service ends up being particularly effective because it does not take account of the fact that the set of symptoms or challenges it is designed to address has been made more complex by its merger with the other set. Even more than students with one or the other condition, the experiences of those impacted by both magnify the importance of supportive learning environments.

In this section we share four stories of students with both trauma histories and neurodevelopmental disabilities whose families were represented by the Education Law Clinic. Each student's narrative is a complicated tapestry; our effort will be to shed light on three common threads that can be seen in all of them: (1) how the attributes of a trauma-sensitive school culture could have benefitted the student, (2) how the elements of an inclusive culture as elucidated in the research on SWND could have benefitted the student, and (3) how school-wide operations were implicated in what was not working well for the student.

Katrina

As an initial example, Katrina's story illustrates profoundly how a *shared understanding of the impacts of trauma* could have made a world of difference for a student with a neurodevelopmental disability. As a third grader, she was diagnosed as having a nonverbal learning disability (NVLD), including difficulties with understanding pragmatic language and social cues and the tendency to form naive judgments (both overly positive and overly negative) about the intentions of peers. Comorbid with her NVLD was mild depression and anxiety that stemmed from the social difficulties she encountered at school and from the severe disapprobation she perceived in the constructive feedback of her teachers. Her school appropriately placed her in a supportive, substantially separate class with other high-functioning students on the autism spectrum and provided counseling and social skills support in her IEP. However, not long after entering her new classroom, she began getting bullied by a male classmate. The bullying took the form of insults followed by verbal manipulation; he would make Katrina feel bad by insulting her and then get her to misbehave as a means of winning back his favor. For the most part, this bullying went under the adults' radar screen. The young man started inviting Katrina to his house to play on the weekends, and her parents were glad to take her, unaware of the bullying and thrilled that for the first time Katrina was getting invited to a peer's home. On one of these weekends, the boy sexually assaulted Katrina. She initially kept this to herself and told no one, though her parents noticed that she started to act differently, becoming hypervigilant and skittish all the time. Eventually, Katrina decompensated entirely under the weight of this secret trauma and had to be hospitalized, at which point she told her parents of the bullying and the assault. Her parents shared this information with the school and asked for Katrina to be placed in a classroom separate from the little boy. School officials refused this request. While they took Katrina's word that the assault had occurred, they argued that there were adults present who could keep her safe from an assault at school; there was no need to separate her from the boy.

Unfortunately, Katrina began refusing to attend school because she did not want to see the boy, and as her parents and school officials became embroiled in an escalating and protracted conflict about her placement, the school itself grew to become a trigger. By refusing to recognize her trauma and promise to keep her safe, the school became for Katrina an extension of the trauma; it became associated in her mind with danger and a loss of safety. She could not enter the school and would decompensate if her parents even drove her down the street it was on. While the school was by no means responsible for the sexual assault she endured (perhaps it did bear some responsibility for not recognizing the initial bullying), the lack of understanding among leadership and staff about the impact this traumatic experience was having on Katrina—a student whose ability to process emotions and relationships was already by definition impaired—contributed greatly to her downward trajectory. Katrina spent more than a year out of school, receiving no education whatsoever, and her parents ultimately had to advocate for her placement in an out-of-district therapeutic school.

Taking a step back, it is clear that the operational functions of the school may have been implicated in barriers that contributed to this problem. It would seem that staff had not had appropriate *professional development*, in that they did not appear to understand that, even if no additional assaults or bullying occurred, Katrina was triggered to feel highly unsafe by the boy's mere presence and unable to focus or learn at all when reminded of the assault. They also did not fully appreciate how at risk Katrina was for being bullied when she entered their class, given her difficulty understanding social situations related to her NVLD. In a "culture of inclusion," the school might have had stronger *policies* in place regarding the prevention of bullying. In a school with an "upstander culture," Katrina's more socially aware peers might have recognized the manipulation and spoken up on her behalf when Katrina could not [33]. Additionally, frequent *communication between Katrina's parents and the school* would have potentially helped recognize the victimization sooner and established a relationship of trust from which Katrina would have benefitted as the adults figured out how best to support her and keep her safe.

Monique

Monique's story highlights the relevance of another trauma-sensitive attribute, as operationalized through the Flexible Framework: the use of *resources and services* to *address students' needs in holistic ways*. Monique was a third grade student who lived with her aunt in a large urban city. She had low-functioning autism and spoke very few words, which made her a target of other youths in the neighborhood. Beginning at age 7, she was repeatedly raped by an older teenaged boy in the neighborhood, who was thought to be trustworthy. Monique did not have the language ability to tell any adults this was happening to her, but her aunt finally became aware of the abuse when a friend walked in one day to find it taking place. She took immediate action to keep Monique safe from the older boy and in short order arranged for her to begin seeing a trauma-informed mental health professional. Predictably, behavioral manifestations of Monique's trauma began to show up at school. Her aggression increased and she engaged in tantrums and meltdowns for no apparent reason. The teachers in her substantially separate autism program were stymied when the ABA-based behavioral supports they had been providing proved inadequate to help re-regulate Monique's explosive behaviors. Her community-based therapist attended many school meetings and explained to Monique's team that her behaviors were rooted in her trauma and the corresponding urge to keep herself safe. She explained that a therapeutic, relational approach to Monique's behavior was necessary. The autism program teachers felt they were neither equipped to understand Monique's trauma-based behavior nor able to adapt the approaches they were using, so the district proposed changing her placement to a substantially separate therapeutic classroom. Monique was not successful in the new class either because, while the teachers there had more training in therapeutic techniques, they did not have expertise in the instructional strategies necessary for advancing the learning of a nearly nonverbal student on the autism spectrum. In short, this school district had separate specialized programs that could each meet *part* of Monique's complicated set of needs, but there was no program that could address all of her needs *holistically*.

When presented with the dilemma of what to do for Monique, district officials did not seem to have any basis for considering what an integrated approach to her needs might consist of. What would a trauma-informed, relational approach to ABA look like? How could therapeutic supports effective for neurotypical children be adapted for lower-functioning students on the spectrum? If the larger culture in either school had been focused on supporting staff to be *flexible and willing to adapt* their approaches to Monique's specific needs, *collaboration with outside resources* might have provided a solution. The community-based therapist could have been contracted to work with Monique's teachers to help adapt established behavioral supports. Or, if the therapeutic classroom better met Monique's academic needs, the school could have contracted with a BCBA from the community to provide ABA services within the therapeutic classroom. Possible solutions like these were not explored. Members of the team seemed stymied by the complexity of Monique's profile, lured into the simplistic hope that plugging her into one of two programs that already existed would suffice. Instead, the reality was that her two discrete sets of needs were interacting to result in something new and complicated, something more than merely the sum of their parts.

Carlos

Carlos, another student who experienced interrelated challenges from traumatic experience and an autism diagnosis, is almost the prototypical example of the importance of *explicitly connecting students to the school community*. His story also particularly highlights the importance of the combined school operations of appropriate *policies and protocols* and *family collaboration*. Carlos was a senior in high school who resided with his single mother. The two of them were living in hiding in a well-to-do suburb, placed there through an innovative domestic violence program that helps victims flee their abusers, change their names and identities, and utilize a centralized mailing address to keep their whereabouts unknown. As a young boy, Carlos had witnessed his mother verbally and physically abused by his father, on several occasions watching the ambulance come and take her to the emergency room. He received special education in substantially separate settings throughout his elementary and middle school years, but when he got to high school, the service delivery model used by his district was almost entirely inclusion-focused. While Carlos had paraprofessional support in his academic classes and two periods per day in a "learning center" with a special educator, he was largely left to navigate the academically difficult and socially treacherous terrain of a large comprehensive high school on his own for the majority of the school day. By the time he got to his senior year, his mother was frantic that he was not acquiring any concrete skills that he would be able to use to secure a job or care for himself in the community after graduation. While the justification for the lack of specialized support in Carlos' IEP was inclusion in the mainstream, his physical proximity to his nondisabled peers did not change that fact that he was tremendously isolated from them socially.

His mother shared one poignant story that captured the cruelty of this isolation. Carlos wanted more than anything to attend the homecoming dance and be one of the "cool kids." Though his mother had qualms about his participation, the guidance counselor at school latched onto this desire as a way to support Carlos' age-appropriate participation in the mainstream life of the school. Especially with the counselor encouraging him, there was no deterring Carlos, so mom helped him get ready. When the dance came, she snuck into the school gym to observe discretely from the corner, only to watch her son taunted and ridiculed by the rest of the student body as he jumped wildly up and down, flailing his arms to the music—his form of dancing. The adult chaperones stood by; they had no idea how to stop the situation they had put in motion, how to reverse a dynamic that was quickly causing Carlos to become the court jester of the homecoming dance.

While some students receive intensive special education supports in cloistered settings that never help them learn how to generalize their skills to the mainstream, Carlos was a victim of the opposite—but equally troubling—problem: he was set adrift in the mainstream environment without adequate structure or scaffolding to help him effectively navigate that environment (*and* without adequate work to help the nondisabled students in the school understand how to appreciate, respect, and include a vulnerable peer). He was physically part of the school community, but his services did not connect him to that community in meaningful ways. Carlos may have been better protected if the counselor had listened to his mother's concerns and *collaborated* on how to provide a more successful and meaningful interaction with peers. *School policies* that emphasized timely and appropriate responses to incidents of bullying may have prevented such a widespread social acceptance of ridiculing a vulnerable classmate. This is a perfect example where the combined implementation of a "culture of inclusion" within a trauma-sensitive school could have best served Carlos and the larger school community. If the entire school, from the principal to the students, took pride in embracing all differences, then Carlos might have been joined by his peers, or at least the chaperones, on the dance floor. It might have been seen as an opportunity to embrace instead of a problem to solve.

Roberta

Finally, Roberta's story is an illustration of how important it is for educators to *embrace teamwork* and share responsibility for all students. As one of four siblings, Roberta grew up in a home with an abusive father who was ultimately incarcerated. The stable, lower middle class life in a small, close-knit Massachusetts town that her mother provided the family was sufficient to buffer many of the negative impacts of the abuse for Roberta's brothers and sister. They attended school, participated in sports and activities, had good friends, were supported by teachers, and graduated. But unlike her siblings, Roberta was diagnosed with a mild intellectual impairment and with autism. When she got to high school, she was flummoxed by the social scene and the increased academic demands. Her family happened to live next door to the high school, and many days her anxiety would skyrocket, and she would bolt from the school and retreat across a busy street to her house. Ultimately, she refused to attend school altogether and simply stayed home for almost two full school years. When school staff finally succeeded at coaxing her back to school, they put in place a more comprehensive IEP, with counseling and speech and language services, both focused on helping her build stronger social skills. The team also made sure she got to participate in chorus and art, two areas of considerable strength for her. A Board Certified Behavior Analyst constructed a behavior plan that identified triggers for her bolting behavior so staff would be able to intervene and calm her down before her anxiety would escalate. On paper, this seemed a very reasonable plan to support Roberta's success. Unfortunately, she continued to flounder and threatened to leave school once again.

Upon accompanying her mother to an IEP meeting, it became immediately apparent what was getting in the way: though a strong team of highly skilled professionals had been assembled around Roberta, *none of them were collaborating with each other*. The chorus teacher had not seen (or been trained in how to implement) the behavior plan. The academic teachers had not received any consultation from the speech and language therapist so they could build on the skills Roberta was learning in her biweekly pullout sessions. There was nothing drawing the *parts* of

Roberta's education plan together into a cohesive *whole*, and as a result she continued to slip through the cracks. Though we endeavored to build more consultation and collaboration into her IEP, the overriding culture of the school was not one of teamwork among the professionals. The *building leadership* did not seem to have set the example or provided the professional space for teamwork to occur. There did not appear to have been any *professional development* around collaboration with specialists or basic behavioral supports for children with autism. Not surprisingly, the words written in the IEP document were not powerful enough to transcend the underlying values and norms—the implicit ways of doing business—in the school building. Roberta's experience demonstrates why *collaboration between school staff and specialists* has been identified as a key component of both a trauma-sensitive school and a "culture of inclusion." Roberta's mother finally had to pursue an out-of-district placement where her daughter received essentially the same services as in her high school but in a smaller setting where the staff worked together cohesively to build a community in which everyone supported Roberta's learning in consistent and coordinated ways.

Trauma-Sensitive, Inclusive Schools for *All* Students

The stories we have shared so far have illustrated the negative consequences for traumatized students and/or those with neurodevelopmental disabilities that can result from the lack of safe and supportive environments in their schools. Equally instructive—and much more inspiring—are stories where the effectiveness of services and supports provided to students was *elevated* by the presence of a safe and supportive context. To be sure, one would not expect to find many such stories in a caseload that by definition consists of families whose children are struggling in school, but there are a few, and we will share one of them here in order to reinforce and extend the learnings generated by the previously shared (and decidedly less positive) stories.

Tyrice

Tyrice was a second grade student living with his single female guardian, Sharon. Sharon had been the upstairs neighbor of Tyrice's biological mother when he was born, and she often babysat for Tyrice when his mother went out. As time went on, Tyrice's mother was gone for longer and longer periods of time; some days she would not come home at all. It soon got to the point that Tyrice was basically living with Sharon. His mother had developed a serious substance abuse problem and increasingly began to neglect many of her son's needs. Ultimately, when she failed to follow through on much-needed medical procedures for Tyrice, Sharon initiated a proceeding in court and eventually was awarded full guardianship. In addition to attachment issues stemming from his mother's neglect and abandonment, Tyrice was also diagnosed with autism. During kindergarten and first grade, he struggled both behaviorally and academically, missing a great deal of school. In second grade, he was fortunate to be placed in a new "inclusion" school being launched by his school district. In this school, each classroom had approximately one-third to one-half students with disabilities and one-half to two-thirds typically developing students. There were two certified teachers in each classroom, at least one of whom was dually certified in regular and special education. The goal was to weave specialized approaches into the regular school day so that students with disabilities could be supported to learn in the mainstream to a much greater degree. In this new setting, Tyrice's aggressive behaviors began to subside, and he began to engage more in his academic work, though his skill levels were still quite far behind.

Prior to enrolling in the new school, Tyrice had been receiving mental health services from a nearby community-based agency. This agency had partnered with local researchers expert in the field of trauma to implement a pilot therapy program where child patients were taught to use sensory integration techniques to help them process and cope with their traumatic experiences. The agency converted an old conference room into a new "sensory integration room": they installed a plastic ball pit, ropes to swing on, cushions to dive in, and padded floors to land on. The basic idea behind this treatment approach is that being engaged in meaningful physical activity during the therapy session, rather than sitting passively in the therapist's office, can engage more of the brain, improve cognitive processing, and help children regulate their emotional states. Tyrice's therapist began using this new approach with him and the improvements were dramatic. He loved all the movement—especially crashing into the pillows—and his therapist reported that he began for the first time to articulate insights during the sensory integration therapy that he had never been able to express to her through other therapy models. "It's like a whole new part of his brain opens up," is how she explained the difference she saw in Tyrice during therapy sessions.

Given the improvements in language and information processing Tyrice experienced during his sensory integration therapy sessions, his therapist understandably recommended that similar trauma-sensitive OT practices be woven throughout his school. In a report to his IEP team, the therapist recommended that the school hire a consultant to advise staff on how to adapt similar techniques for use in the school setting, that the school install a "sensory integration room" similar to the one that had been installed in the clinic (that would be for the benefit of all the students in the school), and that Tyrice have multiple meetings each week with the school-based occupational therapist. As Sharon's lawyers, these recommendations were the focus of our advocacy. At the IEP meeting, however, we were seemingly rebuffed by school officials. Though they were interested in hearing about the ideas behind the new therapy model and accepted the premise that Tyrice's learning could be enhanced through regular, purposeful physical movement, they did not find the therapist's recommendations appropriate. They explained that there was no space in the small school for a special sensory integration room and that the occupational therapist, who was only in the building 2 days a week, did not have room in her schedule for multiple sessions with Tyrice. Instead, they maintained that Tyrice's sensory integration needs could be met by having the classroom teachers and aides weave similar approaches throughout the school day, incorporating physical movement into classroom activities, providing Tyrice with regular opportunities to do heavy physical "work" (like helping move desks to get ready for a whole-group activity), and having the occupational therapist consult with outside providers to develop a sensory diet for Tyrice that could be implemented across all school settings. In fact, many of these approaches, they assured us, were already taking place in the school, not just for Tyrice but for all the students. "We are not going to implement *your* recommendations," they seemed to be telling us, "but *trust us*, we are doing these things *in our own way*."

As lawyers who have received similar assurances from many schools as attempts to deflect caregivers' advocacy efforts, we were skeptical about the team's assertions. Two months or so into the school year, we arranged for several of Tyrice's outside evaluators and providers to conduct observations of his classroom to see if the school was living up to its promises. Indeed, each of the observers was completely impressed by what they saw. Tyrice's lead teacher, a former physical education teacher, was incorporating all kinds of movement into her academic instruction. She utilized music and dancing as part of reading and math lessons. The occupational therapist followed through on her commitment to collaborate with Tyrice's outside therapist to develop a "physical movement plan" for him, and she met with all of the key adults he interacted with throughout the school day to be sure they each knew how to help implement this plan. To accommodate for the school's small size and lack of opportunity for outdoor recess, the principal invested in portable indoor play equipment that could be set up in the lunchroom each day for physical activity and then conveniently put away in the storage room. In short, the whole staff embraced a norm that all students should have the opportunity to benefit from physical movement throughout the school day, and they also took responsibility for understanding Tyrice's particular needs in this regard and for utilizing planned strategies as needed to support these needs no matter where he was in the building.

This story is an example of how integrating supports into the fabric of the school can often accomplish so much more for a student than isolated services that do not connect to the rest of the school community. In addition, weaving such approaches throughout the school's programming provides an opportunity for all students to benefit from them, even those who do not have a particular set of specialized needs. While the indoor play equipment might have addressed a particular disability-related need of Tyrice's, there is no student in the school who did not benefit from the restoration of recess to the daily schedule. Every adult in the building from the principal on down understood and subscribed to the goal of adjusting the mainstream learning environment so that it could bend to meet the needs of a larger variety of students. This commitment to an inclusive culture also paved the way for the school to become more trauma-sensitive, even though this was not the stated objective. If the premises underlying Tyrice's special sensory integration therapy are correct, then incorporating similar types of opportunities for movement throughout the school day no doubt helped other traumatized students in the school who may not have been as fortunate as Tyrice to participate in a cutting edge pilot initiative outside of school. In addition, the teamwork and consistency among the staff necessary to implement this kind of cohesive approach engendered a sense of safety and stability in the building that could serve as a foundation for all students' learning and success.

We began the chapter with two stories that showed how the lack of "ecological fit" between a student and his or her context can work to sap the effectiveness of well-intended and expertly delivered special education supports and services. We end with this final story in the hope that it persuasively conveys the opposite: how the presence of a safe and supportive context can *amplify* individualized interventions for particular students and even extend their benefits to others in the school community. Our additional hope is that all of the stories taken together make a compelling case about the universality of the need for trauma-sensitive, inclusive school cultures. The seven students we have briefly profiled here come from diverse racial and ethnic backgrounds. Some are boys and some are girls. Some are from urban and some from suburban communities. They have experienced many different types of adversity in their young lives, with the traumatic response from these events impacting different aspects of their school functioning. Some of these students also had neurodevelopmental disabilities, while others did not. All of them, however, needed to feel safe in their school settings, to feel a sense of belonging and inclusion in the school community, to have educators rally around them as a team to support their unique needs. While there are certainly many types of students not represented in these few stories (including those who unjustly receive no or very low-quality special education services), our descriptions of both the positive and negative aspects of the cultures in these schools will hopefully seem relevant to others' experiences as well. The imperative to reconceptualize education from the perspective of a new paradigm that emphasizes the importance of context and "ecological fit" may be particularly urgent for students with needs who are similar to those we have described here, but all students can benefit from inclusive, trauma-sensitive school cultures that emphasize safety and belonging as a foundation for learning.

Conclusion and Policy Implications

While educators and building leaders have an important role to play in translating the new paradigm we have described into educational reality for students, we cannot expect them to do this hard work alone. Just as the culture within a school building serves as a foundation for students' learning, the culture of the larger education system is the foundation for educators' professional practice. If we are to expect educators to engage in the collective inquiry, planning and reflection that underlie the creation of trauma-sensitive, inclusive school cultures, then laws and policies must set conditions that support them to do so [1].

Mandating that educators create trauma-sensitive, inclusive schools would be unlikely to generate the results we might desire. On the contrary, tempting as such an approach might seem, it would likely only lead to the development of a compliance mentality, in which conscientious rule-following would likely serve as a pale substitute for the kind of genuine urgency and motivation that must underlie the process of transforming schools' cultures in trauma-sensitive, inclusive ways. Similarly, attempts to diminish or sidestep the individual legal rights and entitlements that students have would also likely come to little avail. It is not that students need supportive educational contexts *instead of* high-quality, state-of-the-art educational services and thoughtfully constructed IEPs; as the stories we have shared make clear, they need these environments *in addition to* the critical services and supports to which they are already entitled.

Fortunately, there are many other ways in which education laws and policies can support the paradigm change for which we advocate in this chapter.[8] First and foremost, education and government leaders can publicly prioritize the creation of safe and supportive schools and share their own sense of urgency about this issue. Second, policymakers can organize new laws and policies according to the school operations outlined in the Flexible Framework, so that they more closely reflect the way schools actually "do business" and therefore become easier to implement on the ground. Third, systems of education can ensure professional development opportunities—at both the pre-service and in-service levels—designed to deepen educators' understanding about the importance of school culture and the educational needs of students impacted by trauma and by neurodevelopmental disabilities. Fourth, schools and outside agencies can be incentivized to collaborate to ensure that appropriate and coordinated services are available to individual students and families as needed (while respecting confidentiality and the right to privacy). Fifth, policymakers can ensure that districts and schools have access to the leadership and staffing capacity necessary to engage in the process of whole-school culture transformation described in this chapter. Sixth, laws and policies that require the use of evidence-based approaches can be revised to make clear they allow schools to engage in locally based, staff-driven evaluative inquiry where educators play a role in determining the kind of evidence that is relevant for demonstrating the effectiveness of their efforts. Seventh, accountability regimes can be refined in a way that rewards schools for taking positive steps to transform their cultures in trauma-sensitive, inclusive ways. Eighth, executive agencies at the federal, state, and regional levels can create communities of practice—through conferences, technical assistance, sharing of materials and best practices, and other activities—that support educators to learn from each other about how to engage effectively in this work. And finally, funding can be made available—both through grant programs and as part of schools' and districts' foundation budgets—to support the relatively minor costs associated with the time and effort involved when staff develop and implement action plans at the local level.[9]

---

[8] The recommendations that follow are adapted from policy recommendations articulated elsewhere by TLPI. See Cole et al. [5], pp. 88–93.

[9] Many of these approaches are reflected in the Safe and Supportive Schools Framework Statute advocated for by TLPI and passed into law by Massachusetts in 2014. See MGL c. 69, § 1P, available online at https://malegislature.gov/Laws/GeneralLaws/PartI/TitleXII/Chapter69/Section1P.

Taking such steps to support educators in the creation of trauma-sensitive, inclusive whole-school cultures is imperative for students such as those we have described in this chapter. To repeat, it is not that we should set aside for one moment our obligation to keep striving for appropriate individualized supports—services, accommodations, teaching approaches, and placements—for traumatized students and for SWND. We must continue to meet our legal and moral obligations to these students. (And where these obligations are not being met, lawyers, advocates, policymakers, and families should continue to pressure school districts and state governments and seek to hold them accountable.) However, *alongside* these imperative advocacy efforts, we must also think of creative ways to educate policymakers about the importance of safe and supportive school cultures so that they can take positive action to unlock the full value of our collective investment in individualized student services and ensure educational success for all our students.

References

1. Cole S. Implementing legal strategies for creating safe and supportive school environments. J Appl Res Child Informing Pol Child Risk. 2014;5(2):1–22.
2. Harvey MR. An ecological view of psychological trauma and trauma recovery. J Trauma Stress. 1996;9(1):3–23.
3. Cole S, et al. Helping traumatized children learn, vol. 1: supportive school environments for students traumatized by family violence. Boston: Massachusetts Advocates for Children; 2005.
4. Kinniburgh JK, Blaustein M, Spinazzola J, van der Kolk B. Attachment, regulation and competency: a comprehensive intervention framework for children with complex trauma. Psychiatr Ann. 2005;35(5):424–30.
5. Cole S, et al. Helping traumatized children learn, vol. 2: creating and advocating for Trauma-Sensitive Schools. Boston: Massachusetts Advocates for Children; 2013.
6. Anda RF, et al. The enduring effects of abuse and related adverse experiences in childhood: a convergence of evidence from neurobiology and epidemiology. Eur Arch Psychiatry Clin Neurosci. 2006;256(3):174–86.
7. Anda RF, et al. Building a framework for global surveillance of the public health implications of adverse childhood experiences. Am J Prev Med. 2010;39(1):93–8.
8. Bethell CD, et al. Adverse childhood experiences: assessing the impact on health and school engagement and the mitigating role of resilience. Health Aff. 2014;33(12):2106–15.
9. Danese A, et al. Adverse childhood experiences and adult risk factors for age-related disease: depression, inflammation and clustering of metabolic risk markers. Arch Pediatr Adolesc Med. 2009;163(12):1135–43.
10. Felitti VJ, et al. Relationship of childhood abuse and household dysfunction to many of the leading causes of death in adults: The Adverse Childhood Experiences (ACE) Study. Am J Prev Med. 1998;14(4):245–58.
11. National Scientific Council on the Developing Child. The timing and quality of early experiences combine to shape brain architecture: working paper no. 5. Cambridge: Center on the Developing Child at Harvard University; 2007.
12. Perry BD. Incubated in terror: neurodevelopmental factors in the 'cycle of violence'. In: Osofsky JD, editor. Children in a violent society. New York: Guilford Press; 1997. p. 124–49.
13. Perry BD. Neurodevelopmental impact of violence in childhood. In: Schetky DH, Benedek EP, editors. Principles and practice of child and adolescent forensic psychiatry. Washington, DC: American Psychiatric Publishing, Inc.; 2002. p. 191–203.

14. Gruenert S, Whitaker T. School culture rewired: how to define, assess and transform it. Alexandria: ASCD; 2015.
15. UNESCO. Salamanca statement and framework for action on special needs education. 1994.
16. U.S. Department of Education, National Center for Education Statistics. Digest of education statistics, 2015 (NCES 2016-014), chapter 2. Table 204.64. 2016. https://nces.ed.gov/fastfacts/display.asp?id=59
17. Christensen DL, Baio J, Van Braun K, et al. Prevalence and characteristics of autism spectrum disorder among children aged 8 years—autism and developmental disabilities monitoring network, 11 sites, United States, 2012. MMWR Surveill Summ. 2016;65(3):1–23.
18. Shogren K, Gross J, Forber-Pratt A, Grancis G, Sattter A, Blue-Banning M, Hill C. The perspectives of students with and without disabilities on inclusive schools. Res Pract Persons Severe Disabil. 2015;40(4):243–60. https://doi.org/10.1177/1540796915583493.
19. Hebron J, Oldfield J, Humphrey N. Cumulative risk effects in the bullying of children and young people with autism spectrum conditions. Autism. 2017;21(3):291–300.
20. McMaster C. Building inclusion from the ground up: a review of whole school programmes for sustaining inclusive change. Int J Whole Schooling. 2013;9(2):1–24.
21. Zollers NJ, Ramanathan AK, Yu M. The relationship between school culture and inclusion: how an inclusive culture supports inclusive education. Int J Qual Stud Educ. 1999;12(2):157–74. https://doi.org/10.1080/095183999236231.
22. Iadarola S, Hetherington S, Clinton C, Dean M, Reisinger E, Huynh L, Kasari C. Services for children with autism spectrum disorder in three, large urban school districts: perspectives of parents and educators. Autism. 2015;19(6):694–703. https://doi.org/10.1177/1362361314548078.
23. Kurth J, Lyon K, Shogren K. Supporting students with severe disabilities in inclusive schools: a descriptive account from schools implementing inclusive practices. Res Pract Persons Severe Disabil. 2015;40(4):261–74. https://doi.org/10.1177/1540796915594160.
24. Roberts J, Simpson K. A review of research into stakeholder perspectives on inclusion of students with autism in mainstream schools. Int J Incl Educ. 2016;20(10):1084–96. https://doi.org/10.1080/13603116.2016.1145267.
25. Yang C, Rusli E. Teacher training in using effective strategies for preschool children with disabilities in inclusive classrooms. J Coll Teach Learn. 2012;9(1):53–64. https://doi.org/10.19030/tlc.v9i1.6715.
26. Harding S. Successful inclusion models for students with disabilities require strong site leadership: autism and behavioral disorders create many challenges for the learning environment. Int J Learn. 2009;16(3):1447–9494.
27. Horrocks JL, White G, Roberts L. Principals' attitudes regarding inclusion of children with autism in Pennsylvania public schools. J Autism Dev Disord. 2008;38:1462–73.
28. Haines S, Gross J, Blue-Banning M, Francis G, Turnbull A. Fostering family-school and community-school partnerships in inclusive schools: using practice as a guide. Res Pract Persons Severe Disabil. 2015;40(3):227–39.
29. Peck CA, Staub D, Gallucci C, Schwartz I. Parent perception of the impacts of inclusion on their nondisabled child. Res Pract Persons Severe Disabil. 2004;29(2):135–43.
30. Hebron JS, Humphrey N. Exposure to bullying among students with autism spectrum conditions: a multi-inform-ant analysis of risk and protective factors. Autism. 2013;18(6):618–30. https://doi.org/10.1177/1362361313495965.
31. Freeman R, Eber L, Anderson C, Irvin L, Horner R, Bounds M, Dunlap G. Building inclusive school cultures using school-wide positive behavior support: designing effective individual support systems for students with significant disabilities. Res Pract Persons Severe Disabil. 2006;31(1):4–17.
32. Trauma and Learning Policy Initiative. Dr. Mary E. Curtis on trauma-sensitive professional development for educators. 2014. www.traumasensitiveschools.org.
33. Wood L, et al. Engaging upstanders: class-wide approach to promoting positive bystander behavior. Sch Psychol Forum. 2016;10(1):66–77.
34. Harvey MR. Towards and ecological understanding of resilience in trauma survivors: implications for theory, research, and practice. J Aggress Maltreat Trauma. 2007;14(1/2):9–32.

Chapter 13
Assessment and Recommendations

Randall A. Phelps and Jason M. Fogler

> Sometimes I even envy the gardener who inhabits a restricted plot of ground. It discourages foolishness.
>
> —Roy Barrette

> My green thumb came only as a result of the mistakes I made while learning to see things from the plant's point of view.
>
> —H. Fred Dale

> Plants respond far better to moderate but consistent care than they do to occasional bouts of heroic intervention.
>
> —Martha Stewart

The roots are tangled. Can we prune the ramifications? As has been mentioned many times throughout this book, a diagnosis of autism can help a child to access valuable services, including habilitative therapies, family supports and respite, and funding. Given the power vested by our healthcare system in the ASD label, it is not surprising that wait lists for autism diagnostic assessments are intolerably long. As a result, children with ASD wait unacceptably long intervals to access the medical diagnosis, a key to crucial services. Meanwhile, many children without ASD, who have screened positively or who have various red flags, also wait in this long line, only not to be told they do not meet diagnostic criteria for ASD. Even those children

R. A. Phelps (✉)
Oregon Health & Science University, Eugene, OR, USA
e-mail: phelpsr@ohsu.edu

J. M. Fogler
Developmental Medical Center, Boston Children's Hospital, Boston, MA, USA
e-mail: Jason.Fogler@childrens.harvard.edu

J. M. Fogler, R. A. Phelps (eds.), *Trauma, Autism, and Neurodevelopmental Disorders*, https://doi.org/10.1007/978-3-030-00503-0_13

who do not end up being diagnosed with ASD have significant difficulty with development and/or behavior, often with serious accompanying impacts on family functioning. In most cases, they will likely receive a diagnosis, and with this new diagnosis, they will usually be given some direction to go for assistance. Often, the diagnostic referral centers which provide ASD assessments are able to provide some interventions targeting this new diagnosis. Frequently, however, new referrals will be generated, and then there will be new lines to wait in, for different diagnostic assessments. This can be a very painful, trying experience for families, who may well have hoped, even expected, that they were nearing some diagnostic certainty at the end of their long wait. *Finally*, they thought, they would have a definitive diagnosis, and that diagnosis will finally open the vault to services their child has needed for a *very* long time. So, the question remains: can we improve this experience for our patients and families? Realistically, obtaining a diagnostic assessment for a child with developmental and behavioral problems is never going to be a "walk in the park." But can we alleviate some of the confusion and discomfort, maybe prune back some of the hazardous low-hanging branches?

Tolerating Diagnostic Uncertainty

At some point in our careers, most if not all of us will come face to face with the frustrated parent, incredulous that a year's wait, 4–8 h of testing, and a seemingly interminable flow of paperwork and copays have resulted in an "Unspecified," "Provisional," or "Rule-Out" diagnosis. If they don't say it in words, their faces broadcast the message loud and clear: "That's it?? All that time spent and you don't *know*?? What kind of doctor are you?!" The early career clinician will feel keenly stung by this rebuke, and who can blame them? Anyone who enters the healthcare professions wants to be helpful and provide useful information. Seasoned clinicians want these things too, of course, but we learn to judge our worth by the clarity of our analysis and communications, not necessarily by how they are received.

At the end of the day, neuropsychiatric diagnosis is a well-informed guess or hunch about the most parsimonious way to explain a child's presenting clinical phenomena. We connect psychometric data to behavioral observations to history and arrive at the best formulation we can. That formulation will by necessity be a moving target. Children will grow into and out of all manner of strengths and challenges, not all of them diagnosable or even apparent until a sensitive period of development, and interventions are especially impactful when children are young. We must be humble about the limits of our soft science: we are "making a case" not uncovering Truth with a capital T. Clinicians looking at the same data will come to different conclusions based on their particular frame of reference. We do not yet have the satisfying certainty of biomarkers or the equivalent of a blood test for most neurodevelopmental disorders. As perceptive and insightful as we might be, we may jump to unwarranted conclusions. Unlike our colleagues in radiology, pathology, and phlebotomy, our diagnostic process requires the patient's disclosure, rapport, and trust.

This is in no way meant to diminish the artful skill of distracting a child enough to get a tears-free blood sample or X-ray, but rather speaks to how helpless we would be as diagnosticians without a willing, or at least active, participant in the process.

One Solution: Rejecting the Diagnostic Model for Disability and Embracing the Function Model

Healthcare providers have long sought sensible ways of classifying and labeling disease to enable clear description of specific illnesses for the purposes of facilitation of clear communication between healthcare providers about patients; defining the salient characteristics of a given disease in order to be able to study a disease, to better understand its natural history, and to be able to test interventions and treatments; and communicating with payers, to justify and enable consistent payment for diagnostic assessments and therapeutic procedures. Obviously, with all of these good reasons for creating diagnostic labels for various illnesses, it is a worthy goal to create manuals that define and categorize various illnesses and diseases. Over the years, the World Health Organization has developed serial iterations and improvements in the International Classification of Disease (ICD). The most recent version, the ICD-10, was published in 1999, but not fully implemented in the United States until 2015 [1].

One problem, however, is that disabilities do not fit neatly into this diagnostic model. On the one hand, it is helpful to define disabilities for all of the reasons listed above that we define diseases. Just as with diseases, it is helpful for healthcare providers to be able to communicate with one another about different disabilities. It is important for scientists to be able to communicate clearly about disabilities in order to study these conditions, to increase understanding, and to discover new treatments. It is necessary to communicate clearly with payers about patients who have disabilities, in order to justify payment for diagnostic, habilitative, and rehabilitative services for these patients. On the other hand, disabilities differ markedly from diseases in important ways. Disability advocates criticized the WHO for the equation of disability and disease implied by the inclusion of disabilities right alongside diseases in the ICD-9. One objection of particular relevance to this book was that people born with developmental disabilities may always have those developmental disabilities for their entire lives. Does this mean that such people are continuously "diseased"? Understandably, disability advocates object to this view. However, what is the solution? It is well established that it is helpful to define and classify various conditions. How do we describe disability in a way that is not offensive to people with disabilities?

Out of this productive conversation between disability advocates and the WHO emerged a framework for the description of individuals and their functioning, which greatly improves upon the old diagnosis-centered model. The International Classification of Functioning, Disability, and Health (ICF) [2] has multiple advantages over the old model [3, 4]. It emphasizes function over diagnostic labels, which enables the identification of strengths as well as deficits. Furthermore, the ICF locates the person being described in his or her own social context, not the clinical context.

The ICF describes a person on three levels: at the level of Body Structure and Function (how we traditionally locate and talk about disability), at the level of Activities that a person desires to participate in, and at the level of Participation in those activities. Furthermore, the ICF describes the person in context, describing how Health Conditions, Environmental Factors, and Personal Factors act to mediate a person's functioning. We all have variations in our Body Structures and Functions. Variations which depart significantly from typical structures and functions are termed "impairments." Some of us are born with or may acquire impairments of Body Functions and Structures as the result of various Health Conditions. At some point in our lives, all of us experience at least some impairments. According to the ICF model, impairments may or may not result in difficulty performing certain daily Activities, depending on the presence or absence of various Environmental or Personal Factors. Treatments, technologies, accommodations, or supports from other people, or even animals, enable us to perform various Activities, which Impairments in our Body Structures and Functions might otherwise prevent. The ICF model recognizes that our ability or disability to perform various Activities is thus an interaction between Body Functions and Structures and Environmental or Personal Factors. In other words, though impairments of Body Functions and Structures are intrinsic to us as individuals, Ability or Disability is *not* intrinsic but is a product of interaction between impairments, environment, and personal factors. Similarly, Disabilities may or may not translate into restriction in societal Participation, depending on the presence of various barriers or facilitators, such as Environmental or Personal Factors.

To illustrate these abstract concepts with a concrete example, consider a person—we'll call him "Bud"—who has the Health Condition of diabetes mellitus. Diabetes is a health condition that results in nerve damage in the feet and legs. Unfortunately for Bud, this, in turn, leads to untreated infections, which result in gangrene. Ultimately, Bud ends up with bilateral below-the-knee amputations. The amputations result in impairments of Bud's Body Structures, specifically his legs. After the amputations, the daily Activity of walking presents quite a challenge. One way that this impairment and resultant disability might be addressed is by fitting Bud with prosthetic limbs, which help to directly remediate the impairment. That would seem to be the obvious solution, at least in the traditional medical model. However, if recurrent gangrenous sores preclude fitting Bud with prosthetics, other solutions may need to be explored, at least temporarily. Providing Bud with a wheelchair, an Environmental solution, does not restore the specific Activity of walking, but it does restore mobility. Now the question becomes to what extent is mobility restored such that Bud can resume desired levels of Participation. This depends on various Environmental and Personal Factors. Environmental factors would include the arrangement of Bud's home—for example, do his furnishings and toilet or bathing facilities accommodate wheelchair transfers or allow access from a seated position? Other Environmental factors might include whether there are people who live with Bud and assist him as he adjusts to his new realities. How about community

Participation? Are the sidewalks, public transportation, and buildings in Bud's community wheelchair accessible? In addition to the built environment, how is the attitudinal environment in Bud's community? Are there personal supports Bud can rely on? In addition to Environmental Factors, Personal Factors also have to be considered. Following the amputations, is Bud eager to get back into the community, or does self-consciousness about being out in the community in a wheelchair pose its own barrier to Participation?

Our goal, as healthcare providers to individuals with disabilities, is to promote Participation, or, in other words, to increase community inclusion of people with disabilities. The most effective and enduring way to achieve this goal is to use all of our modalities of intervention, including the following: (1) medical interventions to prevent and treat impairments and/or to prevent or treat comorbid health conditions in people with disabilities; (2) Environmental modifications, such as assuring accessibility of the built environment and providing assistive technology, personal supports, and assistance; and (3) addressing any barriers of Personal Factors, such as motivation.

The ICF framework, applied to acquired physical disabilities, as illustrated with the example of Bud, above, is equally applicable to developmental disabilities. For example, children with ASD have impairments in Mental Functions included in the ICF as Body Functions and Structures, such as Attention, Emotional, Perceptual, and Language functions. These impairments tend to translate to disabilities of such daily Activities as making eye contact, responding appropriately to social overtures, initiating and concluding conversations appropriately, and inhibiting self-stimulatory behaviors in public, to name some examples. These disabilities tend to translate into restrictions in Participation, such as not engaging in social activities, clubs, and sports or even being able to successfully attend school. As illustrated above, however, the impairments do not inevitably translate to disabilities in Activities or restriction in Participation. Interventions targeted at any of the three levels—Body Function and Structure, Activities, and Participation—can help to ameliorate the effects of the impairments intrinsic to ASD on a person. For example, an important intervention for children with ASD is the teaching of social skills. Despite impairment in innate skill in recognizing social cues, the appropriate recognition of and response to social cues can be taught, for example, with social stories. In addition to working with the child with ASD directly to enhance particular skills, environmental modifications, such as classrooms that are less noxious for children with sensory sensitivities, can be crucial to promoting successful school Participation. A powerful intervention to promote inclusion is to teach classmates more about autism, to modify the attitudes of the classmates to be more accepting and understanding (see the previous chapter for outstanding examples of such school-based environmental modifications for children with primary trauma and stressor related disorders). Personal factors may certainly come into play in developing an effective treatment plan. Children with ASDs tend to be highly motivated to pursue their intense, intrusive interests or repetitive activities. Earning protected time to engage in these activities in exchange for participation, for example, in a less-desired (but therapeutically necessary) social skills group can be used as a powerful motivator for participation in group therapy. Finally, in addition to helping organize a treatment plan around the remediation of deficits, a big advantage of the ICF framework is that, because it is not about diagnostic labels but about the description of aspects of functioning, the ICF can be used to describe strengths as well as deficits. This is crucial, as any assessment and any treatment plan should always keep strengths and interests in mind, as participation in activities of interest and high proficiency is one of the most likely keys to promoting inclusion and to promoting healthy self-esteem.

The point has been made in this book that it is important to differentiate ASD and TSRD in order to identify appropriate interventions. Indeed, diagnoses do matter, as they can help to inform a treatment plan, as described extensively in previous chapters. However, we do think the use of diagnoses as keys to the allocation of resources is problematic and is contributing to diagnostic confusion by creating incentives for professionals and families to embrace certain diagnostic categories and to reject other categories. One possible solution may be to shift clinicians', scientists', and payers' attention and emphasis to functional assessments. Children who have severe restriction in Participation owing to severe emotional and behavioral disorders should be able to access whatever treatment and family supports they and their families need to alleviate suffering and stress and to promote inclusion, regardless of whether the underlying diagnosis is ASD or TSRD. Such an emphasis, on Community Participation, also would help us shift from narrow-minded "parent-blaming" to a broader perspective on the context in which our patients function.

Another Solution: Research Domain Criteria

Another solution comes from the Research Domain Criteria (RDoC) initiative, which explicitly seeks common brain mechanisms (and their potential biomarkers) as treatment targets rather than drawing (often arbitrary) distinctions between overlapping criterion symptoms [5, 6]. TSRD, with its associated and neurobiologically mediated features of emotional dysregulation, negative self-concept, disrupted attachment, dissociation, and learning and executive functioning deficits, is a particularly important diagnostic entity to study from an RDoC perspective. Furthermore, with its requirement of a Criterion A event, TSRD offers some degree of precision for those interested in studying gene × environment interactions, for example, or the Polyvagal theory. Understanding the underlying mechanisms of traumatic stress, or the highly heritable traits that drive neurodevelopmental disorders, can advance mental health treatment as a whole, agnostic to diagnosis.

In Conclusion

As noted throughout the book, many providers have stretched diagnostic criteria when, in their judgment, the services that can be accessed by that maneuver might outweigh any disadvantages such stretching might pose to "the Greater Good" of future research or mental health policy. Yet, as we also point out, there can be serious consequences to making the wrong diagnosis, including exacerbating a child's symptoms and distress. This kind of exacerbation is especially likely to occur in cases of TSRD when a well-intentioned intervention is inadvertently triggering or re-traumatizing and in the case of neurodevelopmental disorders when the demands of treatment exceed the child's ability to understand or comply with what is expected. So, how can we support families in need of, for example, respite services, without making diagnostic contortions? We suggest that more widespread use and acceptance of functional assessment, using the ICF framework, could provide a solution to the dilemma that currently faces diagnosticians [7]. With the ICF, diagnosticians don't have to choose between the needs of the stressed families sitting in front of them and upholding two important cornerstones of our field: valid and reliable diagnosis and targeted, evidence-based treatment. Instead of qualification for support hinging on a particular diagnostic label, which just ends up causing that label to be overused and artificially inflated, a particular threshold of functional challenges could be used to determine access to needed services. Such an approach would have the additional benefit of lessening the problem of cultural biases or gender-based biases, which may cause diagnoses to be overlooked, as discussed by Benavides-Rawson and Grinker and by Chavez, Huang-Storms, and Zuckerman, in their respective chapters.

In our ideal world, use of such strategies as Applied Behavioral Analysis would not be restricted to the treatment of autism. Indeed, ABA was never intended to be specific to the treatment of autism (http://abaappliedbehavioranalysis.weebly.com/facts-and-statistics.html). Functional behavioral analyses would be deployed appropriately for the problem at hand, not for any diagnostic label. We would no longer make arbitrary distinctions between ADHD or PTSD, but instead ask nuanced questions about the conditions under which a child would benefit from executive functioning support, trauma-sensitive emotional support, or both. For these reasons, we are inspired by the broad vision and universal design perspective of the Trauma Sensitive Schools Initiative, as illustrated by Gregory and Nichols, and would celebrate this kind of thinking applied widely to research and intervention for children with trauma and neurodevelopmental disorders. As pointed out by Munger, Loi, and Roth, all children benefit from community investments which help them to build "regulatory capital," no matter whether a child's elevated risk of dysregulation stems from ASD or TSRD.

References

1. Centers of Disease Control and Prevention. International classification of diseases, (ICD-10-CM/PCS) transition—background. https://www.cdc.gov/nchs/icd/icd10cm_pcs_background.htmICD-10. Accessed 12 Feb 2017.
2. World Health Organization. International classification of functioning, disease, and health (ICF). http://www.who.int/classifications/icf/en/. Accessed 12 Feb 2017.
3. Feldman H. Redesigning health care for children with disabilities. Baltimore: Brookes; 2013. p. 70–71.

4. Lollar D. Launching into adulthood. Baltimore: Brookes; 2010. p. 52, 117.
5. Cuthbert BN. The RDoC framework: facilitating transition from ICD/DSM to dimensional approaches that integrate neuroscience and psychopathology. World Psychiatry. 2014;13(1):28–35. https://doi.org/10.1002/wps.20087.
6. Young G. PTSD, endophenotypes, the RDoC, and the DSM-5. Psychol Inj Law. 2014;7(1): 75–91. https://doi.org/10.1007/s12207-014-9187-x.
7. World Health Organization. Towards a common language for functioning disability and health. Geneva: WHO; 2002. p. 9. Retrieved from http://www.who.int/classifications/icf/training/icf-beginnersguide.pdf; adapted by permission.

Afterword: Precision Mental Health and the Twilight of Categories

Joseph Gonzalez-Heydrich and Matcheri Keshavan

This wonderful book takes us leagues towards understanding a polarizing rift in our field that continues to play itself out in consultation rooms throughout the world, but the work of understanding is not done and we have a ways to go before the rift is healed. The rift is between presumed biological and presumed psychological causation for major psychiatric disorders in children, including Autism Spectrum Disorders (ASD) and Trauma Stress Related Disorders (TSRD) such as PTSD. The authors take us along a historical journey though the last several decades at the end of which, as more of the biology of neurodevelopmental disorders has been understood, the boundaries of influence have moved, but are still demarcated according to the categories of our current nosology. ASD, which in the hay day of psychological causation was blamed on mothers, has fallen to the shock troops of neuropsychiatry and is now conceptualized as a biological and neurologically mediated disorder. TSRD has so far resisted the siege of biological insights and is still conceptualized as a set of disorders caused by the psychological environment. Patients are seen as falling on one or the other side of this divide and must make due with the resources and interventions that have fastened themselves to one or the other of these categories. This is true even though at this juncture treatments on both sides of this divide are essentially psychologically based treatments, Applied Behavioral Analysis (ABA) and its various offspring for ASD and some form of Trauma-Focused Cognitive Behavioral Therapy (TF-CBT) or trauma sensitive support for TSRD. This leads to the high stakes arguments described throughout this book. Arguments that ultimately do not optimally serve patients, families, or systems of care.

The authors have clearly seen this. In the conclusion of this book, Fogler and Phelps point out that the two cornerstones of our field have been reliable diagnosis and targeted evidence based treatments. However, these corner stones have thus far been largely interdependent as the reliable diagnoses have been categorical and the evidence for treatment has been accrued for separate categories. As has been increasingly apparent, reliability is not synonymous with validity. The corner stone of reliable diagnostic category was laid on the shifting quick sands of clinical phenotypic

J. M. Fogler, R. A. Phelps (eds.), *Trauma, Autism, and Neurodevelopmental Disorders*, https://doi.org/10.1007/978-3-030-00503-0

observation and studies of treatments for dimensions of psychopathology that are expressed across various categorical diagnoses have been discouraged. However, change is afoot.

The human genome has been sequenced and the tools to apply genomic science to clinical populations increasingly have come on line. The genetic architecture of categories such as ASD has been found overlap considerably with that psychotic disorders but also mood disorders. Where strong genetic causation has been found for ASD, pleiotropy and heterogeneity rule. A given genetic mutation can give rise to a broad range of clinical manifestations (pleiotropy) and any given clinical manifestation can arise from a plethora of genetic variation (etiologic heterogeneity). Additionally, imaging, psychophysiological, and psychological studies have found overlap between children who survived severe early neglect and those with ASD. These and other observations have loosened the iron grip of the Diagnostic and Statistical Manual (DSM). The scales have fallen from our eyes and as a field we can now consider more fully if symptoms which are common between categories are due to commonalities in brain circuits affected. This begs the question, have we as a field been taking dimensional constructs that are inherently intertwined and inseparable and tried to fit them into our categorical diagnoses? Accumulating evidence suggests this is the case.

Consider a child with a genetic variation that markedly increases the risk for ASD like Fragile X disorder. The biology of Fragile X disorder increases brain excitability relative to inhibition. Anxiety is markedly elevated in response to many stimuli and it is entirely plausible that the threshold for severe trauma and other life changes, to induce brain changes is markedly lower in children with Fragile X Disorder. Major attachment relationships are in danger of being affected by the ASD itself and compound it. A given patient with Fragile X may have a great deal of ASD symptomatology and trauma related symptoms intertwined and benefit from elements of both ABA and developmentally appropriate TF-CBT or trauma sensitive support. Conversely consider that the developmental effects on the brain of the very low-stimulation, and cold and inconsistent parenting experienced by children raised in extremely neglectful institutional or home environments during critical periods of brain plasticity overlap those seen in ASD arising from a strong genetic causation. Clinically these children may show similar cognitive, language and behavioral deficits because of overlapping effects on brain connectivity. They both may benefit from both ABA and TF-CBT. Fogler and Phelps argue correctly that the time has come for therapeutics to be guided by functional assessment rather than categories. In planning treatment one might ask to what extent is the child's functioning is impacted by autism spectrum symptoms, by reactivity due to traumatic exposures or neglect, and by relational problems with care givers and each domain addressed regardless of which DSM category fits best.

Clearly the paradigms are shifting, but what next? We believe that that even the currently best conceived symptom dimensions (arguably the RDoC dimensions Fogler and Phelps cite) will ultimately be found to be artificial approximations at best. Categories will continue to be redefined as the specific genetic vulnerability to specific environmental adversities at specific points in development are increasing described. The ubiquity and utility of genetic tools will increase and their cost will decrease. Our ability to measure brain circuit involvement in vivo and with minimal risk to the patient will increase. We will get to the point that we will start to understand the gene by environment interactions in an individual child. Categories will be replaced by detailed developmental pathways. A greater understanding of the psychobiology of pathways will be translated into novel treatments. The evidence base will develop for treatments targeted to mechanisms active in a given child rather than to a diagnoses. The cornerstones of our field will increasingly sit on the firmer ground of precision mental health and appreciation for the individuality of each patient and family. Our academic arguments pitting biological against psychological causation will be a footnote of historical interest and to the extent that we are able to capitalize on increasing knowledge and technology, children and families will be better served. Finally, and to the benefit of the patients and their families, the decisions as to who may benefit from what treatment, and how treatment resources may most optimally be allocated to those in need, will be based on measurable physiological and behavioral constructs rather than labels based on symptom clusters of limited validity. The insights in this volume are not unique to developmental disorders alone, but translate broadly to all of mental health, as exemplified by accruing evidence that the boundaries between psychotic, bipolar and major depressive disorders are increasingly blurred. Time is ripe for a trans-diagnostic reconceptualization of all of psychiatry across neurobiologic and behavioral continua, which may have positive implications for more effective approaches to diagnosis and treatments in the future.

Index

A
Aberrant great vessels, 99
Addiction, 28, 30
Advocating Success for Kids (ASK), 242
Alcohol-related birth defects (ARBD), 95, 96, 98, 99
Alcohol related neurodevelopmental disorder (ARND), 95, 96, 98, 112
American Academy of Pediatrics (AAP), 179
American Psychiatric Association (APA), 207
Anaclitic depression, 7
Animal-assisted therapy, 135
Anxiety disorder, 150
Applied Behavioral Analysis (ABA), 275
Asperger's disorder, 172, 173
Assessment
  data gathering, 64
  ICF framework, 273, 275
  observations and formal, 75
  personal assessment approach, 64
  primary purpose, 65
  questionnaire-based, 84
  re-experiencing, 68
  science and craft, 63–65
  and therapy, 67
  tools, 83, 84
  traumatic stress symptoms, 62
  and treatment plan, 274
  validity scale, 68
Atrial septal defects, 99
Attachment disorder, 61
Attachment therapy, 56
Attention deficit hyperactivity disorder (ADHD), 164, 222
  children and adolescents, 226, 228
  country/region of assessment, 228
  DSM-IV, 226
  predictors, 228, 229
  symptoms, 226
  United States children, 228
Auditory processing disorder, 57
Autism
  ascription, 6
  diagnosis, use of, 7
  Emma's, 6
  evidence-based intervention, 11
  historical context (*see* Historical context)
  "Refrigerator Mom" concept, 6
Autism diagnostic observation schedule (ADOS), 163, 195
Autism spectrum disorder (ASD), 243
  ADOS, 163
  ascertainment and diagnostic bias, 169
  behavioral, cognitive and developmental patterns, 170
  children and families, 17
  comorbid mental disorders, 164
  conceptualization, 82
  diagnosis, 82
  diagnostic feedback, to families, 86
  diagnostic label, 87
  differential diagnosis (*see* Differential diagnosis)
  DSM-5, 82
  etiologic protective factors, 170
  family perspective, 181–182
  female, 167–170
  histories, 10
  increased prevalence, 81–83
  individuals, 164
  intellectual disability, 83, 163
  intervention methods, 87

J. M. Fogler, R. A. Phelps (eds.), *Trauma, Autism, and Neurodevelopmental Disorders*, https://doi.org/10.1007/978-3-030-00503-0

Autism spectrum disorder (ASD) *(Cont.)*
Maria, 15 year-old Latina girl, 161–163
practice and policy, 182–184
predictors, 229
prevalence, 164–165, 229
public health relevance
behavioral factors, 177
chronic condition of adulthood, 176
healthcare and larger systems perspective, 176–177
pre-diagnosis stage, 177–179
service utilization, 179–181
racial and ethnic disparities
ADHD, 172
ascertainment bias in children, 172
Asian/PI and American Indian, 173
case of Early Intevention, 173
definition, 171
hormonal and genetic etiological associations, 171
measurement, 174–175
Medicaid-eligible children, 172
middle-class Black population, 173
over-identification, 172
in Pennsylvania, 173
research, 171
SES, 175
the US Census, 171
variability, 171
racial and ethnic minority people, 164
sex differential biological factors, 166–167
sex-differential genetic and hormonal factors, 170
sex ratio, 165–166
social communication and interaction, 229
supports, 88
therapeutic pre-schools, 88
and trauma, 169–170
treatment, 87, 89
youths, 199

B
Behavioral phenotype, 94, 104
Bereavement related disorder (BRD), 215, 224, 225, 233
Bettelheim
Austrian Jews, 8
autism, causes, 6, 7
nazism, 8
parent-blaming bias, 12
Biological markers, 57
Biomarkers, 10
Bucharest Early Intervention Project, 141
Bud's community, 272, 273

C
Camptodactyly, 101
Caregivers, 255
Central amygdala (CeA), 24
Central nervous system (CNS), 96, 99, 102–105
Childhood abuse, 31, 35, 39
Childhood trauma, 21, 33, 36, 38–40
Childhood trauma treatment (CCT), 135
Child-parent psychotherapy (CPP), 128, 131–132
Child Protective Services (CPS), 124
Children's relief nursery (CRN), 135
Children with special health care needs (CSHCN), 174
Civilian PTSD
child abuse, 33
childhood trauma, 36
and co-morbidities, 34
criminal justice system, 33–37
cycle of trauma, 36
financial costs, 31
man-made disasters, 32
natural disasters, 32
prison sentences, 36, 37
social support and community cohesion, 33, 34
trauma, rates, 32
violent assault, 32
Cognitive behavioral therapy (CBT), 201
Community cohesion, 33, 34
Comorbidity
ADHD, 231
National Comorbidity Study-Adolescent Replication, 212
PTSD, 231, 233
Comprehensive diagnostic assessment
diagnostic concerns, 74, 75
diagnostic formulation, 75
evaluation, 76
giving feedback, 76
observations and formal assessments, 75
patient's behavior, 74
patient's history, 73
social history, 74
Comprehensive psychological assessment, 56, 58
Conduct disorder, 15, 150
Conotruncal heart defects, 99
Cortisol, 30, 39, 41–43
Coventry Child and Adolescent Mental Health Services (CAMHS), 157
Coventry Grid, 79
Craniofacial dysmorphology, 104
Cross-cultural, 154

Cruel guards, 8

D

Depression, 6, 7
Developmental delay (DD), 178
Developmental disability services, 197
Developmental Medicine Center (DMC), 242
Developmental trauma, 56
Developmental trauma disorder (DTD), 111
Development and wellbeing assessment-reactive attachment disorder (DAWBA-RAD), 224, 225
Diabetes, 272
Diagnosis
- diagnostic model, 271
- ICF framework, 273
- modalities of intervention, 273
- neuropsychiatric, 270
- RDoC, 274

Diagnostic and statistical manual of mental disorders, fifth edition (DSM-5), 164
Differential diagnosis
- attachment disorders, 80
- attachment problems, 78
- Coventry Grid, 79
- difficulties, 78
- DSM-5, 78
- early life experiences, children's, 79
- gender prevalence, 79
- RAD and DSED, 77
- symptoms, 77
- tool, 79

Disabilities, 271–273
Disinhibited social engagement disorder (DSED), 77, 215, 224, 225, 233
Distant mothering, 9
"Doorknob comment", 66, 67, 69
Dysmorphic craniofacial features, 96, 99, 101, 112

E

Early Childhood Inventory-4, 85
Early childhood special education (ECSE), 128
Early intervention (EI), 128
Early intervention/early childhood special education (EI/ECSE), 128
Ecological fit, 246, 253, 265
Electroencephalogram (EEG), 141
Emotional learning, 41
Epicanthal folds, 101
Epidemic, 12, 13
Epidemiology
- attention deficit hyperactivity disorder, 227
- autism spectrum disorder, 229
- posttraumatic stress disorder, 217–220
- public health, 206
- traumatic events, 208–211

Executive functioning (EF), 65, 70
Exploratory factor analysis (EFA), 224
Eye anomalies, 99

F

Facial dysmorphology, 96, 101
Family supports, 269, 274
Family therapy, 88
Fear
- and addiction circuitries, 28
- and anxiety behaviors, 29
- circuitry and behavior with PTSD, 27, 28
- human fear circuitry, 25–27
- rodent fear circuitry, 23, 24
- in rodents, 23

Fetal alcohol spectrum disorders (FASDs), 202
- alcohol-related defects throughout pregnancy, 97
- alcohol related neurodevelopmental disorder, 112
- child trauma, 95, 96
- CNS abnormalities, 102–105
- cognitive and behavioral phenotype, 94
- diagnosis, 94, 98–100
- epigenetics, 97
- facial characteristics, 102
- facial features, 101
- FAS facial features, 103
- growth restriction, 102
- intrauterine alcohol exposure, 96–97
- justice system, 113
- lip/philtrum morphology, 103
- long-term morbidities, 95
- mental health services, 112
- minor features, 101–102, 104
- neurobehavioral profile, children, 106–111
- neurocognitive and behavioral deficits, 107–109
- neurodevelopmental disorders, 111–112
- NIAAA Expert Consensus Diagnostic Guidelines, 105
- overview, 95
- prenatal alcohol exposure, 95, 99–101, 105–106, 113–115

Fetal alcohol syndrome (FAS)
children, 95
diagnosis, 98
facial features, 95
FASDs (*see* Fetal alcohol spectrum disorders (FASDs))
p-FAS, 95, 98
Fictitious epidemic, 12, 13
FKBP5 (FK506 Binding Protein-5), 40, 42, 43
Functional magnetic resonance imaging (fMRI), 141
Funding, 269

G
Gene by environment (G x E), 21, 40, 43
Genetic
G x E interaction, 43
PTSD, 21
transgenerational transmission, trauma, 40
Genome wide association studies (GWAS), 40

H
Habilitative therapies, 269
Historical context
ASD and TSRD
actions of parents, 11
caregiver, interview of, 10, 11
on clinical interview and examination, 10
diagnosis of autism, 11
diagnostic assessments, 10
IQ test, 13
fictitious epidemic, 12
Kanner and Bettelheim, 8
Nazi naturism *vs.* Freudian nurturism, 7–9
History gathering, 58, 60, 67
Human resilience, 80
Hypertelorism, 102
Hypoplastic fingernails, 101
Hypotelorism, 102
Hypothalamic-pituitary-adrenal (HPA), 135, 136, 142–145

I
ICF framework, 273–275
ICF model, 272
Individualized Educational Program (IEP), 162, 243
Individuals with Disabilities Education Act (IDEA), 12, 198, 243
Injury, 15
Institutional rearing, 41
Intellectual disability (ID), 83, 178
Intergenerational transmission, 39, 40
The International Classification of Functioning, Disability, and Health (ICF), 272–275
Intervention
Bucharest Early Intervention Project, 141
Circle of Security, 133
EI/ECSE, 128
TBRI®, 128, 134
Intrauterine alcohol exposure, 96–97
IQ test, 13

K
Kanner
Austrian Jews, 8
autism, causes, 7
career, 8
naturism, 9
nurturism, 9
parent-blaming bias, 12
as pseudodiagnostic wastebasket, 12
"Refrigerator Mom" concept, 6
syndrome, 13

L
Lip and philtrum morphology, 101

M
Magnetic resonance imaging (MRI) study, 140
Massachusetts Advocates for Children (MAC), 242
Mental health policy, 274
Midface hypoplasia, 101
Minnesota Multi-Phasic Personality Inventory (MMPI), 153
Mongolism, 13

N
National Child Traumatic Stress Network, 57
National Study of Adolescents (NSA), 216
Naturism, 8, 9
Nazism, 8, 9
Neurobehavioral disorder associated with prenatal alcohol exposure (ND-PAE), 112
Neurocognitive testing, 55
Neurodevelopmental disabilities, 203, 265
ASD, 243

ASK, 242
DMC, 242
educational approach, 242
MAC, 242
policy implications
collective investment, 267
evidence-based approaches, 266
professional development opportunities, 266
school culture, 265
school culture (*see* School culture)
special education, 241
TLPI, 242, 247–253, 255, 256
and trauma, 256
ABA services, 259
Autism Spectrum Disorder, 261
cognitive behavioral therapy, 257
culture of inclusion, 258, 261, 262
Education Law Clinic, 256
educational linchpin, 256
Monique's explosive behaviors, 259
NVLD, 257
paraprofessional support, 260
school culture, 257
special education, 260
speech and language therapist, 261
trauma-sensitive schools (*see* Trauma-sensitive schools)
Neurodevelopmental disorder, 57, 58, 63, 69, 95, 98, 111–112, 270, 274, 275
ADHD and ASD, 233
public health, 233
and trauma-related, 207, 226, 233
Neuropsychiatric diagnosis, 270
Neuropsychological assessment, 58
NIAAA Expert Consensus Diagnostic Guidelines, 98, 104
Non-human primate models, 41
Non-verbal learning disability (NVLD), 150, 257
Nurturism, 8, 9

O

Obsessive-compulsive disorder, 150
Occipitofrontal circumference (OFC), 98, 102
Operational functions, 249

P

Parent-child interaction therapy (PCIT), 132–133, 200
Parent management training (PMT), 200
Partial fetal alcohol syndrome (p-FAS), 96, 98, 99, 101, 104
Polyvictimization, 214
Population-based research, 206, 212
Posttraumatic stress disorder (PTSD), 75, 76, 131, 141, 164, 170
childhood maltreatment, 21
civilian (*see* Civilian PTSD)
demographics, 221
family factors, 222
lifetime rates, 21
mental and behavioral health conditions, 215
mental health, 222
neural networks, in threat responses
fear and addiction circuitries, 28
fear circuitry and behavior, 27, 28
human fear circuitry, 25–27
rodent fear circuitry, 23, 24
rodent models, 23
stress response system, 29, 30
prevalence, 216, 220
risk and resilience, 38
characteristics, in parents and children, 38, 39
childhood critical periods, 41
FKBP5, 42, 43
transgenerational transmission, trauma, 40
substance abuse, 22
symptom clusters, 20
trauma exposure, 215, 221, 222, 231–232
Potentially traumatic events (PTEs), 207, 212–215, 223
Prenatal alcohol exposure
adolescence and adulthood, 110
adverse effects, 95
brain development, 110
brain regions, 105–106
cardinal facial features, 98
child's caregivers, 101
facial characteristics, 102
FASD, 99
gestural communication, 110
individuals, 114
infancy, 106
intrauterine, 95
ND-PAE, 112
neurobehavioral deficits, 99
neurobehavioral phenotype, 104
pregnancy, 96
preschool, 109
query, 115
SNV, 97
suspicion, 95
trauma often co-exist, 95

Preschoolers
biological outcomes, 135–136
immune function, 145
TF-CBT, 131
trauma treatment, 127, 130
trauma's adverse consequences, 146
Prevalence estimates, 223, 226–228
Primary care provider (PCP), 196
Program for the Education and Enrichment of Relational Skills (PEERS), 201
Psychiatry, 20, 40
Psychodynamic theory, 152, 154
Psychometric testing, 61, 63, 67
PTSD before age 6, 131, 132
Public health
acute stress disorder, 222–223
ADHD (*see* Attention deficit hyperactivity disorder (ADHD))
ASD (*see* Autism spectrum disorder (ASD))
BRD, 224
children's exposure, 207–213
clinician, 206
epidemiologic research, 207
epidemiologic studies, 233
and neurodevelopmental disorders, 230–231
prevention programs, 233
PTSD (*see* Posttraumatic stress disorder (PTSD))
RAD and DSED, 224, 225
trauma exposure
demographic characteristics, 213, 214
epidemiologic studies, 214
family and peer relationships, 215
mental health, 214
victimization, 214
trauma-related sequelae, 233

R
Radioulnar synostosis, 99
Ramifications, 13, 18
Reactive attachment disorder (RAD), 6, 7, 12, 15, 77, 111, 112, 205, 206, 215, 224, 225, 233
vs. ASD
American Psychiatric Association, 154
behavioral phenotype, 155
diagnosis, 158
DSM-5 guidelines, 151–154
Korea, 150, 151
Latin American parents, 155
management and care of individuals, 158
mother-child relationship, 154
non-Hispanic White children, 155
non-minority children, 155
perpetual childhood, 155
psycho-diagnostic assessment, 156–158
psychodynamic conceptualization, 154
SES, 155
Spain, 149, 150
underdiagnosis, 154
Renal anomalies, 99
Research Domain Criteria (RDoC), 274
Respite services, 269, 275
Risk factors, 224, 225

S
School culture, 251, 255, 265–267
autism and inappropriate approaches, 255
behavioral disruptions, 254
culture of inclusion, 252–255
disability-rights community, 253
ecological fit, 252
neurodiverse population, 252
outcomes, 256
physical school environment, 254
problematic behaviors, 254
social skills, 254
special education, 252
SWND, 253
TLPI, 256
ubiquitous factor, 255
universal design, 256
Scoliosis, 99
Semi-structured interviews, 85
Sensory integration room, 263
Sensory-motor affect regulation therapy (SMART), 135
Services, 13, 14
Sex discrepancies
ascertainment and diagnostic bias, 169
female ASD phenotype, 167–169
prevalence in males and females, 164–165
racial and ethnic variables, ASD sex ratio, 165–166
sex differential biological factors, 166–167
trauma in females, 169–170
Social support, 33, 34, 38
Socio-economic status (SES), 174
Special education, 242, 243, 245, 246, 252, 253, 260, 263, 265
Stress response systems, 29, 30

Students with neurodevelopmental disabilities (SWND), 252–257, 267
Substance abuse disorder (SUD), 34, 38

T
Theraplay®, 128, 134
Threat
  and anxiety, 22
  neural networks, examination
    and behavior with PTSD, 27, 28
    fear and addiction circuitries, 28
    human fear circuitry, 25–27
    rodent fear circuitry, 23, 24
    rodent models, 23
  threatening stimuli, 22
Toxic stress, 80
Transitional issues
  behavioral assessment, 195
  eye contact and facial expressions, 196
  fundamental problems, 202, 203
  Office of Developmental Disability Services, 196
  primary care provider, 196
  psychiatric care, 197
  self-cutting behaviors, 196
  sex-offenders, 195
  stress and trauma, 197
  trauma-inflicted injuries, 203
  youth
    developmental disabilities, 197–198
    mental health care, 199
    treatment, 199–202
Trauma, 19
  assessment (*see* Assessment)
  disclosures, 66, 67
  dynamic, 66
  on neurocognitive functioning, 61–63
  PTSD (*see* Posttraumatic stress disorder (PTSD))
  survivor, 65
  treatment needs, 69–70
  TSRD, 20
Trauma-focused cognitive behavioral therapy (TF-CBT), 129, 131, 202
Trauma histories, *see* Neurodevelopmental disabilities
Trauma and Learning Policy Initiative (TLPI), 242, 256
Trauma-related disorders
  and neurodevelopmental disorders, 226, 230–231
  incidence and prevalence, 231
Trauma-sensitive schools, 246, 250, 255, 257, 261, 262
  attributes, 248
  concretize efforts, 250
  definition, 247, 248
  direction and welfare, 249
  ecological fit, 245, 246, 265
  flexible framework, 249
  four iterative questions, 250
  IDEA, 243
  inquiry-based process, 251
  operational functions, 249
  physical movement plan, 264
  pilot therapy program, 263
  productive learning, 251
  safe and supportive, 262
  school culture, 248, 250
  screening tool, 249
  sensory integration room, 263
  special education, 243, 244, 246, 263, 265
  TLPI, 247
  Tyrice, 263
  universal design, 247
Trauma and stressor related disorders (TSRDs), 20–22, 25, 29, 30, 44, 58, 164, 179, 180, 184, 215
  adaptive concerns, 128
  vs. ADHD, 62
  APGAR score, 125
  ASD, 123, 126
  assessment tools and tendency, 85
  biological correlation, 145–146
  biological outcomes, 135–136
  body-based treatments, 135
  brain, 136, 140, 141
  challenge, in assessment, 83–85
  childhood cancers, 146
  children's acquisition, 146
  children with TSRD, 59
  circle of security, 133
  in the classroom, 124
  constructing and integrating trauma, 129–130
  co-occurring diagnoses, 58
  coping skills, 130
  CPP, 131, 132
  CPS, 123
  developmental concerns, 128–129
  diagnostic feedback, to families, 86
  differential diagnosis (*see* Differential diagnosis)
  DSM-5 criteria, 125
  Early Childhood Inventory-4, 85

Trauma and stressor related disorders (TSRDs) *(Cont.)*
early life trauma, 136–146
environmental stress, 84
family therapy, 88
genes, 144
historical events, 60
history gathering, 60
hypothalamic-pituitary-adrenal axis, 142–144
immune system, 145
intervention methods, 87
maternal grandmother, 124
methamphetamines and heroin, 123
motor and language skills, 126
neurobiological basis of impairment, 80–81
parent-child relationships and parenting skills, 127
PCIT, 132, 133
pediatricians, 126
physical play, 125
preschoolers, 127, 130
public school kindergarten, 124
repetitive behaviors, 124
restoring felt safety, 129
safety, 64
semi-structured interviews, 85
social security support, 88
supplemental supports, 133–135
symptom domains, 58, 59
team's medical social worker, 126
TF-CBT, 131
therapeutic pre-schools, 88
therapeutic preschools and childcare, 135
Theraplay®, 134–135
treatment, 87
trust-based relational intervention, 134
Traumatic experiences
childhood experiences, 57
symptoms, 56
trauma and toxic stress, 56
Traumatic stress, 85, 104
assessment, 68
children with co-occurring developmental delays/disabilities, 69
history of, 62
on neuropsychological functions, 61
professional support network, 69
symptoms, 63
Trier Social Stress Test for Children (TSST-C), 144
Trust-based Relational Intervention® (TBRI®), 134

U
UNESCO's Salamanca Statement, 252

V
Ventricular septal defects, 99
Vertebral segmentation defects, 99
Victimization, 57
Violence
domestic, 36
and high stress communities, 34
physical and sexual, 36
in prison, 36

Y
Young adulthood, ASD, 201

GPSR Compliance
The European Union's (EU) General Product Safety Regulation (GPSR) is a set of rules that requires consumer products to be safe and our obligations to ensure this.

If you have any concerns about our products, you can contact us on

ProductSafety@springernature.com

In case Publisher is established outside the EU, the EU authorized representative is:

Springer Nature Customer Service Center GmbH
Europaplatz 3
69115 Heidelberg, Germany

www.ingramcontent.com/pod-product-compliance
Ingram Content Group UK Ltd.
Pitfield, Milton Keynes, MK11 3LW, UK
UKHW022213051026
15624UKWH00001B/141
9783030005023